Essentials of Medicine and Surgery for Dental Students

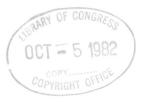

Churchill Livingstone Dental Series

ESSENTIALS OF ORAL BIOLOGY
D. Adams

A MANUAL OF PAEDODONTICS
R. J. Andlaw and W. P. Rock

ESSENTIALS OF DENTAL SURGERY AND PATHOLOGY,
Third edition
R. A. Cawson

CLINICAL PHARMACOLOGY IN DENTISTRY,
Second edition
R. A. Cawson and R. G. Spector

NOTES ON DENTAL MATERIALS,
Fourth edition
E. C. Combe

DENTISTRY FOR THE ADOLESCENT,
J. A. Hargreaves

THE MANAGEMENT OF TRAUMATIZED ANTERIOR TEETH IN
CHILDREN
Second edition
J. A. Hargreaves, J. W. Craig and H. L. Needleman

THE IMPACTED WISDOM TOOTH,
Second edition
H. C. Killey and L. W. Kay

THE PREVENTION OF COMPLICATIONS IN DENTAL SURGERY,
Second edition
H. C. Killey and L. W. Kay

BENIGN CYSTIC LESIONS OF THE JAWS, THEIR DIAGNOSIS AND
TREATMENT,
Third edition
H. C. Killey, L. W. Kay and G. R. Seward

PRACTICAL DENTAL ANAESTHESIA
A. Kilpatrick

ANATOMY FOR STUDENTS OF DENTISTRY
Fourth edition
J. H. Scott and A. D. Dixon

INTRODUCTION TO DENTAL ANATOMY,
Eighth edition
J. H. Scott and N. B. B. Symons

PRINCIPLES OF PATHOLOGY FOR DENTAL STUDENTS,
Fourth edition
J. B. Walter, M. C. Hamilton and M. S. Israel

BASIC AND APPLIED DENTAL BIOCHEMISTRY
R. A. D. Williams and J. C. Elliott

Essentials of
Medicine and Surgery
for Dental Students

A. C. Kennedy

M.D., F.R.C.P. Lond., Edin. and Glasg.
Muirhead Professor of Medicine,
University Department of Medicine,
The Royal Infirmary, Glasgow

L. H. Blumgart

B.D.S., M.D., F.R.C.S. Eng., Edin. and Glasg.
Director and Professor of Surgery, Royal Postgraduate
Medical School, Hammersmith Hospital, London;
previously St Mungo Professor of Surgery,
The Royal Infirmary, Glasgow

FOURTH EDITION

CHURCHILL LIVINGSTONE
EDINBURGH LONDON MELBOURNE AND NEW YORK 1982

CHURCHILL LIVINGSTONE
Medical Division of Longman Group Limited

Distributed in the United States of America by
Churchill Livingstone Inc., 19 West 44th Street, New
York, N.Y. 10036, and by associated companies,
branches and representatives throughout the world.

© Longman Group Limited 1977, 1982

Third edition 1977
Fourth edition 1982
First two editions published under the title *Essentials of
Medicine for Dental Students* by A. C. Kennedy

ISBN 0 443 02534 7

British Library Cataloguing in Publication Data
Kennedy, A. C.
  Essentials of medicine and surgery for dental
  students.—4th ed.
  1. Diseases 2. Wounds
  I. Title II. Blumgart, L. H.
  616′.00246176 RB111

Library of Congress Catalog Card Number 81–68802

Printed in Singapore by Selector Printing Co Pte Ltd

Preface

In 1960 one of the authors (A.C.K.) published the first edition of *Essentials of Medicine for Dental Students*. The reception accorded to the book indicated that it was of value to dental students in Glasgow and throughout the country and it became quite widely used.

When faced with the question of producing a third edition in 1977 a decision was made to incorporate the elements of surgery, and in that year a volume combining the essentials of medicine and surgery for dental students was written under our joint authorship. It is relevant to note that L.H.B., in addition to being a practising surgeon, is also qualified in dentistry. In that edition we expressed our hope that the work would prove acceptable to dental students and would provide them with the essentials of medicine and surgery necessary for their studies. The sales of the book indicated that it clearly met a need and a reprint was required in 1979/1980.

The fourth edition is based on the original text but all the medical and surgical material has been thoroughly revised and brought up to date. Many new illustrations are incorporated throughout the text and the sections on shock, injuries and surgical operations have been considerably amplified in response to comments from reviewers of the third edition. A new chapter has been added giving a brief account of some common psychiatric problems.

The original intention to present a simplified account of the various medical and surgical disorders has been maintained. Many of the details which are required by the doctor for the actual practice of medicine or surgery are omitted and in particular details of management which are firmly within the realm of medical, as opposed to dental, practice. The description of many of the diseases is, of necessity, incomplete but as before we have tried to avoid statements which are incorrect. Disorders such as facial pain, haemophilia, swellings about the face, and surgical conditions related to the mouth are dealt with at rather greater length since the dentist should have a full knowledge of such matters.

The majority of the chapters and sections open with a brief description of the relevant anatomy and physiology, as we have found, in the course of teaching, that most students welcome a brief refresher in these pre-clinical subjects. Line drawings, tables, and illustrative clinical photographs and X-rays are included throughout the text. It is our belief that these will be of considerable value and interest to the student.

The burden of the secretarial work fell on Miss Margaret Nicol and Miss S.J. Fenwick to whom we are greatly indebted. Lastly, it is a pleasure to record the help given to us by the publishers.

Glasgow, 1982   A.C.K.
                                                                 L.H.B.

Contents

1

Diseases due to infection—medical aspects

GENERAL CONSIDERATIONS

Infection of man with pathogenic microorganisms has been an extremely important cause of disease since antiquity but it is only within the last hundred years that we have gained precise knowledge regarding the causal agents. Bacteriological knowledge has been followed by truly remarkable advances in the prevention and treatment of the infectious disorders and, in consequence, several diseases, which were previously widespread, have been almost eliminated from many countries, e.g., diphtheria, or even more remarkable, as in the case of smallpox, eliminated throughout the world. Despite such striking achievements there is still much to be done; this is especially so in the tropical and semi-tropical areas of the world but it is also true in the temperate zones. Indeed, having regard to the laws of nature, it is almost certain that man will never be free from the risk of infection with pathogenic organisms, although he may possess increasingly effective remedies.

In this chapter a brief account will first be given of some general principles applicable to all the infectious diseases and this will be followed by a description of several of the commoner diseases grouped according to the causal organism. Those infectious diseases which produce effects predominantly on one organ or system of the body are dealt with under that system.

Pathogens and commensals

According to their ability to produce disease in the human, the microorganisms may be grouped as follows:

1. Active pathogens which almost invariably cause disease when they gain access to the body in sufficient numbers unless the individual has a high degree of natural or acquired immunity.
2. Commensals which multiply on the skin and mucous membrane surfaces of the body, and within the body (e.g. in the intestines), without causing damage.

The division into these two groups is, however, not a rigid one and many commensals are capable of causing disease under certain circumstances. Thus the pneumococcus, which is usually present in the normal flora of the mouth and throat, may cause bronchopneumonia if the resistance is lowered by diseases such as measles or influenza. Another example of a potential pathogen is the production of subacute bacterial endocarditis by the usually harmless *Streptococcus viridans*.

Results of infection
Infection of the tissues of the body with pathogenic organisms is not necessarily followed by recognizable disease. The outcome depends on the balance between the resistance of the individual and the intensity of the infection. Factors favourably influencing resistance are natural immunity from previous contact with the organism, artificial immunity as a result of prophylactic vaccination, etc., and a satisfactory state of the general health and nutrition. Factors influencing the intensity of the infection are the number of organisms concerned, their virulence which is not a constant for any given species, and the portal of entry. Depending on the resultant of these various factors there may be produced:

1. A subclinical infection.
2. A clinical infection, of varying severity, but with recovery.
3. A clinical infection which proves fatal.

Sources of infection
The infection may be derived from the excreta of cases or carriers of the disease, both human and animal.

An important factor favouring the spread of infection from cases is the high infectivity of many of these diseases in the earliest stages, often before a diagnosis has been reached and preventive measures and treatment instituted. Spread of the upper respiratory tract infections, such as the common cold, is facilitated by the widespread custom of continuing one's ordinary activities during the illness.

A *carrier* is an apparently healthy individual who harbours a pathogenic organism. In some instances this follows a clinical attack of the disease, but in others this is not so. Perhaps the best known example is the typhoid carrier who may excrete pathogenic organisms in the faeces and urine for several years and be responsible for many cases of typhoid particularly if engaged in the preparation or handling of food.

Modes of transmission

A healthy individual may become infected with pathogenic organisms in the following ways:

1. By *direct contact* with someone suffering from the disease, e.g. the venereal diseases, impetigo.

2. By *contact with some intermediate object* such as improperly sterilized syringes, needles, and other instruments, and common articles of cutlery and crockery.

3. By *airborne transmission* of the organisms. Many organisms are sprayed into the atmosphere during speaking, coughing and sneezing, and they may remain airborne, in fine droplet form, for considerable periods and thus be inhaled by several individuals. Even after the droplets have dried the risk is not over for the fine particles of dust which are formed may contain resistant organisms such as the tubercle bacilli. Airborne transmission is the principal mode of spread in many of the common infectious diseases of childhood, e.g. measles, whooping cough.

4. By *ingestion* of infected food and water. This may be responsible for large scale outbreaks of typhoid fever, bacillary dysentery, and cholera.

5. By *vectors* including the house fly, which is responsible for the mechanical transmission of many organisms, the body louse (epidemic typhus) and the mosquito (malaria).

Prevention and control

The principal measures employed to prevent and control the infectious diseases may be grouped as follows:

1. *Isolation of cases* is vitally important in the highly infectious disorders such as smallpox, cholera, and dysentery. Isolation used to be standard practice in Britain for the majority of children suffering from the common infectious diseases such as measles, scarlet fever, etc., and many special hospitals were built for this purpose. Due to the wide scale use of immunization, the reduced virulence of some of the organisms, the improvement in living standards, and the introduction of the antibiotics, these diseases are now much less frequent and less dangerous. Isolation is still carried out in the occasional cases of diphtheria which occur but otherwise hospital admission is usually necessary only when the home circumstances are very unsatisfactory, or the attack is particularly severe.

2. Detection and treatment of *carriers*.

3. Maintenance of a *clean water and food* supply, and control of sewage.

4. Control of *vectors* such as flies, lice, and mosquitoes.

5. The production of *active immunity* in vulnerable individuals by the use of vaccines and toxoids. A vaccine is a preparation of killed or attenuated bacteria or viruses which retain their antigenic properties, i.e. stimulate the production of antibodies, but are no longer capable of producing disease. A toxoid is a toxin artificially modified so that it is no longer poisonous but remains antigenic.

Prophylactic immunization is now widely practised and in Britain it is usual to advise immunization of young children against diphtheria, tetanus, pertussis (with the so-called triple vaccine), smallpox, and poliomyelitis. Immunization against many other diseases is also available and may be required in the special circumstances of war or in the tropics—e.g. against typhoid and paratyphoid fever, and yellow fever.

6. *Passive immunity*, which is short-lived, may be conferred on susceptible individuals before or just after infection has taken place, by the injection of serum or gamma globulin containing antibodies to the organism concerned. Examples are the use of antitoxic serum in actual or suspected cases of tetanus, gas gangrene, and diphtheria.

It may be noted in passing that the infant has a natural passive immunity, of some months duration, to many infectious diseases, derived from the transplacental passage of antibodies from the mother during intrauterine life.

Clinical features

Many of the infectious diseases have clinical features in common. The onset is usually sudden after an incubation period ranging from a day or two to several weeks, but which is relatively constant for a given organism. In general, the patient feels unwell, has a poor appetite, may vomit, has a coated tongue, a rapid pulse, and an elevated temperature. A lesion may be present at the portal of entry of the organism. In several instances, skin rashes occur and these may be sufficiently distinctive to be of diagnostic value. Symptoms otherwise largely depend on the localization of the organism, e.g. in the liver in cases of infective hepatitis, or in the lung in lobar pneumonia.

A leucocytosis develops due to a polymorphonuclear increase in the bacterial infections and there is an increase in lymphocytes in viral infections.

VIRAL INFECTIONS

Viruses are the smallest microorganisms known to cause disease. Electron microscopy is necessary for their visualization. As far as is known, they multiply only within living cells. Certain viral infections such as poliomyelitis and smallpox produce a long-lasting immunity whereas in others such as the common cold and influenza, the immunity is, unfortunately, short-lived.

Among the more important viral diseases are the common cold, influenza, poliomyelitis, infective hepatitis, infectious mononucleosis (these are described elsewhere), and measles, German measles, mumps, chickenpox, herpes zoster, and smallpox.

Measles

The incubation period of measles is 10 days to the onset of the first symptoms, and 14 days to the development of the rash. It is spread by droplet infection.

The illness starts with an upper respiratory tract infection and, during this stage, the child appears as if he has an extremely severe head cold. In addition, the conjuctivae are usually injected ('pink eye'), while examination of the buccal mucosa at this stage will reveal the presence of Koplik's spots which are small, whitish-grey, spots set on an erythematous base. They are most often seen along the line of closure of the molar teeth. After three or four days a blotchy, purplish rash develops particularly on the face and trunk; it is often first apparent behind the ears. In most cases fever lessens and the rash begins to fade in a further three or four days.

The main complications are secondary bacterial infection spreading to the middle ear (otitis media), and bronchopneumonia, both of which are less frequent and serious since the introduction of antibiotics.

Gamma globulin derived from the plasma of individuals who have had measles may be used to give passive immunity to children for whom an attack of measles might be particularly dangerous.

German measles (*rubella*)

The incubation period is two to three weeks.

It is usually a relatively mild febrile illness associated with rhinitis, tender enlargement of the cervical lymph glands, and a transient rash which is often maximal behind the ears. Koplik's spots do not occur.

The condition is of little importance except in pregnant women, when it may cause congenital heart disease and other defects in the offspring.

Mumps (*epidemic parotitis*)

The incubation period of mumps is two to three weeks.

The characteristic feature is tender swelling of the parotid glands with inflammation of the orifice of the duct. Occasionally the other salivary glands are also involved.

The main complications of mumps are inflammation of the pancreas (pancreatitis), and the testes (orchitis). These are more liable to occur in adults.

There is no specific treatment for mumps. A fluid diet is usually required until the acute parotid swelling subsides. Oral hygiene is important.

Chickenpox (*varicella*)

This is caused by a virus which has an incubation period of two to three weeks.

The infection usually causes relatively little general upset. The characteristic feature is the occurence of many small blisters, or vesicles, filled with a clear fluid, on the skin, particularly of the trunk, and on the mucous membranes. The lesions are superficial, intensely itchy, and they occur in successive crops. Secondary infection of the vesicles may occur due to scratching and may cause small permanent scars.

The principal object of treatment is to prevent secondary infection of the vesicles.

Herpes zoster (*shingles*)

The virus of herpes zoster is identical to that of chickenpox and the illness may occur in those in contact with chickenpox, and vice versa. It has a predilection for the posterior nerve roots particularly those of the trunk and for the fifth cranial nerve. The condition is always unilateral.

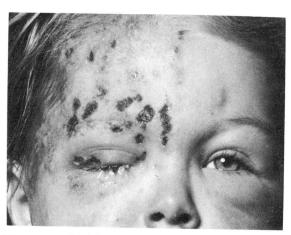

Fig. 1.1 Herpes zoster of ophthalmic division of trigeminal nerve.

The infection starts with three or four days during which the individual feels unwell, has mild fever, and experiences pain, which is often severe, in the sensory area of the affected posterior nerve root. A red rash then develops along the sensory distribution of the affected nerve followed by the occurrence of small vesicles filled with a clear fluid. These vesicles usually last for about one week and if secondarily infected they may leave a permanent scar. The discomfort and pain produced by the vesicles is often extreme. If the fifth cranial nerve is involved (Fig. 1.1) the lesions may occur on the eye causing corneal scarring with resultant impairment of vision. After the condition has cleared there may be persistent pain in the affected area. Postherpetic neuralgia is commoner in the elderly (see also p. 306).

The vesicles should be kept dry and free from infection and analgesics are given to relieve pain.

Small pox (*variola*)
This is due to a virus with an incubation period of about 12 days. Smallpox used to be common in Britain and in the Middle Ages it is said that a woman could lay some claims to beauty if she possessed a skin unblemished by its ravages. The prefix 'small' was used to distinguish it from the 'great' pox, syphilis.

There is a short prodromal stage of malaise and fever followed by an extensive rash which is at first papular, then vesicular, and then pustular. The great majority of the lesions occur at the one time and not in successive crops as in chickenpox. They are maximal on the peripheral parts of the body, e.g. the face and the distal parts of the limbs. The pustules rupture, or dry up, with the formation of scabs; when these separate they may leave very disfiguring scars. The mortality rate is considerable in severe infections.

In the late eighteenth century Jenner, an English country doctor, noted that persons who had been infected with a rather similar illness affecting cows (cowpox) either did not develop smallpox, or at least got it in a mild form. This inspired clinical observation led to vaccination and a subsequent marked reduction of smallpox in countries where vaccination was widely practised. A small quantity of lymph containing the cowpox virus is placed on the skin (usually the shoulder area) and, either by multiple pressure or by scarification, is introduced into the deeper layers of the skin. A localized reaction develops which goes through the same stages as the lesions of smallpox, namely, vesiculation with a clear fluid, pustulation, scab formation, and permanent scar. Vaccination produces an active immunity which gives protection against smallpox for approximately seven years. Vaccination may, therefore, have to be repeated at time of special risk.

RICKETTSIAL INFECTIONS

The rickettsiae are microorganisms which are intermediate between viruses and bacteria. They occur naturally in various arthropods, which act as vectors of infection.

Rickettsial infections are still widespread in many parts of the North American continent and in the Pacific area although their incidence has been much reduced by insecticides to control the vectors. Examples are scrub typhus and Rocky Mountain spotted fever.

Epidemic typhus (gaol fever or camp fever). This is the most serious of the rickettsial infections. The vector is the human body louse, *Pediculus corporis.* Typhus was common in Europe until the end of the nineteenth century and was again a scourge in Russia and Eastern Europe during and shortly after the First World War. An outbreak in Naples during the Second World War was prevented from spreading by prompt application of strict hygienic measures. Chloramphenicol and tetracycline are effective remedies for rickettsial infections.

BACTERIAL INFECTIONS

The number of bacteria which are actively or potentially pathogenic to man is very large. They are usually grouped according to their reaction to Gram staining.

1. Gram-positive bacteria—streptococci, staphylococci, pneumococci, diphtheria bacilli, tubercle bacilli, tetanus bacilli, and gas gangrene bacilli (*Cl. welchii*).
2. Gram-negative bacteria—gonococci, meningococci, *H. pertussis*, *E. coli*, members of the typhoid and dysentery group, *V. cholerae*, and the plague bacilli (*P. pestis*).

Streptococcal infections

The haemolytic streptococci are very important pathogens responsible for several infectious diseases. In addition, an immunological reaction to streptococcal infection is generally considered to be the cause of rheumatic fever, chorea, and acute nephritis.

Penicillin has greatly facilitated the treatment of streptococcal infections.

Streptococcal sore throat. Infection of the throat with the haemolytic streptococcus is a common ailment. The infectivity is high and the incubation period short. It occurs more frequently in the autumn and winter months and affects particularly children and young adults. Small epidemics may occur.

The throat shows evidence of acute inflammation and is fiery red on inspection. The tonsils, if present, are enlarged and points of pus may be visible on the surface; in some cases a thin, yellowish membrane, which is easily removed, covers the tonsillar area. The cervical lymph glands are enlarged and tender. Constitutional upset shown by fever, tachycardia, malaise, and leucocytosis is usually associated and, in severe infections, may be marked.

Mild cases usually respond to symptomatic treatment while in more severe cases sulphonamides or penicillin are given.

The infection may cause an abscess in the tonsillar area (quinsy throat) requiring incision to permit drainage; this complication is now infrequent.

Scarlet fever (scarlatina). This is due to infection of the throat with strains of haemolytic streptococci which possess a toxin capable of producing a red rash in susceptible individuals. The disease is now much milder than it used to be and cases occur where the rash is slight or absent. The incubation period is a few days.

The essential clinical feature is acute inflammation of the throat as described under streptococcal tonsillitis. When present, the red rash is widespread but it does not involve the area around the lips which appears pale relative to the rest of the face (circumoral pallor). The tongue is thickly coated with a white fur in the early stages. Later this peels off leaving a red tongue with engorged papillae, sometimes referred to as a strawberry tongue.

The infection may spread to the ears, causing otitis media, while rheumatic fever and acute nephritis should be remembered as possible complications.

Erysipelas. This is a local infection of the deeper layers of the skin and the subcutaneous tissues with haemolytic streptococci. The incubation period is a few days.

The affected area is red, oedematous, has a raised border, and spreads rapidly. The face and legs are the commonest sites.

Impetigo. This is due to infection of the superficial layer of the skin with streptococci alone or in combination with staphylococci. It is most often seen on the faces of poorly cared for children who may also harbour head lice and have scabies.

The lesions commence as small vesicles filled with yellow pus which forms honey-coloured crusts or scabs. Impetigo is highly contagious.

The principal aspects of treatment are initial cleansing to remove the crusts, application of penicillin or ammoniated mercury ointment, and attention to the general health and hygiene.

Puerperal fever. Childbed fever, due to streptococcal infection, used to be a dreaded complication in maternity hospitals and was responsible for many maternal deaths. Fortunately, it is now very rare.

Staphylococcal infections

Many of the infections due to staphylococci are essentially surgical problems and are dealt with in Chapter 2.

Sycosis barbae (barber's rash). This is a staphylococcal infection of the hair follicles in the beard area in men. Numerous small yellow pustules develop and close inspection reveals that each is centred by a hair. The condition is very contagious but fortunately it usually responds to local antibiotic applications. The patient may have to stop shaving for a few days.

Diphtheria

This is due to infection with the *Corynebacterium diphtheriae.* The incubation period is short (two to seven days). Fortunately, the incidence of diphtheria has been greatly reduced following the widespread adoption of immunization of children. Despite the small number of cases now occurring, it is important that the immunization programme is maintained.

The child with diphtheria is usually extremely ill and toxic. Examination of the throat shows a grey-yellowish membrane covering the tonsillar area; the membrane is very adherent and, if it is forcibly removed, small bleeding points are left. The throat is not fiery red as in streptococcal infections. Enlargement of the cervical lymph glands is present.

Diphtheria is an extremely serious illness as the toxin produced by the organism may produce myocarditis and various forms of paralysis, the commonest being paralysis of the soft palate. Furthermore, the membrane in the throat may be so extensive as to obstruct the airway necessitating tracheotomy to prevent asphyxiation.

In actual, or suspected, cases diphtheria antitoxin is given promptly and penicillin is administered in full dosage.

Whooping cough (*pertussis*)

This is caused by the organism *Haemophilus pertussis.* The incubation period varies from one to almost three weeks.

The illness starts with what appears to be a severe upper respiratory tract infection, associated often with conjunctivitis. After a short period it is noted that the child is having paroxysms of severe cough with an inspiratory whoop at the end of each paroxysm. The whoop is due to forced inspiration through a glottis which is in spasm. Vomiting not infrequently occurs at the end of each severe paroxysm and, if this is prolonged, it may lead to serious malnutrition. The paroxysms of coughing may cause ulceration of the fraenum of the tongue.

Whooping cough may be complicated by bronchopneumonia and, in some instances, there is collapse of small portions of lung tissue with danger in the future of bronchiectasis.

Antibiotics are required in full dosage if any of these respiratory complications occur.

Bacillary dysentery

This bowel infection is caused by a group of bacilli which bear the names of some of the most distinguished bacteriologists (Sonne, Flexner, and Shiga). The incubation period is short. The usual mode of infection is by contamination of food and drink. Cases occur mainly in the tropics but it is by no means uncommon in Britain. Serious epidemics were a scourge of many military campaigns in the past and there is an old reference to the disease as 'the bloody flux which decimated armies'.

The main features of the illness are colicky, abdominal pains associated with intense diarrhoea with blood and mucus in the stools, and a high fever. The condition is extremely infective. In severe cases there may be serious dehydration and shock.

Poorly absorbed sulphonamide drugs such as phthalylsulphathiazole are very valuable in the treatment of bacillary dysentery.

Typhoid and paratyphoid fever

Typhoid and paratyphoid fever, or the enteric fevers, are caused by bacteria of the Salmonella group which produce acute inflammation of the small intestine. The infection is transmitted in a similar way to bacillary dysentery, but in the first few days the microbes enter the blood stream, from which they may be isolated.

There is a prodromal period of toxaemia and pyrexia before severe diarrhoea develops. At this stage rose-coloured spots occur on the trunk and the spleen becomes enlarged. After several days of extreme illness the temperature gradually falls. The main complications are perforation of the gut and intestinal haemorrhage.

Chloramphenicol has greatly improved the prognosis and ampicillin is also of value.

SPIROCHAETAL INFECTIONS

The spirochaetes are elongated, spiral organisms which, although motile, do not possess flagella. The major systemic spirochaetal diseases are syphilis (page 24), Weil's disease, yaws, and relapsing fever. Vincent's infection of the buccal cavity is due to the combined effects of fusiform bacilli and a spirochaete.

Weil's disease (*Leptospirosis icterohaemorrhagiae*)

The usual mode of infection is contamination of minor skin abrasions with water to which rats, which are carriers of the spirochaete, have had access. Sewage workers are mainly affected. The disease is a serious one and is characterized by severe liver damage with jaundice and a tendency to haemorrhage. Cases of moderate severity usually respond to penicillin, but acute liver failure or acute renal failure may occur in very severe cases.

FUNGAL INFECTIONS

The fungi are multicellular microorganisms often forming long branching filaments. Localized infections of the skin, such as athlete's foot, and of the mucous membranes, such as thrush are quite common. Systemic fungal infections are rare in Britain but not infrequent in America.

Ringworm (*tinea*)

This is a general term which includes several varieties of localized infection of the skin and adnexae caused by closely related fungi.

One of the commonest sites is between the toes (athlete's foot) where the skin becomes thickened and sodden, small blisters develop, and an offensive odour results. This infection may secondarily involve the fingers and other parts of the body such as the groins.

Other varieties include ringworm of the scalp (tinea capitis) which causes scaly areas on the scalp associated with a patchy loss of hair, and tinea circinata characterized by reddish, ring-shaped lesions on the skin.

Actinomycosis.

This is dealt with in Chapter 2.

PROTOZOAL INFECTIONS

Protozoa are unicellular parasites which are extremely important causes of disease in tropical and semitropical countries. The most important protozoal infections of man are malaria, amoebiasis, trypanosomiasis or sleeping sickness, and leishmaniasis or kala-azar.

Malaria

This is caused by a protozoal parasite of the genus Plasmodium. The parasite has two stages in its life cycle, one being passed in the mosquito and the other in the red blood cells and reticuloendothelial system of man.

The classical feature in benign tertian malaria, which is one of the common forms, is recurring bouts of fever occurring every 48 hours. At the start of each bout the individual feels intensely cold, has a rigor, and experiences aching in the muscles; he then becomes extremely hot and the temperature rises quickly; the third stage is that of profuse sweating with fall of temperature; thereafter he usually falls into a sleep. Enlargement of the spleen is a characteristic finding. In chronic cases anaemia develops.

The traditional drug used in the treatment of malaria is quinine, but there are now also many synthetic preparations, such as primaquine and chloroquine available both for the treatment and prophylaxis of malaria. The main step in the eradication of the disease is control of the mosquito and, in particular, destruction of its breeding grounds.

Amoebic dysentery

This is caused by a protozoan parasite known as the *Entamoeba histolytica*. The illness is usually less acute than bacillary dysentery. Diarrhoea, weight loss, and pyrexia occur. There is a tendency for chronic infection to be established in the bowel and for spread to occur to the liver, producing amoebic hepatitis or amoebic abscess.

The main therapeutic agents are emetine or, more recently, metronidazole and chloroquine.

METAZOAL INFECTIONS

The metazoa are multicellular, invertebrate animals, several of which are parasitic to man.

Examples which may be seen in Western countries are threadworms and tapeworms. Other parasitic worms of great importance include schistosomal infection of the intestine and bladder which is common in the Middle East, fluke infection of the liver and lungs seen especially in the Far East, and hydatid disease caused by the larval stage of the tapeworm Echinococcus which is encountered particularly in Australia.

Threadworms

Infection of the gut with threadworms is quite common in Western countries especially in children. The adult worms measure about 1 cm in length and are actively motile.

No symptoms are produced by the presence of the worms in the gut, but the female worm emerges from the bowel at night to lay eggs in the perianal region and this causes intense local itching. The fingers of the individual commonly become infected with the eggs due to scratching and subsequent reinfection through the mouth is common. Threadworms are popularly believed to cause children to grind their teeth at nights but it is doubtful if this is so.

The main steps in treatment are improved hygiene to prevent reinfection and the use of a drug which has a lethal action on the worms.

Tapeworms

The beef tapeworm, *Taenia saginata*, is a commoner intestinal parasite than the pork tapeworm. *Taenia solium*. Infestation arises from eating undercooked meat or pork which contains the worms in cyst form. The worms lodge in the small intestine, being attached to the mucosa by a row of suckers on the head, and may grow to many feet in length. Ripe segments which contain eggs, become detached from the terminal portion of the parasite and are passed with the faeces. Treatment consists in the administration of drugs which have a toxic action on the worm.

THE ARTHROPODS

The arthropods are a special group of metazoa including flies, fleas, lice, the parasite of scabies, spiders, and scorpions. They may cause disease in man by transmitting infection, by parasitic infestation, or by injection of poisons.

Lice

Only the head louse, *Pediculus capitis*, and the body louse, *Pediculus corporis*, will be described.

The head louse is most likely to be seen in the hair of ill-cared for children and adults. The ova, or nits, are small white oval objects firmly atached to the hairs by a special cement. The adult lice are larger, flat, and mobile. The ova hatch within one week and mature in two weeks so multiplication takes place at a great rate. Head lice produce considerable irritation of the scalp and secondary infection of the resultant scratch marks is common; chronically infested individuals, however, appear able to harbour vast numbers of lice without discomfort.

The body louse, which is rather larger than the head louse, lives on non-hairy skin and usually chooses the seams of clothes as a site for depositing the ova. Irritation of the skin leads to scratching, excoriation, and secondary infection. The body louse is of great importance in the transmission of typhus.

Proper hygiene is the main factor in the prevention of louse infestation. Ova may be removed from the hair by the use of a fine comb dipped repeatedly in weak acetic acid which loosens the cement. Malathion, applied locally, is an effective insecticide for the adult lice.

Scabies

Scabies, which is caused by a parasite known as the *Acarus scabiei*, is spread by close contact. The female acarus burrows under the horny layer of the skin to lay its eggs. The small tell-tale burrows are seen especially around skin folds such as between the fingers, at the wrists and in the axillae and groins. Scabies causes intense itching, especially at night, and scratch marks and secondary infection are commonly present. Benzyl benzoate ointment, applied liberally to the whole body after hot baths, is a common remedy. Clean clothes and improved hygiene are indicated.

TUBERCULOSIS

Incidence

Tuberculosis has been known since the earliest days of medicine and has been variously termed the 'captain of the men of death', consumption and phthisis; these latter terms were descriptive of the wasting which is a striking feature of the advanced forms of the disease.

The incidence of tuberculosis was very high in Britain in the nineteenth century when it was a major cause of death. The poor social conditions which were commonplace during the Industrial Revolution were largely responsible for the prevalence of the infection. The marked improvement in living standards which has occurred since the nineteenth century contributed greatly to the

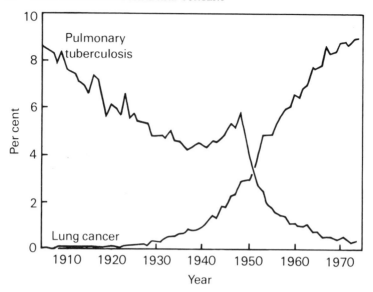

Fig. 1.2 Deaths from pulmonary tuberculosis and lung cancer in men in Scotland as a percentage of deaths from all causes (prepared by Professor A. J. Haddow from material derived from the Registrar General's returns).

decline in the incidence of tuberculosis and the advent of anti-tuberculosis drugs accelerated the fall. Fig. 1.2 shows the striking fall in the mortality figures in the present century; these contrast markedly with the increasing mortality rate for bronchogenic carcinoma.

Tuberculosis is still far from being a rare disease, however, and there is no room for complacency. Many thousands of new cases of respiratory tuberculosis are detected annually in Britain. The incidence is higher where social conditions are poor and in the coloured immigrant population.

The maximum age incidence of the disease is in children and young adults. Cases may occur also in older people and may go undiagnosed for many years constituting an important source of infection.

Bacteriology

The tubercle bacillus was discovered by Koch in 1882. It is a rod-shaped organism with certain individual staining characteristics which are of great importance in its recognition; with the Ziehl-Neelsen technique the bacillus is stained red and this colour is not removed by acid, hence the term acid-fast bacillus. The tubercle bacillus has a high resistance, and will live for weeks outside the body under certain conditions, e.g. in dust. It is, however, killed by exposure to strong daylight, by boiling for at least two minutes, and by autoclaving.

There are two types of tubercle bacillus of importance to man. The human variety, which is endemic in man, causes pulmonary tuberculosis and most cases of bone and joint tuberculosis, genitourinary tuberculosis, and meningeal tuberculosis. The bovine variety, which is endemic in cattle, causes most cases of alimentary and lymph gland tuberculosis.

Mode of spread
The majority of cases due to the human strain of the organism are spread by droplet spray from the lungs of patients with 'open' pulmonary tuberculosis. The dentist is, by nature of his work, particularly prone to this form of infection.

The bovine variety of the organism is spread to man by ingestion of milk from an infected cow unless the tubercle bacilli have been killed by pasteurization or boiling.

Pathology of pulmonary tuberculosis
The tubercle bacilli are inhaled, settle in the lungs and cause a small local reaction known as the primary focus, or Ghon focus. The main histological features of the 'tubercle' are a central area of coagulative necrosis, termed caseation, and a cellular rection in which epithelioid and giant cells are characteristic. The lymph glands at the hilum also become infected. The term primary complex is used to describe the lung lesion plus the associated lymph gland lesion.

1. In most cases firm healing of both the lung and the gland components takes place, at first by fibrous tissue and later by the deposition of calcium salts. Small healed, calcified areas are quite commonly seen in the chest X-ray of adults who give no past history of pulmonary tuberculosis. The individual is now sensitized to tuberculin (see below) and has acquired a partial immunity.
2. In some individuals the infection persists and spreads in the lungs to produce either local, or diffuse tuberculosis of all degrees of severity. The lesions may vary from a single small area of caseation to multiple lesions, with large cavity formation, throughout both lungs. The disease may manifest itself soon, or many years after the primary infection has taken place.

3. In a minority of cases blood spread occurs to the bones and joints, the kidneys, the nervous system, and throughout the lungs themselves.
4. There may be recrudescence of activity from an apparently healed primary focus under conditions of impaired resistance or following prolonged steroid therapy.

Tuberculin sensitivity

Within a few weeks of a person becoming infected with tubercle bacilli he develops a sensitivity to tuberculin which may be revealed by a positive reaction to the intradermal inoculation of a very small amount of the diluted substance, as in the Mantoux technique. Tuberculin sensitivity is an extremely valuable phenomenon as it enables us to separate those who have been infected with tubercle bacilli from those who have not. A positive Mantoux reaction is not to be taken as an indication that someone is suffering from tuberculosis but only that at some time in the past he has been infected with tubercle bacilli.

Clinical features of tuberculosis

Active tuberculous infection is associated with lassitude, malaise, loss of appetite, and loss of weight. The pulse is rapid, there is a tendency to evening pyrexia associated with night sweats, and the erythrocyte sedimentation rate is elevated. In addition there may be local features depending on the organ involved.

Pulmonary tuberculosis

Pulmonary tuberculosis may take several forms (Figs. 1.3–1.6).

1. *The primary complex.* The individual may be quite unaware of the primary infection, there may be a vague illness which passes undiagnosed, or there may be evidence of 'tuberculous toxaemia' as described in the preceding section.

2. Occasionally the primary infection causes a brisk pleural reaction with the formation of a straw-coloured effusion containing lymphocytes.

3. *Acute spread* through the lungs. In some unfortunate individuals the tubercle bacilli spread rapidly through the lungs producing a very active, extensive, lesion almost like a pneumonia in its rate of spread. This is the variety which used to be termed 'galloping consumption'.

4. *Fibrocaseous pulmonary tuberculosis.* This is the commonest form of tuberculosis of the lungs. The lesions are most often at the apices and in the absence of treatment progressive caseation causes

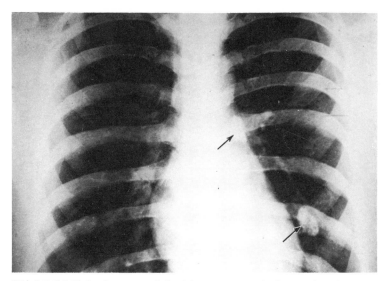

Fig. 1.3 Calcified pulmonary and glandular component of primary tuberculous complex.

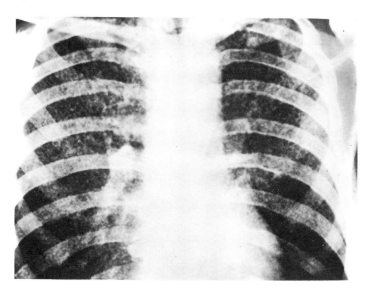

Fig. 1.4 Snowstorm appearance in miliary tuberculosis.

much tissue destruction and cavities develop. Cough and spit, haemoptysis, breathlessness and discomfort in the chest may all be present in addition to the features of toxaemia described above. A chest X-ray is an essential step in diagnosis. Finger clubbing occurs in chronic cases where there is much suppuration.

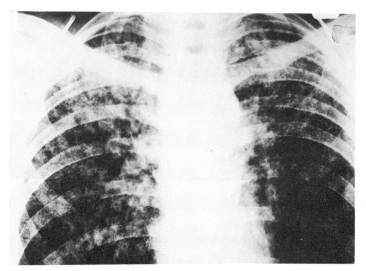

Fig. 1.5 Bilateral active tuberculosis.

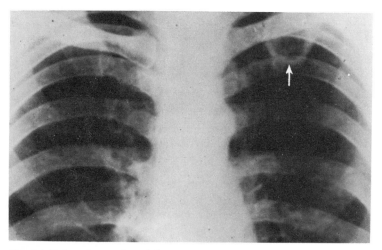

Fig. 1.6 Tuberculous cavity at left apex.

5. *Miliary tuberculosis.* This is caused by the haematogenous spread of the organism, and in the lungs it is represented by the presence of literally thousands of small tubercles which, on chest X-ray, give the appearance of a 'snow storm' lung.

Alimentary tuberculosis
This may be a primary infection due to ingestion of milk infected with bovine tubercle bacilli or it may result from swallowing infected sputum in chronic pulmonary cases.

1. Lesions of the buccal cavity are uncommon. Superficial painful ulceration of the tongue may occur in chronic pulmonary cases with infected sputum.

2. The ileocaecal region is the part of the alimentary tract most frequently affected as the temporary hold-up in intestinal contents at this site gives the tubercle bacilli a greater opportunity to invade the lymphatic tissue in the wall of the gut. Diarrhoea is the principal symptom.

3. The infection may spread from the gut to the abdominal lymph nodes and peritoneum causing ascites. The swollen abdomen contrasts with the general wasting which occurs.

Tuberculous lymphadenitis

The two main sites for tuberculous lymphadenitis are the neck and abdomen. The latter has already been described. Disease in the neck is usually fairly well localized and is more common in the upper cervical region where it is the result of tonsillar infection reaching the jugulodigastric node but later extending to other nodes. The lesion is a primary focus and not secondary to tuberculosis elsewhere. However, infection of the lower cervical glands can occur, and this is always secondary to disease elsewhere, usually the apex of the lung. Very rarely there is a diffuse enlargement of the cervical nodes related to blood spread of tuberculosis. Following the initial reaction resolution may occur or the lesion proceed to caseation, the necrotic tissue extending towards the surface and perforating the ensheathing layer of deep cervical fascia and then later the skin (collar stud abscess).

Bone and joint tuberculosis

The main sites of skeletal involvement are the vertebrae, the hip joints, and the knee joints. Local bone destruction occurs producing pain, deformity and impaired joint function. Severe hunchback deformity can result from involvement of the spine and there may be cold abscess formation with pressure on adjacent structures, e.g., the spinal cord.

Genetourinary tuberculosis

Involvement of the kidneys and bladder is always secondary to tuberculosis in some other site. Frequency of micturition is a common symptom. Microscopic examination of the urine commonly reveals pus and blood.

Tuberculous meningitis

Involvement of the covering membranes of the brain and spinal cord is seen especially in children. It is due to blood spread from the primary site of infection. The child becomes drowsy, irritable and obviously ill. Evidence of meningeal irritation is shown by stiffness of the neck. Examination of the cerebrospinal fluid, obtained by means of lumbar puncture, is the main diagnostic step.

Diagnosis

From the *clinical* point of view the main points to be considered are the family history, the individual's personal history regarding any of the symptoms mentioned in the preceding sections, physical examination, and the result of the Mantoux reaction.

Radiological examination of the lungs, bones and joints, of the kidneys etc., is essential if tuberculosis of these sites is suspected.

The *bacteriological* demonstration of the organism is the final proof of diagnosis. It may be found in the sputum, the urine, the faeces, the cerebrospinal fluid, and in pus or scrapings direct from lesions. It should be looked for in direct smears after staining by the Ziehl-Neelsen technique, by culture, and, if these measures are negative, by guinea pig inoculation. The bacteriologist can also give very valuable information regarding the sensitivity of the organism to the anti-tuberculous drugs.

Prophylaxis

The main aspects of prophylaxis are

1. The eradication of undesirable *social factors* such as poor housing, overcrowding, and faulty nutrition.

2. The *early diagnosis and treatment* of active tuberculosis. If cases can be detected early, and treated effectively, then the reservoir of infection will obviously be steadily reduced. Even in very advanced cases, where cure is not possible, the patient may be rendered non-infective by chemotherapy. The X-ray survey carried out in Glasgow in 1957 may be quoted as an example of the value of such campaigns. A total of 2,842 active cases of tuberculosis and 5,379 cases requiring observation was discovered out of 714,915 persons X-rayed in a five-week period.

3. *Elimination of tuberculous milk* may be achieved by the build-up of herds of cattle which are free from infection and, secondly, by the pasteurization of milk so that if any tubercle bacilli should be present they are rendered harmless.

4. The *protection of uninfected individuals* who are particularly at risk by a vaccine prepared from an attenuated, avirulent, strain of tubercle bacilli such as the bacillus Calmette Guérin (BCG). This procedure is especially valuable for children, and for nurses,

medical students, and dental students. Only those who are 'Mantoux negative' should be vaccinated, i.e. those who have not been infected. BCG vaccination does not give complete protection but there is now ample statistical evidence as to its worth in reducing the incidence of the disease in vulnerable groups of the population.

Treatment

Treatment of tuberculosis may be considered briefly under four aspects.

1. The patient's *natural resistance* to the disease should be built up as far as possible by means of rest, fresh air, and nutritious food. At one time this was the main form of treatment available and special centres, or sanatoria, were built in country and mountainous districts where these measures could be employed to the greatest advantage.

2. The provision of *local rest* to the diseased part is a basic principle in the treatment of any inflammatory condition. In the case of extensive pulmonary tuberculosis the work of the affected lung or lungs may be reduced by a variety of measures including injection or section of the phrenic nerve to partially paralyse the diaphragm, and by pneumothorax, but such procedures are now much less frequently required in consequence of the beneficial role of antituberculous drugs. In bone and joint tuberculosis prolonged immobilization in plaster casts is usually required.

3. The use of *antituberculous drugs* has revolutionized treatment and has very materially reduced the morbidity, mortality and incidence of the disease. Classical antituberculous chemotherapy for pulmonary tuberculosis consists of the triad of streptomycin intramuscularly and isoniazid and para-amino-salicylic acid (PAS) given orally for 6–12 weeks followed by isoniazid and PAS orally to a total of 18–24 months. Alternative drugs are rifampicin and ethambutol. It is essential that more than one drug is used at a time otherwise drug resistance is very rapidly induced.

4. *Surgical removal* of hopelessly diseased portions of tissue is an essential step in certain advanced cases, e.g. removal of a lobe of a lung (lobectomy) or removal of one kidney (nephrectomy).

Dental considerations

From the immediate practical point of view the dentist should remember the following important points:

1. The possibility of encountering tuberculous lesions of the buccal cavity.

2. The personal risk to himself should he undertake treatment in someone who has pulmonary tuberculosis.

3. The necessity for proper sterilization of instruments after dealing with anyone suspected to have tuberculosis.

THE VENEREAL DISEASES

In the great majority of cases venereal diseases are spread by sexual intercourse. It is important to realise that, in many instances, the persons suffering from the disorder may be unaware that they are a source of infection.

There is a risk that the dentist, doctor, or nurse may accidentally acquire the infection through examination of the mouth of a patient who is suffering from the secondary stage of syphilis. Syphilis may be transmitted from the mother *in utero*. Gonococcal infection of the eyes of the newborn child may occur at the time of birth if the mother is suffering from an active stage of gonorrhoea.

The venereal diseases represent a considerable social problem in practically all countries both in times of peace and, even more, in times of war when promiscuous sexual activity tends to increase.

Syphilis

Historical aspects
There is some doubt about the precise origin of syphilis, or lues, but it is generally believed that the infection was carried back by the sailors of Columbus from the New World since when it has been an unwelcome feature of civilization. It is likely, however, that the infection was present many hundreds of years before this time, and certain Biblical references to illnesses associated with extensive skin rashes may refer to what we now know as syphilis.

The causal organism was detected in 1905 and three years later an extremely valuable serological test was introduced by Wassermann.

Bacteriology
Syphilis is caused by a spirochaete, the *Treponema pallidum*. It is a delicate organism with a corkscrew shape, slightly greater in length than the diameter of a red blood corpuscle. It is able to penetrate the intact skin. It may be seen readily by dark-ground illumination after staining with a silver impregnation method but it does not stain with ordinary dyes. It has a low resistance outside the body and is relatively readily killed by antiseptics.

Natural history of the infection
On an average, some three to four weeks elapse from the time of acquiring the infection to the first sign of disease in the absence of treatment. The effects of the infection can most readily be understood if the disease is considered in three stages—primary, secondary, and tertiary—although it should be appreciated that the process is a continuous one and that the rate of progress from one stage to the other may show considerable individual variation.

Primary syphilis
The characteristic lesion of primary syphilis is termed the primary chancre, or hard sore. It develops some three to four weeks after infection and is usually situated on the genitalia. The lesion starts as a small, firm, raised swelling which breaks down in the centre to form an indurated ulcer which has a firm, rubbery, feel. It is not painful unless secondary infection occurs. The lymph nodes in the area of drainage (usually the groin) become firm, and slightly enlarged. In the absence of treatment the primary chancre will gradually heal and may or may not leave a fine scar. By this time, however, the spirochaetes have invaded the rest of the body.

Extragenital chancres may develop on the lips, or other anterior parts of the buccal cavity, from kissing a person suffering from the secondary stage of the disorder, or on the fingers of dentists, etc., who inadvertently examine the buccal cavity of an individual with secondary syphilis.

Secondary syphilis
The manifestations of secondary syphilis usually appear a few months after the primary stage. In the absence of treatment they may last from one to two years. The individual shows evidence of a general constitutional upset, the main features being irregular pyrexia, anorexia, headache, and limb pains. Skin rashes are common on the trunk and limbs and may be very varied in type; perhaps the most characteristic rashes are a coppery, macular eruption, and a deep red, papular eruption. Lesions of the buccal cavity are of considerable dental importance. They may take the form of mucous patches of sodden, greyish epithelium or superficial 'snail-track' ulcers. Both are extremely infective. Infective lesions also occur in the perineum (condylomata lata). The hair tends to fall out (alopecia), usually in a patchy distribution. Slight enlargement of the superficial lymph glands is commonly present.

Tertiary syphilis
The tertiary manifestations of syphilis may develop as early as 2

and as late as 25 or more years after the primary infection. The characteristic feature of this stage is a proliferative endarteritis of the small arteries resulting in their partial obliteration. This causes diminished blood supply to the affected organ, tissue destruction, and replacement fibrosis.

The two main *cardiovascular lesions* of tertiary syphilis are aneurysms of the aorta and incompetence of the aortic valve. In both instances the basic change is fibrous tissue replacement of the middle coat of the aorta so that stretching of the wall of the aorta occurs. Aortic aneurysms, which are now rarely seen, may be considerable in size and cause pressure on adjacent structures such as the bronchi, the left recurrent laryngeal nerve, and the oesophagus. The valve lesion, which is less uncommon, produces the same effects on the heart as aortic incompetence of rheumatic origin.

The major *central nervous system lesions* of tertiary syphilis are tabes dorsalis and general paralysis of the insane. Tabes dorsalis, which is also known as locomotor ataxia, is due to involvement of the posterior nerve roots of the spinal cord. It is characterized by difficulty in walking, loss of tendon reflexes, shooting or lightning pains in the limbs and trunk, loss of sensation in the deep structures of the legs, a painless arthritis (Charcot's joints), and loss of bladder control. The pupils are smaller than normal, irregular, and do not contract when stimulated by light (Argyll Robertson pupils). General paralysis of the insane is characterized pathologically by extensive invasion of the cerebral hemispheres by the spirochaete with subsequent death of brain tissue and fibrous tissue replacement. Delusions of grandeur are followed by progressive dementia and paralysis.

A *gumma* is the term given to the mass of granulation tissue which is produced as a reaction to the localization, in the tertiary stage of the disease, of spirochaetes in various tissues. Clinically the lesion usually takes the form of a hard, painless lump. Gummata may occur anywhere in the body but the commoner sites are in the skin and subcutaneous tissues, bone, palate, nasal septum, liver, and brain. Gummata situated in a superficial site tend to breakdown with the formation of indurated ulcers with 'punched-out' edges and a yellow, 'wash-leather' slough on the floor.

Latent syphilis
The term latent syphilis is used where there is no obvious clinical lesion to be found in the individual but the Wassermann reaction is positive. This type of case is seen not infrequently following treatment with antisyphilitic remedies.

Congenital syphilis

Congenital syphilis is due to infection passed from the mother to the foetus in utero via the placental circulation. It is much less common nowadays because a high proportion of pregnant women attend antenatal clinics where Wassermann reactions are routinely determined; patients with a positive reaction receive immediate treatment.

If the infection of the foetus is very severe death in utero will occur; if the infection is less pronounced a live, but infected, child will be born.

The syphilitic lesions which are commonest in the early months of life are inflammation of the mucous membranes of the nose producing 'snuffles', destruction of the nasal cartilages leading in later years to a saddle-nose deformity, moist papules at the angles of the mouth which heal leaving fine radiating scars known as rhagades, a papular rash especially over the buttocks, poor general health, anaemia, and enlargement of the liver and spleen.

In later childhood characteristic changes occur in the permanent teeth. The incisors become widely spaced, taper from the base to the cutting edge, and frequently show a notch on the margin (Hutchison's teeth). The first molar teeth tend to show rounding or doming (Moon's molars). Involvement of the corneal tissues of the eyes (interstitial keratitis) produces a ground glass appearance of the cornea with visual deterioration and possibly blindness. Other lesions that may occur include involvement of the eight nerve producing deafness, painless joint effusions (Clutton's joints), and the periostitis of the tibia leading to a sabre deformity.

Diagnosis

A history of exposure to infection is very helpful in suspected cases of syphilis but there may be reluctance to inquire; and the patient may attempt to conceal his indiscretion.

Regarding the clinical aspects of individual lesions one should remember that syphilis has been termed 'the great imitator', as it may produce a very wide variety of lesions which may mimic many other diseases. Suspicion should always be raised in the presence of painless firm ulcers, superficial ulcerated lesions in the mouth not apparently due to Vincent's infection, and in skin rashes which do not readily fit the pattern of the common skin disorders.

In all suspected cases a specimen of clotted blood (5 to 10 ml is sufficient) should be referred for laboratory examination. The serological reactions for syphilis may be negative very early in the infection and in a proportion of later cases but, in general, they are positive in the majority of cases. If syphilitic disease of the nervous system is suspected the cerebrospinal fluid should be examined.

The spirochaete may be demonstrated in scrapings from ulcerated lesions such as the primary chancre, or the secondary lesions of the buccal cavity. Since the organism is readily killed by antiseptics these must not be applied to the lesion prior to the samples being taken.

Prognosis
The prognosis in syphilis has been much improved since the introduction of penicillin. It is still essential, nevertheless, to make the diagnosis as early as possible because, once extensive tissue involvement has taken place, e.g. of the brain, complete cure cannot occur.

Treatment
Prior to the introduction of penicillin the main drugs used in the treatment of syphilis were organic arsenic, bismuth, and potassium iodide, and repeated courses of arsenic and bismuth, usually extending over months and often years were required, and even then many cases were not completely cured. Furthermore, these drugs, especially arsenic, were not without danger and very strict supervision of the treatment was essential.

Penicillin is a powerful spirochaeticidal drug and is largely free from side effects. There is some variation in the schemes of treatment currently in use, but the following is representative

In early cases of syphilis an intensive course of penicillin (e.g., 600,000 units daily for 14 days) is given and thereafter the patient is observed at frequent intervals, a blood Wassermann reaction being performed on each occasion; some authorities also prefer to have at least one examination of the cerebrospinal fluid performed during the first two years. If there is any clinical or serological sign of relapse further courses of penicillin are given. In chronic cases there is a possibility that the penicillin may lead to an anaphylactoid reaction (Herxheimer's reaction) due to the sudden liberation of much foreign protein from the dead spirochaetes into the circulation; this reaction is characterized by tachycardia, hypotension, and collapse. In most cases of late syphilis more than one course of penicillin is required before the infection is controlled.

In the case of congenital syphilis it may be stated categorically that 'the time to treat the infection is before the child is born'. If an expectant mother is found to have any evidence of syphilis, then a course of penicillin similar to that described above should be given and a careful follow-up instituted. If a child is born with any evidence of syphilis, penicillin is again the drug of choice.

Gonorrhoea

Gonorrhoea is caused by the gonococcus, a Gram-negative diplococcus which is mainly intracellular. The incubation period is usually about four to five days.

Clinical features

The main feature of the illness in the male is acute inflammation of the anterior urinary passages causing a purulent discharge and considerable discomfort. In chronic cases the infection may become established in the posterior urinary passages and related structures. Gonococcal arthritis, which is usually monoarticular, is a relatively uncommon complication due to blood spread. The temporomandibular joint may be affected. In the female there is a purulent vaginal and urethral discharge, often of relatively slight degree.

Diagnosis and treatment

The diagnosis is established by the demonstration of the organism in stained smears of the discharge.

Acute cases usually respond well to prompt treatment with penicillin. If the organism is resistant to penicillin, either cotrimoxazole or spectinomycin hydrochloride may be used. The latter drug does not mask incubating syphilis and may be useful in cases where both diseases are suspected.

2

Diseases due to infection—surgical aspects

INFLAMMATION

The response of tissue to infection, usually of bacterial origin, is known as inflammation. Bacteria cause inflammation as a result of cellular damage with disruption of the cells and lysozyme release. A complex chain of events is initiated including antigen antibody reactions with activation of complement and a sequential series of tissue reactions characterised by an accumulation of inflammatory cells. The bacteria also secrete toxins (exotoxins) or release toxins from disintegrating bacteria (endotoxins).

The course of the illness produced is the result of the balance between the number, multiplication and virulence of the bacteria and the defence mechanisms of the host. In addition to the immune mechanisms mentioned in Chapter 1, defence of the host includes the intact epithelial linings of the skin, alimentary, respiratory and urinary tracts, and the local acute inflammation which follows breach of the body's defences. Acute inflammation results in vascular dilation, the passage of exudate into the tissues and the migration of polymorphonuclear leucocytes. The inflamed part becomes red, hot, swollen, tense and painful, and there is some loss of function. Surrounding muscles may go into spasm to protect the part. Thus, in inflammation of the appendix, the abdominal wall muscles are held tense.

The exudate containing antibodies (and administered chemotherapeutic agents) together with the inflammatory cells prevent multiplication or destroy the organisms but these reactions are not as effective in the elderly patient, in the malnourished, if there is severe anaemia or in some concomitant diseases such as diabetes and renal failure. Poor blood supply to a part is also an adverse factor.

The extent of the original bacterial invasion and the virulence of these bacteria are two important components in determining the outcome and some bacteria (for example, *Clostridium tetani*) produce extremely serious effects as a result of exotoxin secretion and yet remain localized at the site of infection.

It is also extremely important to recognize that healthy tissues with a good blood supply do not harbour bacteria readily. On the other hand, in the presence of haematomata, dead tissue or collections of fluid, organisms thrive much more readily. It is an important surgical principle in the prevention of infection to keep such areas to a minimum and to provide drainage following operations which result in collections of serous fluid or haematoma.

Should the body's defences predominate and the infection resolves, this may be accompanied, if the resolution process is slow, by the formation of scar tissue and fibrosis. On the other hand, the infection may progress, invading venous walls and causing infected clot formation (thrombophlebitis). Bacteria then seed into the blood stream and the result is the dangerous condition of bacteraemia. This is diagnosed by obtaining culture of bacteria from blood samples.

Cellulitis

Local progression of the infection results in inflammation of the connective tissue termed cellulitis. This may be subcutaneous (erysipelas, p. 9) but may also occur in other connective tissues such as those in the pelvis, the orbit and the retroperitoneum. Cellulitis is almost always accompanied by a degree of lymphangitis. This can be seen in the skin as red streaks along the lymphatic channels and the regional glands become enlarged and tender (lymphadenitis).

Abscess

Pyogenic organisms tend to form pus. This is composed of dead and dying polymorphs, liquified necrotic tissue and the organisms themselves. Surrounding acute inflammatory reaction walls off the abscess. Septic thrombosis may occur in adjacent small blood vessels and detachment of small infected thrombi can result in septic embolization with abscesses forming at distant sites in the body. The abscess is initially hard, red and painful but later, as the result of formation of much pus, softens and becomes fluctuant. The patient is feverish and there is anorexia, malaise and a polymorphonuclear leucocytosis. If not drained at this stage, it would discharge spontaneously either through the skin, forming a sinus, or internally into a viscus or serous cavity.

The treatment of abscesses is by drainage. Antibiotics without drainage are not only valueless but may be dangerous since the chemotherapeutic agents cannot sterilize the abscess completely which remains as a source of toxaemia and becomes surrounded by an increasingly dense mass of reactive fibrous tissue.

A *boil* (or *furuncle*) is a small abscess arising in a hair follicle and due to the *Staphylococcus pyogenes*. Boils may lead to the formation of distant abscesses and when they occur on the face may spread via the facial veins to the cavernous sinus within the brain, resulting in septic cavernous sinus thrombosis (p. 116).

A *carbuncle* is an area of subcutaneous pyogenic infection resulting in necrosis and discharging to the skin through multiple sinuses. It may commence with the formation of a boil with subsequent spread to surrounding hair follicles. Carbuncles generally occur on the shoulders, back of the neck or on the dorsum of the hands, and the condition is more common in diabetic patients.

Acute osteomyelitis

This infection of bone is most often due to *Staphylococcus aureus*. The infection is usually blood-borne but occasionally comes from an overlying soft tissue wound or compound fracture. The bones most often affected are the tibia or lower end of the femur and the disease occurs mainly in children.

The inflammation and pus spread through the bony canals and raises the periosteum. The tension within the bone occludes the local nutrient arteries producing thrombosis of small vessels and necrosis of bone which finally separates as a *sequestrum*. The elevated periosteum forms new bone (*involucrum*). As the disease progresses, the pus tracks to the surface forming one or more sinuses.

The disease is characterized by the sudden onset of severe pain in a limb accompanied by high fever and toxaemia. There is tenderness and swelling over the affected bone, a polymorphonuclear leucocytosis, and blood culture may reveal the causative organism. X-ray is initially quite normal and osteolytic areas with accompanying periosteal elevation and sclerosis are only noted at a much later stage.

Treatment is by high dosage antibiotics usually cloxacillin and by splintage of the affected limb. If there is not a prompt response then surgical drainage of pus is necessary by incision of the subperiosteal abscess and drilling of the bone through to the marrow cavity.

Failure of complete resolution of acute osteomyelitis results in diffuse bone sclerosis and thickening with infected cavities containing sequestrae. There may be multiple sinuses and old puckered scars in the overlying skin. This condition is known as chronic osteomyelitis and although it may be apparently quiescent, it may suddenly become active, even years later. Surgery is the only effective treatment. The bony cavities must be laid open and curetted.

Inflammation in the pulp of a tooth

Inflammation in the pulp of a tooth (pulpitis) results in the same series of changes as those described above and just as in inflammation in the marrow cavity of bone, the resultant swelling of tissue and pressure together with infection, results in ischaemic necrosis of the pulp of the tooth. As the inflamed pulp attempts to swell and expand in the confines of the pulp cavity, there is intense pain and this persists until the pulp dies. Following death of the pulp, the periapical tissues become involved and a periapical abscess forms. If not drained either by removal of the pulp or the tooth, it will discharge spontaneously to the surface (dental sinus) or into one of the soft tissue spaces around the jaws, resulting in a dangerous spreading cellulitis. This may occur in the soft tissues on the floor of the mouth (Ludwig's angina) and spread so as to compromise the airway.

Anaerobic infections

Tetanus

This is caused by the anaerobic spore-forming *Clostridium tetani*. Tetanus organism is present in soil and faecal matter and is a contaminant of dirty wounds. The organism only grows under anaerobic conditions and therefore thrives in deeply penetrating wounds where there is much dead tissue. It may enter the body through quite minute penetrating wounds.

The organism remains confined but secretes a very powerful exotoxin acting specifically on the cerebrospinal motor cells resulting in local severe muscle spasm, particularly in the neck and trunk. There is a painful trismus and spasm of the facial muscles (risus sardonicus). The disease progresses to intense convulsions and death often occurs from exhaustion, from respiratory tract infection, or asphyxiation. Active immunization against tetanus is the best method of prevention and can be obtained by the injection of tetanus toxoid. This is given to children but a booster dose should be given at five-year intervals and after injuries involving contaminated wounds.

An important part of prophylaxis is the adequate cleaning (debridement) of penetrating wounds, together with prophylactic antibiotics (penicillin). This, together with the injection of tetanus toxoid, is considered adequate prophylaxis and safer than passive immunization with antitetanus serum prepared from horses which carries a high risk of anaphylactic reaction. Human antitetanus globulin is now frequently employed in many centres and given at the same time as the toxoid.

Curative treatment involves care of the wound and nursing in a quiet, darkened room under sedation. Anticonvulsants are employed and penicillin in high dosage to destroy the organisms and thus prevent further production of toxin. Antitetanus serum in high dosage is given. Tracheostomy and artificial respiration are often necessary.

Gas gangrene

The *Clostridia welchii septicans* and *oedematiens* are found in faeces and soil. Like the *Clostridium tetani* they are anaerobic and thrive in dirty wounds. The organisms produce an enzyme which facilitates their spread in tissue and in addition to producing gas, they produce powerful exotoxins which may be haemolytic on entering the blood stream.

Clostridial infections tend to complicate large destructive wounds of tissue, but may also occur from contamination arising from the patient's own gastrointestinal tract following some forms of abdominal surgery. There is profound toxaemia often associated with septic shock and frequently haemolysis. The tissues around the wound are crepitant due to the infiltration of gas and as the disease spreads the tissues become discoloured and gangrenous and a foul smelling discharge occurs.

Prophylactic treatment is by adequate and extensive debridement of dead tissue and the administration of prophylactic penicillin. For the established disease, large doses of penicillin are given and the wound is explored and extensively cleaned. Involved muscle is completely excised and amputation of the limb may be necessary. Anti-gasgangrene serum is administered and blood transfusion is usually necessary.

It cannot be emphasized too strongly that tetanus and gas gangrene are serious infections with a grave prognosis and the best method of treatment is the correct management of contaminated wounds.

Yeast and fungal infection

Thrush

Thrush is caused by the *Candida albicans*, a normal mouth commensal, which is also frequently found in the vagina.

The infection tends to occur in the debilitated, and in patients who have been on long-term administration of broad spectrum antibiotics. The infection may spread to involve the lungs and alimentary tract, and occasionally, in severely ill patients, may invade the blood stream. In the latter instance the prognosis is extremely serious.

Nystatin lozenges are specific for the oral form of the disease and more recently new systemic antifungal agents have been discovered which may alter the previously very serious prognosis for pulmonary and systemic infection.

Actinomycosis

Actinomycosis is produced by a mycotic organism, the *Actinomycosis israelii* which is found as a commensal in the mouth. Other varieties of actinomycis (*Actinomycis bovis*) grow on grasses and are not pathogenic to man. The organisms invade usually through a breach in the oral mucosa but infection may occur in the ileocaecal region of the gastrointestinal tract or, following inhalation, in the lungs.

The disease is characterized by the formation of dense fibrous tissue surrounding multiple pockets of pus so that a honeycomb abscess is formed. The pus contains the characteristic 'sulphur granules' (clumps of mycelia) visible in saline suspension or after spreading the pus on a slide. The infection spreads along fascial planes and is difficult to eradicate. Cervico-facial actinomycosis is the most common and is usually around the angle of the jaw. The underlying abscesses perforate, forming multiple sinuses exuding thin pus. A similar change occurs in abdominal actinomycosis, which is usually localized in the region of the appendix. In pulmonary actinomycosis the disease spreads to affect the pleura and chest wall. Treatment is by high dose, long-term administration of penicillin and by local surgery to eradicate slough and abscess cavities.

Hospital and wound infection

A clean surgical wound may become infected. This is more likely if the operation exposes large surfaces and particularly if operation is prolonged. The infection either takes place from an infected focus on the patient himself, from an infected focus or from the nose of a carrier (e.g. one of the attendants) or from the environment (such as infected air disturbed by blankets, or dirty instruments). Some wounds are particularly liable to infection and this occurs when the operation entails opening infected viscera.

Antibiotics have made a vast change in the prognosis of infection but have not prevented hospital infections. Modern surgery has led to more prolonged operations and many seriously ill patients are kept alive by drugs which reduce body reaction to infection (steroids, anti-cancer drugs). Furthermore, prolonged use of antibiotics in hospital has led to the emergence of bacteria which are often resistant to antibiotics and indeed may be of great virulence.

An outbreak of infection in a hospital must be rigorously investigated and this entails an examination of environmental factors, personnel and procedures such as the carrying out of dressings and the conduct of operations. Such investigations are facilitated by good record keeping within a hospital so that wound infections are documented, the pus from wounds cultured and the organisms typed. In this way outbreaks of infection are traced early, and can be dealt with.

Wound infection
Wound infection is characterized by malaise, fever and local signs related to the wound. The wound may be swollen, fluctuant and the surrounding skin red. Pus may exude between sutures, or on removal of sutures pus can be located with a sinus forcep and allowed to drain away. If this is done and the pus sent for culture then the organisms can be identified and specific antibiotic sensitivities obtained. Antibiotics may not be necessary if free drainage is provided.

3

Wounds and surgical operations

A wound may be described as any forcible disruption of the continuity of tissues. A clean cut made by a very sharp instrument is known as an *incised wound*, whereas the ragged wound made by an instrument which tears at the tissue is known as a *laceration*. Surgical wounds are all of an incised nature, the tissue being deliberately opened in a clean cut fashion. Lacerations may also occur by the forcible stretching of tissue over an underlying structure (such as a tear over the shin following a severe kick). Scrapes against rough surfaces resulting in complete or partial skin loss are called *abrasions*. *Penetrating wounds* occur when a sharp instrument penetrates deeply into the body or are caused by bullets or other trajectories.

A *haematoma* is an extravasion of blood in the tissues from blood vessels disrupted by a blow. It may be superficial, appearing as an obvious bruise, and is very common after minor injury. However, very severe damage may be caused to deeply lying tissues and viscera, without disruption of the overlying skin, by heavy blows from a blunt object. Examples are rupture of the spleen or deep lacerations of liver following a severe blow in the upper abdomen as in an automobile accident.

PATHO-PHYSIOLOGY OF WOUND HEALING

Following disruption of a tissue there is *haemorrhage* into the wound. This may be continuous and severe (Ch. 4), may be followed by shock and lead to death if the bleeding is not arrested. However, once the bleeding has been arrested by a process of contraction of cut vessels and by blood clotting the wound fills with *haematoma*. An acute inflammatory reaction develops quickly in the surrounding tissue and new blood vessels and fibroblasts begin to grow into the haematoma which is absorbed. This new tissue is called *granulation tissue* and its presence signifies a healthy healing wound. The haematoma is eventually completely replaced by granulation tissue which then begins to mature, collagen fibres being laid down. As this process continues, epithelium grows in from the sides of the wound and covers the defect. The growing epithelium can be seen as a fine, blue, filmy layer growing in at the edges. Once epithelial continuity is restored, collagen formation proceeds and the new fibrous tissue contracts drawing the edges of the wound together. This contracted tissue is relatively avascular and covered by firm epithelium and is known as a *scar*. The smaller the area of the wound the less scar tissue formed and consequently the less deformity. Thus an incised wound leaves a much smaller residual deformity than a large lacerated wound which caused much loss of tissue.

Factors affecting healing
Many factors affect healing and these may be local or general. The state of nutrition of the patient, and in particular, an adequate level of albumin and vitamin C in the blood are known to be important. By the same token patients who have malnutrition, those with deep jaundice, liver disease and with certain cancers do not heal as well as do normal individuals. It has been suggested that environmental temperature may be important and that wounds heal more quickly and easily in warm climates. Local factors are extremely important and good coaption of the wound margins without intervening dead tissue or foreign bodies are in favour of rapid healing. However, the most important local factors are the presence of a good blood supply and the absence of infection. Fortunately the blood supply is particularly rich in the head and neck and not often affected by disease but it is important in plastic reconstructive procedures about the jaws to ensure that flaps are adequately nourished.

The presence of infection in a wound leads to a continued inflammatory process with the formation of pus. The granulation tissue at the base continues to grow progressively but is impeded by areas of dead tissue (slough). Epithelial growth is inhibited and the wound will not heal until the infection has been treated or subsides. This process of healing can be slow and leads to the production of much scar tissue.

A further local factor affecting wound healing is immobility of the part concerned and rest is important. Sometimes elevation helps by allowing accumulated transudate and oedema to drain away. This knowledge is made use of in the treatment of wounds of the hand which is often elevated during the healing period.

The treatment of wounds
The treatment of wounds can be considered under the following headings.

1. Arrest of haemorrhage
Any large bleeding vessels are individually clipped and ligated. Should these vessels be essential to the blood supply of the part and if they are large, then reconstruction can be carried out. The same applies to the severance of large nerves which can be sutured and may regenerate in time.

2. Debridement
This refers to the removal of debris and dead tissues from the wound. This is a most important step and the wound must be cut back to reveal clean, viable tissue. The presence of debris within the wound leads to slow healing, the formation of slough and the danger of tetanus or gas gangrene.

3. Prevention of tetanus and gas gangrene
This is important in dirty, contaminated wounds, particularly if deep and accompanied by tissue destruction. Debridement is of the first importance and following this further cleansing of the wound with saline. If the patient has been immunized against tetanus then a booster dose of tetanus toxoid plus an injection of soluble penicillin is adequate. Anti-tetanus serum carries the risk of allergic reaction but can be used once in conjunction with an initial dose of tetanus toxoid and an injection of antibiotics. Human tetanus immunoglobulin is now available in the United Kingdom and wherever possible should be used instead of anti-tetanus serum. If the wound is deep then it is best not closed. A secondary suture can, if necessary, be performed at a later date.

4. Closure of the wound
If the edges can be brought together without undue tension then the wound is closed in layers using absorbable catgut in the deep tissues and interrupted everting silk sutures for the skin. Wounds on the face heal quickly and the skin sutures can be removed by the third or fourth day. For wounds in the mucous membrane catgut is frequently used for suture of all layers but silk can be of value also.

5. Provision of skin cover by skin grafts and skin flaps
Skin grafts and skin flaps are used to provide cover for large open wounds whose margins cannot be coapted or granulating areas in order to assist and hasten healing and to avoid contracture of tissues as a result of excess scar tissue formation during prolonged healing. In addition, grafts and flaps may be necessary to repair defects originating as a result of trauma or surgical operations. For example, after excision of a portion of the tongue and oral cav-

ity for the treatment of oral cancer, a flap of skin may be rotated from the forehead or from the chest wall in order to provide a lining for the floor of the mouth and to repair the defect left by operation. Similarly, after excision of a portion of the mucosa of the mouth it is possible to place skin within the oral cavity to repair the defect.

Skin grafts refer to skin removed from donor sites and then placed in a new site elsewhere in the body. They are of two varieties. Split skin grafts consist of the epidermis and a partial thickness of the dermis and are widely used, especially in the treatment of burns. The resulting defect need not be covered with fresh skin since the skin will regenerate from the remaining dermis of the donor site. Suitable dressings are applied until this occurs.

Full thickness grafts on the other hand consist of the epidermis and the dermis, and the resultant defect can be closed either by direct suture if the donor area is small, by rotational skin flaps created from adjacent areas of skin, or by application of a split skin graft to the area from which the full thickness graft has been removed.

Skin flaps, on the other hand, consist of the epidermis, the dermis and the subcutaneous tissues together with an appropriate blood supply. The latter is important and dictates the length and shape of grafts that can be elevated. Such flaps can be moved on a rotational basis to new sites or can be tubed into the form of a pedicle (Fig. 3.1). The area from which the graft is taken must be

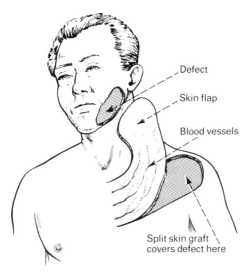

Fig. 3.1 A skin flap raised from the pectoral area to cover a large defect on the face

repaired and this is usually done with a split skin graft taken from a donor site elsewhere. Skin flaps are extremely useful to repair defects created by surgical manoeuvres, particularly in the head and neck and in the management of large defects elsewhere on the body, and in particular on the limbs.

Similar principles to those used in the creation of skin flaps are used in the creation of plastic repairs to internal organs such as the bladder, the pelvis of the kidney and some other internal organs. The dentist may occasionally be called upon to form a small rotational flap of oral mucosa to close a persistent oral-antral fistula.

6. Dressing the wound

A minimum of dressings is desirable and usually of the dry variety. Antibiotics are only used in the prophylaxis of tetanus as described above and sometimes in the prevention of gas gangrene after amputation of the thigh in elderly patients with poor peripheral circulation.

Burns. Burns are a special kind of wound and may be caused by chemicals, by heat and by electricity. A burn is classified as superficial if all layers of the skin are not damaged so that regrowth of skin is possible. Deep burns destroy all the layers of the skin which cannot regrow from skin elements remaining but must heal from the edges or the defect must be closed by a skin graft. Following a severe burn there is a complex initial phase of shock. This is caused partly by the pain of the burn but largely as a result of loss of tissue fluid from the surface of the burn and by destruction of tissue such as muscle. If infection supervenes this can be a major additional factor.

Treatment of burns is directed towards relief of the pain and the replacement of the vast quantities of fluid that can be lost. Attempts are made to prevent infection and the burned area is either treated with a moist dressing or allowed to form a dry eschar. Skin grafting can be done either early or later after the dry crusted eschar separates.

SURGICAL OPERATIONS

Surgical operations are carried out to correct deformity, to remove diseased tissue or to repair defects in tissues caused by trauma or disease.

Incisions are made, if possible, along lines in the skin which will leave a minimum of scarring and will not lead to limitation in the movement of joints or muscles. Incisions in the abdominal or chest wall are made in such a way as to cause minimum muscle damage so as to allow healing with maximum strength.

A number of terms are used to describe various types of operations. Thus the suffix-*otomy* is used to describe operations in which an incision is made into an organ and often that organ is explored but nothing is necessarily removed. Examples are, laparotomy (exploration of the abdomen), thoracotomy (exploration of the chest), craniotomy (opening and exploration of the skull). The suffix-*ectomy* is used to describe operations in which some part of the body is removed. Examples are, appendicectomy, cholecystectomy (removal of the gallbladder) partial thyroidectomy (partial removal of the thyroid gland), glossectomy (removal of the tongue). The suffix-*ostomy* is used to describe operations in which an orifice is made either between an internal organ and the surface or between two internal organs. Examples are, cholecystduodenostomy (creation of an opening between the gallbladder and the duodenum), colostomy (creation of an opening between the colon and the skin —used to relieve intestinal obstruction).

Examples of reconstructive and reparative surgery have already been given (the use of skin grafts) but there are many other examples. Thus, a damaged head of femur can be replaced by a metal prosthesis and of course there are many examples in dentistry from the filling of a cavity in a tooth and the provision of a denture through to the complex reconstructive procedures used to repair defects of the mandible as a result of loss by trauma or surgical removal. Repair of congenital defects such as cleft lip and cleft palate are other well known examples involving the use of plastic surgical techniques. Indeed, this form of reconstructive or reparative surgery is common in the head and neck and elaborate dental prosthesis is often necessary. The plastic surgeon and dentist work as a team.

Excisional and incisional surgery has a very wide range and can be used to treat a variety of disorders of most parts of the body. The operations used include drainage of pus from abscess cavities, selective division of nerves in order to produce specific effects, removal of cancerous growths and total or partial removal of diseased organs. Some structures can be removed with almost total impunity. Thus, the spleen can be sacrificed without undue ill effect and one kidney can be removed provided the other is normal. Indeed the remaining kidney hypertrophies and the patient suffers no significant defect in renal function. On the other hand, organs such as the liver cannot be totally removed but large portions of it can be removed since it has extraordinary regenerative capacity and the remaining liver substance will grow in such a way as to reconstitute the original mass and support life. Large portions of the small bowel may be removed and partial or total gastrectomy can be performed. Removal of some organs leads to a necessity for replacement therapy. Examples of this are the necessity to supply vitamin B_{12} to patients who have had gastrectomy since they lack intrinsic factor and the necessity to supply corticosteroids to patients who have had the adrenal glands removed.

Abdominal operations are frequently used for diseases of the stomach or gut. For example, division of the vagus nerves (vagotomy) is used in the treatment of peptic ulceration because this cuts down gastric acid secretion and allows a duodenal ulcer to heal. Similarly, partial or total gastrectomy can be carried out for gastric ulcer or gastric cancer respectively and the same applies to the colon. Defects in the continuity of the intestinal tract are repaired by direct reconstruction (anastomosis) between the divided ends.

Pre- and postoperative care
It may seem too simple to state that no operation should be carried out unless it is necessary and has a good chance of success. It is, however, important to emphasize that good operative judgement depends on accurate diagnosis. Given precise diagnosis, good judgement and expert technique, the success of an operation depends on the care with which a patient is prepared, the skill of anaesthesia and the attention to detail in the postoperative period.

Preoperative preparation
A history must always be taken. No matter how minor the procedure the surgeon should always enquire as to the patient's general health and previous illnesses. The presence or absence of a productive cough, chest pain or dyspnoea, reflecting cardio-respiratory disease must be sought and any medical history of hypertension or myocardial infarction ascertained. A tendency to bleed easily is of importance and especially bruising or continued haemorrhage from minor wounds. It is also important to take a drug history and to enquire as to allergy regarding particular drugs (for example, a patient on anti-coagulant drugs may bleed heavily if subjected to surgery and a patient sensitive to penicillin may well die of an anaphylactic type reaction if given further penicillin).

Postoperative deep vein thrombosis can complicate any operation no matter how minor (see below). A history of a previous episode of pulmonary embolism is sought and since the contraceptive pill predisposes to deep vein thrombosis enquiries should be made as to whether the patient is taking such a preparation. If this is the case, and the patient is to be submitted to general anaesthesia and so lie recumbent on an operating table for any length of time then she should cease taking the drug for at least one month before surgery.

A full physical examination is carried out with particular reference to cardiac and respiratory status. A chest X-ray and an electrocardiogram may be required. At least a haemoglobin estimation but usually a full blood count is carried out and anaemia corrected before operation. Estimation of the blood urea and electrolytes are performed especially for operations which are likely to be followed by disturbances in fluid balance or by blood loss.

In the case of diabetics appropriate precautions are taken usually consisting of the administration of insulin and covered by dextrose infusion. Should the patient have a bleeding tendency or a disease which predisposes to this then a full coagulation screen is performed and appropriate precautions taken on the basis of the result. Thus for instance, in jaundice, vitamin K_1 is administered before operation.

The anaesthetist is consulted in advance so that an appropriate assessment can be made of the best form of anaesthesia. It is important for the surgeon to select a form of anaesthesia which will allow him to proceed in an adequate manner and not be limited by inadequate anaesthesia as for instance may occur where a local anaesthetic is inappropriately used.

Postoperative management

In the immediate postoperative period the patient must be closely observed until fully recovered from anaesthesia so that obstruction to the airway or inhalation of vomitus or foreign bodies or of pharyngeal secretion does not occur. Respiratory function is of the greatest importance and in some patients who have respiratory embarrassment assisted ventilation by means of an indwelling endotracheal tube or even tracheostomy may be necessary for some days.

The patient's respiratory rate, pulse and blood pressure are monitored. The earliest sign of postoperative bleeding is a sustained rise in the pulse rate and this occurs before obvious signs of collapse occur. Urine output is carefully observed and is the best index of adequate renal perfusion and of adequate fluid intake.

In some patients operations on the gastrointestinal tract necessitate postoperative nasogastric suction in order to keep the gastrointestinal tract, and particularly the stomach, empty, and fluids must be supplied by means of intravenous therapy. Blood transfusion is administered as required and based on repeated estimations of the haemoglobin and haematocrit. The temperature of the patient is measured at least four hourly and a rise in temperature is investigated (see below).

The patient is carefully observed for postoperative complications and these may be specific to the operation performed or more general and likely to complicate any procedure.

Postoperative complications

Respiratory deficiency

Patients with pre-existing respiratory disease (e.g. chronic bronchitis) are more prone to postoperative respiratory problems and in addition operations upon the chest itself or involving upper abdominal incisions predispose to postoperative chest problems. Inhalation of vomitus, pharyngeal secretions or foreign bodies (for example, an inhaled tooth) are certain to be followed by postoperative chest complications (Fig. 3.2 and Ch. 7).

In severe cases the patient is clearly dyspnoeic after operation and cyanosis is evident. The respiratory rate is rapid. Measurement of blood gases is helpful both in assessing severity and progress and in diagnosis of the respiratory defect.

The commonest chest complications are atelectasis (collapse of a

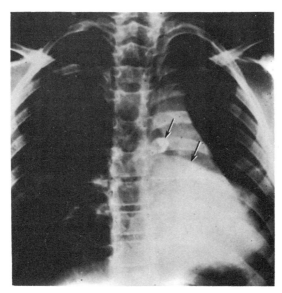

Fig. 3.2 Tooth (upper arrow) in left lower lobe bronchus with collapse of left lower lobe (lower arrow) and mediastinal displacement.

portion of the lung due to plugging of a bronchus or bronchioles) and bronchopneumonia which is particularly liable to occur in the basal areas of the lung in old people confined to bed. Very occasionally lobar pneumonia complicates the postoperative period. A chest X-ray is helpful in differentiating these conditions but they may coexist and are usually accompanied by a rise in temperature. Pulmonary embolism is a further severe postoperative complication which is discussed below.

Management is in the first instance by means of vigorous physiotherapy and encouraging the patient to cough. This must be done together with the provision of adequate analgesia. A specimen of sputum is sent for culture and the patient may then be commenced on antibiotics although many prefer to await the result. It is often found that in the intervening period the condition resolves spontaneously as a result of the simple measures outlined above. Occasionally, bronchial secretions must be removed by means of aspiration through a bronchoscope and very occasionally assisted respiration is necessary. This is also needed in severe chest injuries with disruption of a portion of the chest wall (flail chest) so that paradoxical respiration occurs. In this situation an endotracheal tube is passed and connected to a ventilator. The patient is paralysed with appropriate drugs and ventilated by the machine until such time as he is fit to breathe again himself. Whilst the endotracheal tube is in place the bronchial secretions are aspirated at regular intervals with sterile catheters and humidified air is provided so that the bronchi do not become dried with the formation of crusting which also threatens respiration. An endotracheal tube can be left in place for two or sometimes three days provided that the cuff on the tube is deflated at regular intervals so as not to cause pressure necrosis of the tracheal wall. Should assisted ventilation be necessary for a prolonged period then tracheostomy must be performed.

Tracheostomy. This is an important operation and one which the dentist must understand. It consists of an opening in the trachea below the cricoid cartilage and through the second, third and fourth rings of the trachea so as to allow the insertion of an artificial airway which bypasses the upper respiratory tract. The advantages of tracheostomy are: (i) any obstruction to the respiratory tract in the pharynx or larynx is bypassed, (ii) the dead space is greatly reduced so that respiration is much easier for the patient, and (iii) there is access to the trachea and bronchial tree for toilet and suction as described above.

It is sometimes necessary to perform the operation as an emergency but rarely is it necessary to do so before adequate facilities are at hand. The procedure is not easy and should not be attempted without due preparation unless absolutely essential.

An incision is made in the skin in a transverse manner about two fingers below the lower margin of the thyroid cartilage. Dissection is then proceeded with in the midline and the strap muscles of the neck are retracted or divided. The best guide as to the correct position for a tracheostomy is the isthmus of the thyroid gland and this usually requires division. The trachea is then exposed and either a disc removed from it or a flap hinged forwards and stitched to the lower skin incision. An appropriate tracheostomy tube is inserted and the cuff is then inflated and either connected to a respirator or left open to humidified air. Sterile precautions are necessary and the cuff of the tube must be deflated at regular intervals.

Wound infection
Any wound may become infected. This may arise from pre-existing infection within the patient such as the infection of an appendicectomy wound or may follow secondarily as a result of contamination. Wound infection is characterized by a red, painful and sometimes swollen wound and fluctuation may be present. The patient has an elevated temperature and often an elevated pulse rate. Probing the wound and the removal of stitches results in the drainage of free pus and this should be sent for culture. Antibiotic therapy is not always necessary.

Wound disruption
Failure of the wound to heal may occur for reasons outlined previously. This is treated by either allowing the wound to granulate or by secondary suture.

Other postoperative infections
Apart from infection of the chest and of the wound which are the commonest varieties, infection can also occur elsewhere. Thus, urinary tract infection is common particularly if catheterization has been necessary. Infection of body cavities also occurs and this is particularly common after intra-abdominal operations on infected organs. The usual sites are beneath the diaphragm (subphrenic abscess) or deep within the pelvis (pelvic abscess). These conditions present with fever and local signs of inflammation and are treated by prompt drainage of the accumulated pus to the exterior.

Bacteraemia and septic shock
Very occasionally bacteria enter the blood stream and multiply pro-

ducing toxins leading to profound shock. Septic shock is discussed page 53.

Deep vein thrombosis and pulmonary embolism.
It has been shown that almost 30 per cent of all patients submitted to operation and particularly the elderly, patients with cancer, and women on the pill are at risk. A proportion of patients who develop such thrombi within the legs shed these as emboli which pass in the venous circulation through the right side of the heart and lodge in the lung. A large pulmonary embolus of this character will result in sudden death but multiple small emboli present as chest pain often accompanied by a pleural rub, haemoptysis and fever with typical changes on X-ray.

Deep vein thrombosis may occur with minimal or even without obvious physical signs although leg swelling due to oedema and pain in the calf are not infrequent. An unexplained fever may be the only suggestion of the condition.

Preventive measures are extremely important and amongst these are the maintenance of circulation in the legs during prolonged anaesthesia, early mobilization of the patient and avoidance of operation on women on the contraceptive pill (except in cases of emergency). The use of anti-coagulant drugs and other measures is being investigated.

Treatment of the established condition is by the use of anti-coagulants and by elevation of the legs.

The conditions referred to are the most common general complications of any operation but of course specific operations have their own complications and cannot be covered in detail.

Risks of operation to the surgeon
It is of importance, particularly in dental practice, to recognize that operations carry some risk to the operating surgeon. Of these the most important to mention are the risk of contracting hepatitis as a result of contamination by the patient's blood and the risk of likewise contracting syphilis from an infected case. In addition to these factors penetration of the eyes of the surgeon by infected material or sharp debris is not uncommon and may occur in dental practice.

4

Acute haemorrhage, shock, and severe injury

Haemorrhage may occur as a result of injury or from pathological processes resulting in damage to vessel walls. In addition, severe bleeding may result from apparently trivial injuries in patients who suffer from a haemorrhagic diathesis or who are taking anticoagulant drugs.

The haemorrhage may be external and visible on the surface or from one of the orifices of the body, or internal as when bleeding occurs into a body cavity, into the lumen of hollow viscera or into tissue spaces.

The haemorrhage may be primary and occur at the time of injury or reactionary and occur four to six hours later usually as a result of displacement of clot, dislodgement of a ligature or movement of a dressing. It may be secondary, occurring 7–14 days later associated with infection or separation of a slough.

PATHOPHYSIOLOGY OF HAEMORRHAGE AND OLIGAEMIC SHOCK

Following damage to blood vessel, blood escapes and comes into contact with damaged tissue, platelets become adherent and aggregate, and clot formation is initiated (see Ch. 11). Complete division of a vessel, particularly an artery, results in retraction of the vessel with a tendency to seal off but this does not occur if the vessel is partially divided. As a result of the loss of blood, the blood volume is reduced and consequently the venous return and central venous pressure will fall. There is a tendency for the blood pressure to fall but baro-reflexes operate resulting in tachycardia and peripheral vasoconstriction as a result of sympathetic activity. These factors tend to maintain the blood pressure. Should haemorrhage continue unchecked, then a stage of oligaemic shock results. In this condition despite an increase in the heart rate and maximal peripheral vasoconstriction, the blood pressure falls. In other words, decompensation has occurred. The patient is pale and sweating with a cold clammy skin, there is a rapid pulse rate, hypotension, and rapid shallow breathing. Unless haemorrhage is checked and the blood volume replaced, death results. It should be noted that in a case of progressive haemorrhage, the initial abnormal signs may be only tachycardia and pallor. Once a low blood pressure is present, decompensation has already taken place.

Management of haemorrhage and oligaemic shock

Arrest of haemorrhage

Arterial haemorrhage is to be recognized by the red colour of the blood and the fact that the bleeding occurs in spurts. In venous haemorrhage, on the other hand, the blood is much darker in colour and the bleeding is continuous in nature. Capillary haemorrhage is characterized by an ooze of bright red blood from a broad surface.

The arrest of haemorrhage depends on its nature. Temporary control of arterial bleeding may be obtained by the application of a tourniquet but the only certain way of obtaining control is to ligate both ends of the divided vessel or the main supplying vessel at a proximal point. Thus for severe bleeding from the mouth or face it may be necessary to ligate the external carotid artery. Arterial haemorrhage occurring during operation can be controlled by ligation or clamping of vessels, by firm pressure (packing) or by electrocoagulation.

Venous haemorrhage can be very difficult to control. It may be possible to ligate both ends of a large vein that is bleeding but more often venous haemorrhage is controlled by pressure combined, if possible, with elevation of the wounded part. In the case of venous and arterial haemorrhage, large vessels may sometimes be controlled by patching or suture repair. Capillary haemorrhage usually offers no problem in control unless there is an associated coagulation defect. Bleeding from a ruptured viscus can sometimes be controlled by excision (e.g. splenectomy for splenic rupture).

After extraction of a tooth or operation within the mouth, haemorrhage may occur from vessels in the mucous membrane, periosteum or from within the cancellous bone of the jaws. Control is usually obtained by the insertion of sutures, but occasionally packing may be necessary. Where haemorrhage is anticipated the construction of special splints for the application of gentle pressure may be necessary.

Replacement of blood volume

In addition to arrest of haemorrhage, the management of the patient demands prevention and treatment of shock. The blood pressure and pulse are observed at regular intervals and in the severely ill patient a catheter is inserted to record central venous pressure. This central venous pressure line is of value in monitoring rapid transfusion of fluids used to replace blood volume.

The ideal method of restoring the blood volume is by the transfusion of whole blood compatible with that of the recipient. Donor blood is grouped and cross matched against that of the recipient and must be carefully checked before administration.

While blood is being grouped and cross matched, the patient may be transfused with an electrolyte solution such as Ringer lactate solution or may be given plasma or a plasma substitute such as Dextran. If Dextran is used blood must be taken for grouping and cross matching before its administration. The urine output is monitored and should be maintained at a minimum of 50 ml per hour.

Often surprisingly large quantities of fluid and blood must be transfused in the treatment of haemorrhagic shock and the quantities administered are best guided by reference to the central venous pressure, the heart rate and the urine output.

Blood transfusion

Blood is used to restore depleted blood volume and so permit adequate perfusion of tissues. Occasionally blood transfusion may be used to treat specific defects in the blood such as in the restoration of red cells in some forms of anaemia or in the supply of platelets in thrombocytopenia. Concentrates or specific coagulation factors can be provided (Ch. 11). Blood transfusion is also used widely in some forms of modern surgery such as in the priming of machines for extracorporeal circulation in cardiac surgery.

The recipient blood must be compatible with that of the donor or agglutination and haemolysis occur with dire results. The ABO blood group system contains four primary blood groups based on two antigens denoted A and B (to which antibodies occur naturally). They are found singly, together, or may be entirely absent. The four blood groups which result are given the symbols group

Group	Cells	Serum
O	neither A nor B	anti A
		anti B
A	A	anti B
B	B	anti A
AB	AB	neither
		anti A nor
		anti B

AB, group A, group B and group O, and the blood groups are inherited according to Mendel's law.

Many other blood grouping systems have been discovered but in addition to belonging to one of the four primary blood groups, every individual has or has not in his blood a factor known as Rhesus (Rh). Rh incompatibility can lead to transfusion reactions and whenever possible Rh grouping is undertaken before transfusion is given. Since sensitization to Rh factor can occur, Rh negative patients should whenever possible receive only Rh negative blood.

Complications of blood transfusion

Blood transfusion may be complicated by the dangers associated with the transfusion of any fluid such as infection, fever, allergic reactions, thrombophlebitis, overtransfusion with resultant heart failure and air embolism.

Dangers especially associated with the transfusion of blood include the following:

(a) hypothermia—a rapid transfusion of large quantities of cold blood may lead to reduction in body temperature.

(b) clotting defect—storage of blood results in reduction in platelets and loss of clotting factors. Large transfusions may result in dilution of the recipient's own coagulation factors and a clotting defect.

(c) infection—bacterial contamination or contamination with viruses may result in infection. Thus hepatitis, syphilis and malaria may be transmitted by transfused blood.

(d) biochemical upset—hyperkalaemia or hypocalcaemia may occur in massive blood transfusion.

(e) serological incompatibility—the reactions seen are the result of agglutination and haemolysis. Often the first complaint is of pain in the loins. There may be tachycardia associated with pallor and vasoconstriction of the skin vessels but this may be replaced by flushing. There may be rigors, severe dyspnoea and the patient may collapse. Acute renal failure and also jaundice may develop as a consequence of intravascular haemolysis.

If any of the signs and symptoms referred to above occur, or indeed if there is a brisk reaction to the transfusion in the form of pyrexia, the transfusion should be stopped and samples of the blood in the bottle and of the patient's blood saved for later investigation.

Other forms of shock

In addition of oligaemic shock, which has been dealt with in some detail, the student should be aware of other forms of shock. Some of these are referred to in other chapters.

1. Cardiogenic shock This occurs in myocardial infarction due to failure of the heart as an efficient pump (Ch. 6).

2. Septic shock This is an important form of shock and has shown an increased incidence in recent years, probably due to the increased use of antibiotics (with the development of resistant strains of organism), the fact that operations are conducted on a more extensive scale, occupy longer periods of time and are frequently carried out in the elderly. In addition, surgery is often performed in immunosuppressed patients. The increasing incidence of severe trauma is also a factor.

The condition is due to toxins, usually endotoxins, released from the walls of some bacteria and, in particular, Gram negative organisms such as E. coli, and is characterised by fever, sometimes the development of a classical form of shock but more frequently by the development of warm, dry extremities associated with a decrease in the peripheral resistance, a fall in blood pressure, and by early hyper-ventilation. These features are accompanied by an increased cardiac output in the face of a falling blood volume and it is characteristic that the patient may have an elevated central venous pressure. Arteriovenous shunting occurs in the lungs and there is a decreased peripheral utilisation of oxygen due to the direct effect of the toxins. Blood begins to pool in the periphery and, indeed, clotting may occur in the vessels themselves. Renal function is impaired as a result of hypoperfusion, also possibly as a result of intravascular coagulation.

The condition of septic shock is especially likely to follow procedures which cause infection within the urinary tract, the biliary tree, or after surgery on the large bowel.

Treatment of the condition is by early institution of antibiotic therapy, a good combination being gentamicin and metronidazole, the two antibiotics together coping with most gram negative organisms including the bacteroides. Attempts are made to maintain or even increase the cardiac output and the use of appropriate drugs to stimulate the myocardium, of which dopamine is the most frequently used, is instituted. The administration of digoxin is frequently necessary. Fluid is replaced and blood administered if necessary.

It should be emphasised that septic shock is a highly dangerous condition and the mortality is high, this being inevitable if sepsis is not controlled. Survival depends upon early recognition and appropriate treatment. As mentioned above, the initial therapy is directed at maintaining blood volume and treating the underlying bacteraemia, support of respiration, monitoring of renal function and treatment of the failing myocardium. One of the most important features is the early identification and surgical drainage of abscess collections and of infective fluid. This is mandatory and must be carried out as soon as the initial measures of resuscitation have been instituted.

The most important points to emphasise are the following:

(i) The possibility of preventive measures by the use of prophylactic antibiotics (as, for example, in operations on the infected biliary tree).

(ii) The early recognition of the physical signs.

(iii) The prompt institution of broad spectrum antibiotic cover (without waiting for sensitivities obtained from culture) and supportive measures.

(iv) Adequate drainage of collections of pus (for example, within the peritoneal cavity) if there is to be any real hope of recovery.

3. Anaphylactic shock This results from antigen-antibody reactions in previously sensitized individuals and is the result of the release of a variety of vasoactive substances, mainly histamine. These substances cause intense constriction of small vessels together with increased permeability and constriction of bronchioles resulting in bronchospasm.

4. Neurogenic shock (vasovagal attack) This is the simple faint and is often precipitated by sudden fright, fear or by pain. It is described fully in Chapter 6. It is important to recognize that fainting may occur during anaesthesia and for this reason the administration of anaesthetics in the upright position in the dental chair is associated with danger of cerebral anoxia.

5. Adrenal failure Lack of glucocorticoids due to absence or disease of the adrenals can lead to a clinical state indistinguishable from shock. A similar problem may occur in patients who have been receiving long term steroid therapy with prednisolone or similar preparation; in such individuals atrophy of the adrenal cortex is likely to occur so that the patient is unable to respond in the normal way to the stress of infection, injury, anaesthesia and surgical procedures. In these circumstances patients on steroid therapy may become collapsed, hypotensive and gravely ill.

Assessment and management of severe injury

Severe injury in civilian life is usually due to the effects of road traffic accidents. Multiple injury is frequent with damage to the head, chest, abdomen and limbs. The situation is often complicated by drunkenness in the victims of accidents and perhaps by prior consumption of drugs. Immediate threats to life are usually from obstruction to the airway, haemorrhage and rapidly advancing intracerebral haemorrhage.

The assessment of such injuries and their appropriate management is a complex matter. In general, injuries can be divided into:-

1. Those injuries which are immediately life-threatening. The haemorrhage may be so gross and so rapid that life will be lost if operation is not carried out within a few minutes and there may be obvious obstruction to the airway and impending asphyxia. In such instances immediate control of the airway with, if necessary, the insertion of an endotracheal tube or even an immediate tracheostomy are essential. Haemorrhage must be arrested immediately and blood replaced if life is to be saved. Operation, therefore, may have to be carried out as a dire emergency and possibly even within the Casualty Department.

2. In other injuries, there is no immediate threat to life and there is some time to assess the situation. Most such patients, usually with injury to the chest or abdomen, will require surgery within one to two hours, but there is an opportunity to assess the degree of damage, to group and cross-match blood, and to take essential X-rays. Antibiotics are administered if necessary and the patient is then taken to the operating theatre for appropriate surgery to control haemorrhage and for the removal of damaged tissues or repair of ruptured organs.

3. Occult injury: Such injuries may develop slowly and quietly and there may even be few signs of damage. A high index of suspicion is necessary in the detection of such injuries, which usually involve the abdomen after blunt injury, but also occur in some forms of head injury (see Ch. 18). In such instances there is time for more extensive tests and for assessment of a planned course of action. An example is the delayed presentation which occurs in some ruptures of the spleen and liver. In such instances, the use of angiographic methods or isotope studies may reveal the diagnosis.

In summary, the assessment and management of severe trauma is as follows:-

1. Make sure that the airway is clear. Remove broken teeth, mucus and foreign bodies from the mouth.
2. Arrest obvious haemorrhage.

3. Set up intravenous line for replacement of lost blood.
4. Assess associated injury, particularly:
   a. to the head;
   b. occult injury to the chest and the possible presence of pneumothorax;
   c. injuries to the limbs (compound fractures should be immediately covered with a sterile dressing and temporarily splinted);
   d. assess the presence or absence of haematuria.
5. Pass a catheter to monitor urinary output.
6. Make an assessment of the presence of intoxication, drug consumption or associated disease.

It is important in injury to obtain a good history from the patient if possible, but also from the ambulance driver or police who accompany the patient to the hospital and from any relatives who are either with the patient at the time of admission or who are available at a later stage.

5

Tumours and their management

New growths arising and resembling the tissues of the body are referred to as tumours or neoplasms. They are distinguished from the phenomena of hypertrophy and hyperplasia in that they continue growing independent of the growth or well-being of the host and even after the stimulus which initiated them has been removed. Indeed our understanding of tumours is handicapped in that we know so little of the initiating stimuli. In some instances specific aetiological factors such as hereditary predisposition, chronic mechanical or chemical irritation, infections such as syphilis or response to hormonal stimulation are known to be partially responsible. In most cases, however, the causative factors are obscure.

Neoplasms are classified according to their structure and their behaviour into two groups, benign and malignant. Most tumours can be easily allocated to one or other of these groups but occasionally the distinction is difficult to make and some benign tumours are prone to undergo malignant change.

Differences between benign and malignant tumours

Benign tumours resemble in consistency and in histological characteristics the tissues of the body. In general, they are encapsulated by a compressed layer of connective tissue and displace the surrounding tissues without evidence of invasion. As a result of this, they are well defined and do not readily become attached to surrounding structures. They are generally not dangerous to life but they may grow to a very considerable size and thus interfere with vital structures. In addition, benign tumours may rupture and cause life-threatening haemorrhage or they may secrete abnormal quantities of hormones and thereby cause severe disease.

It is important to recognize that benign tumours do not spread either by direct invasion or by the development of daughter growths to distant parts of the body and are therefore capable of cure by local excision. This is what separates them more than anything else from the malignant tumours which do indeed invade and destroy local tissues and also spread to distant parts of the body by a process known as metastasis.

Malignant tumours, although broadly resembling normal tissue histologically, usually differ considerably from the normal body tissues both in the structure of individual cells and in the architecture of the tissue so that it may be extremely difficult to determine the tissue of origin. Such dedifferentiation is termed anaplasia and the greater it is, the higher the degree of malignancy. The tumours are not encapsulated and have an indefinite growing edge which may involve local blood vessels, nerves or other vital structures. Malignant growths may also compress adjacent tissues or produce abnormal hormone secretion.

In addition, malignant neoplasms are often associated with a progressive deterioration in general health and wasting, referred to as cachexia. The mechanism of malignant cachexia is obscure but may be due to the fact that malignant tumours metabolize excessive quantities of nutrient material to the expense of the host. In addition, they may bleed giving rise to anaemia, they may have an effect on the appetite of the host and, by their situation (e.g. cancer of the stomach) they may lead not only to decreased food intake but to increased protein loss through the gut. Furthermore, secondary infection is undoubtedly an important factor and contributes significantly to a general decline in health.

Spread of malignant tumours

As stated above, malignant tumours invade local tissues and this is referred to as spread in continuity. Closely adjacent structures may also be affected and this is referred to as spread in contiguity. Thus, a carcinoma of the bronchus may affect the surrounding lung tissue and might invade the heart or the nearby oesophagus.

Spread of the tumour to form secondary growths in other parts of the body takes place by a number of methods. Firstly, tumour cells may enter the lymphatics and grow along the lymphatic pathways by a process known as permeation. Alternatively, tumour cells that have entered the lymphatics pass in the lymph flow to the nearest lymph node where they become arrested. This is known as lymphatic embolism. This process is repeated successively until tumour cells pass not only to other local lymph nodes but to subsequent groups of nodes and finally enter the bloodstream.

Secondly, tumour cells may directly invade local blood vessels and such invasion will be followed again by the growth of tumour cells in cords along local blood vessels but more commonly they become detached and embolize along the venous pathways until arrested in the nearest capillary bed. It is for this reason that tumour cells spreading by the bloodstream from cancers of the gut pass in the portal vein and are arrested in the liver, this being the commonest site for daughter growths from the alimentary cancer. On the other hand, tumours associated with or draining into the peripheral venous system shed tumour cells which are arrested in the lungs, which are also a common site of secondary deposits. Not all tumour cells escaping into the lymphatic or bloodstream survive and some tumours seem to have a special predilection for metastasis to certain organs. For instance, secondary tumours in bone tend to be associated with primary growths in the thyroid, breast, kidney, and prostate gland. Some small emboli may succeed in traversing the capillary bed and are then carried from the liver or lungs via the arterial stream to other parts of the body. The process of formation of metastases is of very great importance because prevention of such daughter growths would be a major advance in the treatment of malignant disease.

Thirdly, tumour cells may spread across body cavities by a process known as transcoelomic spread. Thus, a cancer of the stomach may penetrate the wall of the stomach and seed cells into the peritoneal cavity which come to rest on the ovaries within the pelvis. Similar spread takes place in the pleural cavity. Tumours of the central nervous system are a rather special case in that they do not spread outside the meninges but may form daughter growths elsewhere within the central nervous system by spreading within the cerebrospinal fluid.

Fourthly, tumours may grow along pre-existing tubular structures within the body, as for example the growth of a cancer of the renal pelvis down a ureter. Finally, tumour cells contaminating surgical instruments may occasionally be embedded in wounds and grow at their site of implantation.

It is important to differentiate secondary daughter growths from completely new primary tumours within the same organ.

TYPES OF NEOPLASMS

Neoplasms are described depending on the nature of the tissue from which they arise.

Epithelial growths

Such growths may be benign or malignant and originate either in surface epithelium or in glandular structures. The neoplastic tissue is epithelial but there is usually a supporting stroma of connective tissue containing blood vessels and frequently nerve fibres. Benign growths that arise from surface epithelium are known as papillomata and are extremely common. Such small papillomata may occur on the face or in the mouth.

Malignant tumours arising from the epithelium are of importance to the dental surgeon. They may arise from:

Squamous epithelium

Basal cell carcinoma (rodent ulcer) Fig. 5.1 occurs commonly on the lateral side of the nose or at the lateral canthus of the eye. The lesion presents as a small nodule which ultimately forms an ulcer with a rolled, pearly edge.

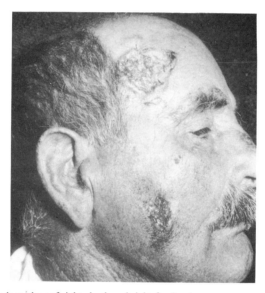

Fig. 5.1 Rodent ulcer of right cheek and right forehead.

Squamous cell carcinoma (epithelioma) occurs widely on the skin of the body and also occurs at the anal canal, on the glans penis, in the squamous lining of the oesophagus and not uncommonly on the lips or in the oral cavity. In this latter situation, it is recognized by the fact that it is commonly ulcerated and has a raised, rolled, everted hard edge and an indurated base.

Glandular epithelium

Carcinomata arising from glandular epithelium are known as adenocarcinomata. Such cancers may arise in solid glandular structures such as the thyroid and adrenal glands but are more common arising from the glandular lining of the gastrointestinal tract (adenocarcinoma of the stomach or colon) or within the breast.

Connective tissue growths

Connective tissue growths may be benign and arise from fatty tissue (lipoma), fibrous tissue (fibroma), bone (osteoma) or cartilage (chondroma). They may contain neural or vascular elements (neurofibroma, haemangioma). Tumours such as simple lipomata are ubiquitous and may be found in relation to the head and neck. Haemangiomata may bleed excessively with trauma and are of importance to dental surgeons since they occur within the oral cavity or even within bone. There is also a group of giant cell tumours known as osteoclastomata which are common in the long bones in the young and are composed of osteoclasts. A variety of benign tumours may arise from tissues of dental origin.

The *malignant* neoplasms of mesodermal origin are referred to as sarcomata and, unlike the carcinomata, are relatively common in children and in the young adult. Like their benign counterparts, they may arise in cartilage, bone, fat or muscle (e.g. liposarcoma).

Such sarcomata are highly malignant and prone to blood-borne metastases, especially to the lungs. They tend to be anaplastic lesions consisting of round or spindle cells. They are common in relation to bone (osteosarcoma) and are highly vascular. Tumours arising from the lymphoid organs (lymphosarcoma) are highly anaplastic growths.

Melanoma

Melanomata arise from the melanin-containing cells of the body and may occur as simple pigmented moles which are extremely common. These moles may be found scattered on the body surface and are quite benign. On the other hand, the malignant melanoma is highly dangerous and metastasizes readily. Should a benign pigmented naevus show an increase in size, change in colour, the development of a surrounding halo of pigment, or bleed, it should be suspected of having undergone malignant change. Malignant melanoma not only occurs in the skin but is also found in the bed of the nails, in the oral cavity, in the oesophagus, and may occur also within the eye. Spread is via the lymphatics and also by means of the blood, multiple liver metastases being very common.

Teratomata

These are neoplasms which contain mixed elements both epithelial and mesodermal in origin. Benign teratomata are extremely rare but occur on occasion and the dermoid cyst of the ovary is an example. It may contain such diverse elements as thyroid gland, cartilage and even teeth and hair. Malignant teratomata, which lead to the formation of metastatic deposits, also occur.

The dermoid cysts which are simple growths found at the lines of embryological fusion, such as at the lateral canthus of the eye, must be distinguished from the teratomata referred to above.

PRESENTING FEATURES OF TUMOURS

Local mass

All tumours, whether benign or malignant, may present as a local swelling. The mass may extremely small so that in the case of malignant tumours the presenting symptom may be from a secondary deposit rather than the primary growth. On the other hand, the local mass may be of very considerable size. Careful examination of the characteristics of the mass is important since benign tumours remain mobile and are not attached to the skin or underlying deep tissues. They tend to grow slowly. Malignant neoplasms on the other hand form local masses which grow steadily in size, are invasive and consequently attached to the surrounding structures and therefore become progressively fixed. These characteristics can be demonstrated on physical examination. Thus, an invasive carcinoma of the breast will produce distortion of the breast and retraction of the nipple due to local invasion and cannot be readily moved on the underlying pectoral muscles when these are contracted.

As tumour grows, it may produce signs and symptoms from pressure on neighbouring structures. Thus, a tumour of the thyroid gland may compress the trachea or oesophagus causing dyspnoea and dysphagia. Such compression may become suddenly more severe if necrosis and haemorrhage occur in the centre of the tumour with consequent rapid increase in size.

The local mass may ulcerate with consequent secondary infection or local abscess formation (Fig. 5.2). In addition, such secondary infection will lead to a reactive change in the draining lymph nodes which should not be mistaken for spread of tumour. The presence of ulceration or central necrosis may be accompanied by local pain.

As the tumour extends locally, the invasive process may involve blood vessels with consequent exsanguinating haemorrhage and this is not uncommon as a terminal event in advanced tumours of the head and neck. Similarly, local nerves may be involved with the production of pain which may be referred to distant sites. The

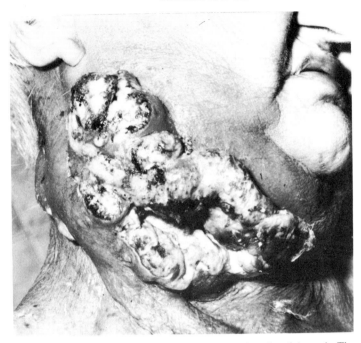

Fig. 5.2 Ulcerating secondary carcinoma involving lymph nodes of the neck. The patient died later from exsanguinating haemorrhage following involvement of the carotid artery

growing tumour may also cause perforation of hollow viscera or fistulate into neighbouring viscera or to the skin. In the case of bone tumours, the local mass may so erode the bone as to result in pathological fracture.

Metastatic tumour

The outstanding characteristic of malignant tumours is the production of metastases (Fig. 5.3) which may be the presenting feature. For example, a patient with primary adenocarcinoma of the colon may present with a painful enlarged liver due to secondary deposits, or a patient with osteosarcoma of bone may be found to have large secondaries in the lung fields on chest X-ray.

Hormonal effects

Benign and malignant tumours may produce abnormal secretion of hormones and present with the clinical effects of excessive hormone production. Thus, for example, patients with insulin-producing tumours of the pancreas may first present with the features of

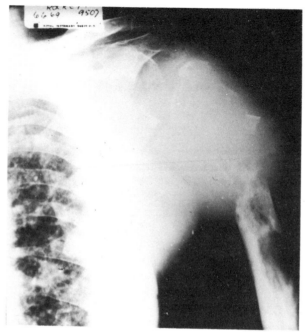

Fig. 5.3 Involvement of the shoulder with lytic deposits from a primary carcinoma of the prostate gland

hypoglycaemia. In a similar way, patients with tumours of the adrenal cortex may present with the clinical features of Cushing's syndrome.

General effects

In addition to the deterioration in general health which has been referred to above, further, more specific systemic affects may be produced in association with tumour growth. Thus, for example, some tumours of the kidney may be associated with fever of unknown origin or with polycythaemia and ill-understood neurological deficits may occur in association with some carcinomata of the bronchus in the absence of demonstrable secondary deposits in the brain.

THE PRINCIPLES OF TREATMENT

In the case of benign tumours, the indications for treatment are the production of pressure effects, abnormal hormone production or if the tumour is unsightly. In addition, many benign tumours are excised for the purposes of histological examination since their nature is in doubt.

In the case of malignant neoplasms, death will result unless the lesion is completely eradicated.

Surgical removal

Removal of a benign tumour results in cure unless small portions of the tumour are left behind, in which case it may recur. Removal is in general not difficult since a tissue plane between the normal and the abnormal tissue can generally be defined. Occasionally, surgical removal is affected by diathermy destruction or the use of cryosurgical methods.

The surgical removal of malignant tumours is not simple since the plane between normal and abnormal tissue cannot be seen with the naked eye. For this reason, wide excision is practised removing a generous portion of surrounding normal tissue. Because of the possibility of spread to local lymph nodes, these are usually excised in continuity although in some instances secondary excision of the lymph nodes is practised if they later show signs of involvement. Local surgery, even with wide excision of the tumour and the related lymph nodes, is bound to be unsuccessful if distant blood-borne metastases or involvement of distant lymph nodes has already occurred. This is the limiting factor in the practice of excisional surgery and much effort is directed towards the definition of the extent of the disease in cancer and in particular to assessment not only of the primary growth and related nodes but of the possibility of the involvement of distant organs.

The wide areas of normal tissue excised along with cancerous growths result in defects which are made good by reparative surgery.

Radiotherapy

Radiotherapy may be applied by irradiation from an external source such as a supervoltage machine or linear accelerator, or less frequently, by irradiation from radioactive material inserted into the tumour substance or administered orally or by injection.

A sufficiently high dosage of X-rays is lethal to all tissues, including all tumours. The use of radiotherapy depends on the fact that firstly some tumours are especially radio-sensitive, their cells being destroyed by radiation dosage which is tolerated by normal tissues and secondly that the X-rays are directed at the tumour as a target. Conventional radiotherapy machines operate at voltages up to 250 kilovolts but supervoltage machines generate radiation of very short wavelength and these have great penetrating powers and thus can be used to deliver larger dosages of the radiation to deeply seated lesions with less risk of damaging overlying tissues. A radioactive isotape of cobalt can provide an alternative source of irradiation, the gamma rays produced being therapeutically effective.

The dosage of radiation is measured in units known as rads, the rad being related to the quantity of absorbed energy in the tissues irradiated. Interstitial irradiation is used in the treatment of some tumours by the insertion of radioactive material in the form of radium needles, radon seeds or by other methods. These procedures are not used as frequently nowadays, having been superseded by better methods of external irradiation, but they still have a place for the treatment of tumours of the tongue, pharynx and bladder. Radioactive iodine (I^{131}) can be administered orally or by injection for the treatment of carcinoma of the thyroid gland but only for such tumours as can be shown to take up iodine.

Indications for radiotherapy

In the treatment of primary tumours, radiotherapy may be used in an attempt to effect a cure and is the treatment of choice for most epitheliomata of the skin, cervix of the uterus, lip and oral cavity, and for basal cell carcinoma of the skin. In addition, radiotherapy and surgical excision can be practised in combination. Thus, in some clinics cancer of the oesophagus is irradiated before surgical excision and the same approach is under investigation in the treatment of carcinoma of the rectum. In the same way, radiotherapy can be used in an attempt to eradicate cells possibly left behind after surgical excision. Thus, for example, in carcinoma of the breast, radiotherapy can be applied to the healed skin flaps and, where there are secondary deposits in the axilla, to the entire remaining lymphatic drainage of the breast in the axilla, supraclavicular and mediastinal nodes.

In the palliative treatment of advanced cancer, radiotherapy is extremely valuable not only for the relief of symptoms from inoperable tumours but for the treatment of metastases. Thus, for example, it is extremely common for patients to develop very painful secondary deposits in bone and the pain can be completely relieved by the skilled application of radiotherapy.

Chemotherapy

Many cytotoxic agents have anticancer effects due to their ability to damage actively dividing cells. They are not specific for malignant tissue and their use therefore produces toxic side effects.

These drugs are currently used mainly for the palliation of advanced malignant disease but they are being employed as adjuvants in cancer surgery or radiotherapy in the hope of yielding a greater cure rate.

The most important toxic effects result from haemopoietic depression but gastrointestinal ulceration and alopecia also occur. Therefore, monitoring of treatment is necessary and frequent estimations of the haemoglobin, white cell and platelet count are necessary. Severe stomatitis, vomiting or diarrhoea may necessitate discontinuing therapy. It is important to bear in mind that the effects of therapy must not be allowed to become more severe than the symptoms of the disease.

Four main groups of cytotoxic agents are in common use:

1. Alkylating agents;
2. Antimetabolites;
3. Alkaloid drugs;
4. Products of microorganisms.

Alkylating agents cause cell death by alteration in essential cellular constituents. Examples of such drugs are the nitrogen mustards or nitrogen mustard analogues such as chlorambucil and cyclophosphamide. The antimetabolites depend on the blocking of enzymatic reactions and fall into two groups, the antipurine drugs and the folic acid antagonists. The best known examples of these are 6-mercaptopurine which is used in the management of leukaemia, and 5-fluorouracil which is finding increasing use in the treatment of metastatic large bowel cancer. The alkaloid drugs such as vinblastine and vincristine have considerable cytotoxic effects and are used in the treatment of Hodgkin's disease, leukaemia and reticulum cell sarcoma.

Chemotherapy using cytotoxic agents may be applied by oral or intravenous injection but high concentrations of anticancer drugs may be delivered to the tumour by intra-arterial perfusion. Such intra-arterial methods have been used in the management of advanced lesions or cancer of the head and neck.

Endocrine therapy
Some tumours are sensitive to changes in their hormonal environment. Such tumours are said to be hormone-dependent and modifications in their growth can be achieved either by additive therapy whereby hormones are prescribed parenterally or orally in an attempt to control the growth of the tumour (e.g. oestrogens in the form of stilboestrol can be given to men with cancer of the pros-

tate) or by ablative therapy whereby major endocrine glands are surgically removed or destroyed by means of irradiation (e.g. hypophysectomy or adrenalectomy in advanced breast cancer). Not all tumours of a particular type are sensitive to their hormonal environment in the same way and research is being directed towards the assessment of sensitivity prior to treatment.

Immunotherapy
The theory that an immune response to cancer occurs is being investigated in many centres and attempts are being made to exploit any possible host reaction to the tumours. The fact that spontaneous regression has been noted in some tumours, particularly in malignant melanomata, has encouraged the investigation of immunotherapy but such methods are not yet established.

Non-specific therapy
It should be remembered that patients suffering from tumours, particularly malignant lesions, require expert nursing, psychological support and, in the advanced stages of the disease, relief from pain. Such measures are of equal importance to attempts at cure. In addition, during the terminal stages of illness, skilled counselling of the patient and family are of considerable importance.

SOME IMPORTANT TUMOURS

It is important that the dentist has a clear appreciation of carcinoma of the tongue, of the lip and, to a lesser extent, of carcinoma of the oesophagus, and these are described below. Carcinoma of the breast is an important tumour which illustrates well many of the points outlined above and is therefore described in some detail.

Tumours of the breast
Both benign and malignant tumours of the breast must be differentiated from cysts of the breast, which are common.

Benign tumours
Papillomata of the ducts of the breast tissue may occur and present with a blood-stained or watery discharge from the nipple.

Fibroadenoma is a benign tumour with epithelial elements derived from the ductules and acini and set in a fibrous stroma. This tumour occurs frequently in young women and is a lump of firm consistency and smooth surface which is well-demarcated and very mobile (breast 'mouse').

Breast cancer

This is the commonest malignancy in women in the United Kingdom. The disease causes over 10,000 deaths annually. Nearly all cancers of the breast arise from the epithelial lining of the duct system. The tumour grows into the breast tissue locally, involving the overlying skin and causing retraction of the nipple and distortion of the breast. Finally the skin ulcerates and satellite nodules may occur involving the whole chest wall. The tumour grows deeply and involves the pectoral muscle with deep attachment. Lymphatic spread extends to the regional nodes of which the axillary nodes are extremely important but, in addition, the mediastinal and supraclavicular nodes become involved. Blood spread tends to occur very early in the disease and the cancer may spread to any tissue. However, the bones are very commonly involved, as are the lungs and liver. Metastases to bone are commonly osteolytic and may be seen on skeletal X-ray but early bony deposits may not be visible although they can be demonstrated by means of radioisotopic scanning techniques.

Diagnosis is based on the clinical finding of a lump in the breast, which may be small and difficult to distinguish from a benign tumour but may be large, with tethering and dimpling of the skin as described above. A lump in the breast must never be regarded as benign on clinical examination alone and excision biopsy is necessary.

Treatment. There is debate as to the treatment of choice for early cancer of the breast. In the United Kingdom, simple mastectomy and biopsy of the axillary nodes is at present the most commonly used method of treatment and radiotherapy is given, should the axillary nodes be involved with tumour. However, these methods of treatment should not be employed if distant metastatic spread is already evident. In this connection, it should be remembered that cancer of the breast may present with a metastasis, the primary tumour being very small. Thus, the patient may complain of a lump in the axilla or may even present with a pathological fracture of a long bone, or indeed of the mandible.

Palliative treatment. In advanced breast cancer, the disease can cause extreme pain and discomfort and effective palliation is extremely important. Radiotherapy can be of great value in treating local recurrence for relief of pain. However, widespread metastatic disease demands more general treatment and alterations in the hormonal environment may affect the course of the disease beneficially. Surgical removal of the ovaries, adrenal or even the pituitary gland, or the administration of sex hormones may be effective.

Cytotoxic chemotherapy is generally reserved for treatment of the disease when it has not responded to the above measures and can given a striking palliation in some patients.

Carcinoma of the tongue

Cancer of the tongue is more likely to be found in patients with poor oral hygiene and has been said to occur more frequently in patients who smoke excessively, who have suffered from syphilis, or who have some form of chronic oral irritation. Leukoplakia, a condition of the oral cavity and some other mucus lined cavities within the body, consists of patches of thickened white mucosal epithelium which are easily recognised and which, on biopsy, have a characteristic appearance. Such leukoplakic patches have a definite pre-cancerous tendency. It is most important that the dentist recognises such areas and their potential malignancy.

A common site for carcinoma of the tongue is in the anterior two-thirds and frequently at its edge (Figure 5.4). The lesion usually presents as a typical malignant ulcer although it may be nodular and occasionally papillary or fissured before becoming ulcerated. The lesion is usually a squamous cell carcinoma and spreads locally to the floor of the mouth, eventually involving the alveolar margin and, in the posterior part of the tongue, the tonsil and palate. Lymphatic dissemination occurs to the submental, submandibular and deep cervical lymph nodes. For tumours at the edge of the tongue, the node involved is generally ipsilateral but in more centrally

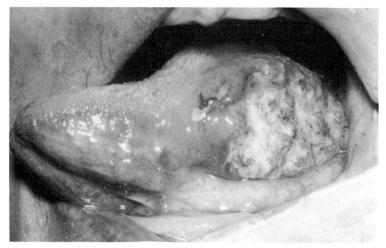

Fig. 5.4 Squamous carcinoma of the tongue. Ulcerated lesion with rolled, everted edges. Note the stitch at the site of biopsy.

placed tumours in the posterior third of the tongue, lymph node involvement may be bilateral. Continuing lymphatic spread involves the mediastinum. Blood spread is unusual.

The presenting symptom is of *a nodule or an ulcer* on the tongue which soon becomes infected and painful. The pain may be referred to the ear or in the distribution of the auriculotemporal nerve. Excessive salivation and halitosis are common and, in the later stages, dysphagia and slurring of speech result from fixation of the tongue. The ulcer is a typical malignant lesion with everted edges and an indurated base. Repeated small haemorrhages, toxic absorption from the infected area and anorexia result in debility and anaemia.

It is essential to examine the neck for palpable lymph nodes which may be enlarged as a result of tumour or infection or both. Indeed, in some growths, glandular involvement in the neck may be the first sign of malignancy.

Death results from general inanition, bronchopneumonia as a result of aspiration of infected material, and in the late stages, sudden haemorrhage from involvement of large vessels.

The differential diagnosis is from other forms of oral ulceration and in particular syphilis and tuberculosis. Suspicion of malignancy is confirmed by biopsy.

Initial management is by good oral toilet and dental extractions may occasionally be required before definitive therapy is commenced. The treatment of choice to the primary lesion is radiotherapy which may be administered in the form of radium needles implanted into the tumour. In the posterior one-third of the tongue, cobalt or supervoltage therapy is preferable.

Surgery is reserved for radioresistant growths and for tumours which recur after irradiation. In addition, in some cases with extensive bone involvement, radiotherapy is impractical and radical surgery is employed. The operation involves removal of the affected tongue following preliminary ligation of the external carotid artery. The excision may need to include a portion of the floor of the mouth and related mandible and suitable prosthetic replacement. Prophylactic surgical or radiotherapeutic treatment of cervical lymph nodes is not necessary if they are impalpable. If, however, on follow-up, lymph nodes become palpable, the treatment of choice is ipsilateral block dissection of the cervical lymph nodes including the sternomastoid muscle, internal jugular vein and posterior belly of the digastric. Should lymph glands in the neck be clearly inoperable, surgery is contraindicated but radiotherapy may afford some palliation.

Cancer of the remainder of the oral cavity presents, in general, the same pathological features, and is managed in a similar fashion although, when surgery is required in carcinoma of the floor of the mouth, monoblock dissection with removal of the primary lesion, related mandible and cervical lymph nodes is more frequently necessary.

Carcinoma of the lip

Cancer of the lip is especially common in individuals who smoke very heavily. It is also very much more common in Caucasian individuals exposed to especially strong sunlight. Management is similar to that of carcinoma of the tongue, consisting of good oral hygiene and treatment of the lesion by means of radiotherapy or by surgery. Operation involves removal of affected lymph nodes, but it is important to be sure that enlarged nodes are not simply the result of lymphadenitis consequent on infection of the primary lesion. As for carcinoma of the tongue, prophylactic removal of lymph nodes is not necessary but should be carried out if such nodes become palpable during follow-up.

The prognosis is worse for lesions on the upper lip and at the angle of the mouth, but in general is better than that for lingual cancer.

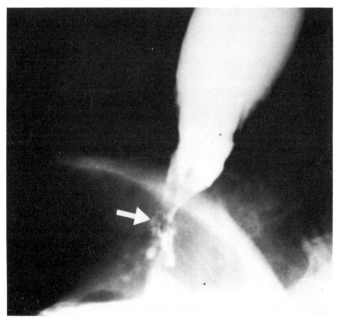

Fig. 5.5 Barium swallow examination showing a carcinoma of the lower end of the oesophagus. There is hold up of barium in the dilated oesophagus above the tumour.

Carcinoma of the oesophagus

This disease is common in elderly men. Some countries have a high incidence, notably among the Bantu populations of South Africa and in South-East Asia and Japan.

The growth is a squamous cell carcinoma, usually of the scirrhous variety but near the lower end of the oesophagus adenocarcinoma may be encountered. The growth infiltrates the submucosa and forms an ulcer in the mucous membrane. The malignant stricture progressively tightens and the cardinal symptom is therefore dysphagia, persistent and progressive, until eventually even fluids cannot be swallowed and are regurgitated. Rapid weight loss results with cachexia and death follows from inhalation pneumonia or perforation of the growth into the pleural cavity.

Barium examination shows the lesion, which has a rigid, irregular outline, and oesophagoscopy with biopsy confirms the diagnosis (Fig. 5.5).

Treatment is by surgery in the distal half of the oesophagus but more proximally radiotherapy is commonly advised.

BONE TUMOURS

Bone tumours may arise from the cells forming the supporting structure of bone (osteocytes, chondrocytes, fibrocytes of the periosteum), from the bone marrow elements or they may be secondary to malignant tumours elsewhere.

Benign bone tumours

Osteomata

are composed of hard and compact bone and are termed 'ivory osteoma'. They are commonly found in the skull and very rarely cause symptoms. Osteomata also occur in the mandible and may occasionally compromise dental extraction or the fitting of dentures.

Chondromata

may be single or multiple. If a chondroma occurs within the bones, it is known as an enchondroma and these are commonly found in the phalanges. Chondromata growing from the surface of bone (ecchondromata) may become very large and are not uncommon on the rib cage. They seldom cause symptoms but by virtue of their size may need treatment. Multiple chondromata are part of an hereditary abnormality known as diaphyseal aclasis. Small caps of cartilage cells become separated from the edges of the growing metaphysis. These continue to grow, forming large exostoses bearing cartilaginous caps. Such exostoses may cause symptoms from pressure and occasionally need removal. Because of the bony element contained within such growths, they are known as osteochondromata.

Solitary bone cysts

usually occur in long bones (humerus or femur). They contain a browny fluid and slowly expand the bony structure, and present as a pathological fracture (Ch. 16). The cause of such bone cysts is not known but they may originate following trauma. They are treated by curettage but, if the bone structure is weak, bone grafting with bone chips may be necessary.

Osteoclastomata

are mostly benign but occasionally malignant forms do occur. The tumour is metaphyseal in origin, usually occurs in young adults, and over 70 per cent of cases occur in the region of the knee joint (femur or tibia). Histologically the tumour is characterized by large multinucleated giant cells of similar appearance to osteoclasts lying in a spindle cell stroma. Haemorrhagic areas are common. There is pain and swelling of the bone, sometimes with pathological fracture. The lesion must be distinguished from osteitis fibrosa cystica in which the serum calcium is raised and the lesions are multiple, and from metastatic tumour. As the tumour grows, the cortex becomes thin and, on palpation, so-called 'eggshell crackling' can be elicited and there is a characteristic radiological appearance. The tumour is usually localized and metastases are uncommon.

A similar enlarging bony mass with eggshell crackling occurs in the jaws, in association with *adamantinoma*. This tumour arises from the enamel organ, is not malignant, but grows in a similar manner to the osteoclastoma. It may present with a swollen jaw, loosening of teeth or pathological fracture of the mandible.

Treatment of osteoclastoma and adamantinoma consists of excision of the tumour, together with an area of normal bone and a graft of bone placed across the gap. Surgical curettage accompanied by X-ray therapy is less mutilating and is effective in many instances.

Malignant bone tumours

It is important to realize that most malignant bone tumours occuring in adults are secondary to malignancy elsewhere. However, there are some important primary malignant tumours of bone, particularly in children and young adults.

Primary malignant bone tumours

Osteosarcoma

This tumour occurs usually in the second decade of life and usually near the actively growing metaphysis of the bone. Occasionally it may occur in late life as a complication of Paget's disease of bone. The tumour arises from osteoblasts with extension along the shaft and through the cortex inwards into the medullary cavity and outwards, raising the periosteum which provides a temporary barrier to the tumour spread. The epiphysis also acts as a barrier to the tumour growth. The tumour is composed of numerous tiny spindle-shaped and round cells lying in a stroma consisting of osteoid and fibrous or cartilaginous tissue. The tumour is very vascular and spread is initially by the bloodstream to the lungs.

The clinical presentation is of a painful, often warm swelling related to bone and near a joint. The knee joint is most commonly affected. On examination, the swelling is bony in texture and tender. Dilated veins may be seen in the overlying skin. The clinical picture may be confused with osteomyelitis.

There are characteristic radiological changes with osteolytic and osteosclerotic areas along the shaft and extending into the soft tissues. Where the periosteum is raised at the edges, there is a characteristic deposition of bone (Codman's triangle) and as the tumour extends outwards, spicules of bone become laid down as the periosteum is pushed away ('sunray' appearance). X-ray of the chest frequently demonstrates secondary deposits. Biopsy is necessary for precise diagnosis. The prognosis is poor and pulmonary metastases may be visible at the time of initial diagnosis. Treatment is by amputation including the whole length of the affected bone. Since amputation followed by subsequent early development of metastases is an avoidable tragedy, it is often advised that radiotherapy be given initially. If 3 months later metastatic spread is not apparent, then amputation is proceeded with. More recently preliminary results of combined chemotherapy followed by amputation have suggested an increased survival in some patients. Adriamycin and methotrexate in combination appear to be the most effective drugs.

Chondrosarcoma

This growth arises usually in the pelvis and ribs but may occur in long bones. The growth is often lobulated and, although consisting largely of cartilage, cystic degeneration and haemorrhage within the tumour are not uncommon. Cartilage cells are apparent but the tumour may be very anaplastic in appearance. The tumour is slow-growing with local destruction and blood spread is much less common than in osteosarcoma. It is important to note that a combination of osteosarcoma and chondrosarcoma (osteochondrosarcoma) may occur.

The tumour occurs in an older age group than the osteosarcoma, usually in adults. Treatment is by wide local excision and amputation may be required. Radiotherapy is not utilised since the tumour is radioresistant.

Ewing's tumour ('onion tumour')

This is a tumour of childhood composed of many small round cells so similar in appearance to the neuroblastoma that for many years the two tumours were confused. Indeed, it is important to make sure that, in cases of apparent Ewing's tumour, there is no neuro-blastoma within an adrenal gland. Clinical presentation is with pain and swelling but the tumour is rapidly growing and fever may occur. Like the osteosarcoma, the lesion can be confused with osteomyelitis although it should be noted that the latter condition is more common near the metaphysis of the bone. The characteristic X-ray appearance shows deposition of layers of bone beneath the raised periosteum. These layers give an onion appearance and biopsy confirms the diagnosis.

The prognosis is poor but the tumour is very radiosensitive and radiotherapy is the treatment of choice.

Bone tumours		
Tumours	Age group	Situation in bone
Chondroma	35+	Epiphysis, fingers
Bone cyst	—	Metaphysis, diaphysis
Osteoclastoma	20–35	Metaphysis (near knee-joint)
Osteogenic sarcoma	10–20 (the elderly is association with Paget's disease)	Metaphysis (region of knee common)
Chondrosarcoma	35–50+	Flat bones (pelvis, scapula)
Ewing's tumour	Childhood	Diaphysis

Secondary tumours of bone

The common tumours which metastasize to bone are the breast, lung, kidney, prostate gland and thyroid gland but bony deposits may ocur in any carcinoma. The metastases are more common in the vertebral bodies, pelvis, upper ends of the femora or humeri, the ribs or in the skull. Occasionally the mandible is involved.

The initial presentation of the primary tumour may be with a secondary lesion in bone. Presentation is with pain at the site of involvement and X-ray often reveals a destructive lesion, although occasionally osteosclerotic lesions (for instance, secondary deposits from carcinoma of the prostate) may be seen. Sometimes lesions are not visible on X-ray and scanning of the skeleton after injection of a suitable isotope may reveal the bony deposit.

Treatment is by palliation only. For localized lesions, radiotherapy is useful but chemotherapy or hormonal therapy may be needed for widespread deposits. Pathological features may be treated by suitable support or by fixation in combination with radiotherapy or chemotherapy.

Final comments

Only some of the tumours which may affect man have been described in this chapter but the general classification and understanding of the mode of spread, the method by which malignant tumours kill and the broad principles of management described are applicable to nearly all tumours. Perhaps the most important factor to appreciate is that accurate diagnosis of the extent of spread of disease in cancer allows planning of rational treatment.

6

Disorders of the heart and blood vessels

ANATOMICAL AND PHYSIOLOGICAL CONSIDERATIONS

The heart lies to the left side of the thorax, being well protected from external damage by the sternum, the ribs, the vertebrae and the chest muscles.

Chambers
The walls of the ventricles, especially the left, are thick and muscular, while the atrial walls are relatively thin. The prime function of the atria is to collect blood while that of the ventricles is to pump the blood into the pulmonary and systemic circulations. The ventricles are divided one from the other by the intraventricular septum, the atria by the intra-atrial septum.

Valves
The flow of blood into and from the various chambers is regulated by the four heart valves, which are formed by folds of endocardium strengthened by fibroelastic tissue (Fig. 6.1). All the valves have

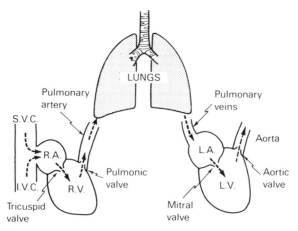

Fig. 6.1 The cardiac chambers, the valves, and the lungs showing the circulation of blood from the right side of the heart to the left.

three cusps except the mitral which has only two. The tricuspid valve regulates the blood flow from right atrium to right ventricle, the pulmonic valve that from the right ventricle into the pulmonary trunk, the mitral valve that from the left atrium to the left ventricle, and the aortic valve that from the left ventricle to the aorta. The pulmonic and aortic valves are attached directly to the walls of the pulmonary trunk and the aorta respectively. The tricuspid and mitral valves have delicate cord-like structures, the chordae tendineae, which pass from the free borders of the valves to the inner walls of the respective ventricles.

Walls of the heart

The walls of the heart are composed of three layers. The inner layer, or endocardium, is a smooth membrane of endothelium which lines the heart chambers and is folded over on itself to form the heart valves. The middle layer, or myocardium, is a very specialized involuntary muscle which, unlike the skeletal muscles, never rests but contracts rhythmically more than once a second from birth to death. The outer layer, or pericardium, is formed by the visceral layer, which is closely attached to the myocardium, and the outer parietal layer.

Conducting system

The heart muscle is intrinsically capable of conducting nervous impulses but there is in addition a very specialized conducting system which forms a pathway through the heart for the rapid transmission of impulses (Fig. 6.2). The starting point of this pathway, the sinoatrial node or pacemaker, is situated in the right atrium near the orifices of the great veins. It initiates each heart beat and regulates the rate and the rhythm of the heart's action. From the sinoatrial node impulses pass down over the atrial walls and are gathered at the atrio-ventricular node which lies between the atria

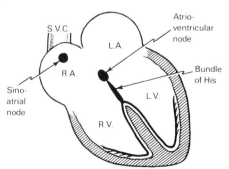

Fig. 6.2 The principal components of the conducting system of the heart.

and the ventricles. It acts as an intermediate collecting and transmitting station from which impulses pass to the bundle of His. In its first part this is a single pathway but it soon divides into the two main branches which go down the left and right side of the intraventricular septum and then ramify over the ventricular walls.

Nerve supply of heart

A cardiac centre lies in the floor of the fourth ventricle and from it impulses are transmitted to the heart by parasympathetic (vagal) and sympathetic nerve pathways. Vagal stimulation leads to slowing, and sympathetic stimulation to acceleration of the heart.

Nutrition of the heart

The heart receives its blood supply from the two coronary arteries which arise directly from the aorta near the aortic valve (Fig. 6.3).

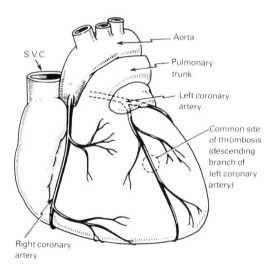

Fig. 6.3 The coronary arteries.

They fill during cardiac diastole. The left is the more important as it is responsible for the blood supply to the greater part of the left ventricle and, in addition, it is more frequently affected by coronary artery disease.

The cardiac cycle

The cardiac cycle occupies three phases:

  1. During *atrial systole* the atria contract simultaneously and

discharge their contained blood into the ventricles through the open tricuspid and mitral valves.

2. At the beginning of *ventricular systole* the tricuspid and mitral valves close, the ventricles contract, and, when the ventricular pressure has risen sufficiently, the aortic and pulmonic valves are forced open and the blood is ejected into the aorta and pulmonary arteries respectively. The aortic and pulmonic valves then close to prevent a reflux of blood into the ventricles.

3. During the third phase of the cardiac cycle, termed *diastole*, the cardiac muscle rests, the coronary arteries fill with blood, the right atrium receives deoxygenated blood from the great veins and the left atrium simultaneously fills with oxygenated blood from the lungs.

INVESTIGATION OF CARDIOVASCULAR DISORDERS

The remarkable technological advances of recent years are of considerable value in the investigation of patients with cardiovascular disorders, but the student should remember that a careful history and physical examination are still of paramount importance.

History
The history that the individual with cardiovascular disease gives in response to an intelligent and patient enquiry is more important than any other single method of investigation. In no other system is the adage more true 'listen to the patient; he is telling you the diagnosis'. The most important symptoms are breathlessness, chest pain, ankle swelling, joint pains, haemoptysis, and palpitation. Regarding past history, enquiry should be made about rheumatic fever, chorea, and sore throats.

General examination
Much information may be gained from a general examination of the patient before a study is made of the cardiovascular system. The presence of cyanosis, oedema, neck vein overfilling (Fig. 6.4), dyspnoea, and finger clubbing can be quite readily detected in the ambulant patient without any special skill.

Pulse
The pulse is normally examined by palpation of the radial artery at the wrist. The student should first become proficient at counting the rate of the pulse and then with determining whether it is regular or irregular. He should then ascertain whether the vessel wall is

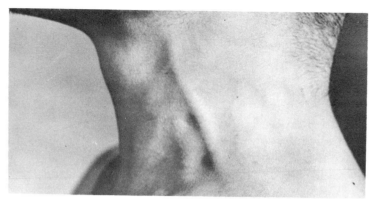

Fig. 6.4 Neck vein congestion.

palpable or not. In young individuals, when the radial artery is emptied of blood, the wall of the vessel cannot be felt but in elderly individuals it is frequently thickened and tortuous due to arteriosclerosis. Appreciation of alterations in the quality of the pulse require more experience but the dentist should be able to recognize the poor quality, thready pulse associated with shock.

Blood pressure
Estimation of the blood pressure is an essential step in the examination of the cardiovascular system. The patient must be relaxed both physically and mentally otherwise falsely high readings may be obtained. The sphygmomanometer consists in essence of an inflatable cuff connected to a mercury manometer. The empty cuff is placed comfortably but firmly round the upper arm and the pressure increased until the radial pulse disappears. This gives an approximate estimate of the systolic blood pressure. The cuff is allowed to empty and, after a few moments, reinflated to a point just above the estimated systolic pressure. The examiner auscultates over the brachial artery in the antecubital fossa and, as he gradually allows the pressure to fall, a distinct beat is heard when the systolic pressure is reached; the pressure is allowed to fall further and on reaching the diastolic blood pressure the sounds quickly fade and become inaudible.

Examination of the heart
Clinical examination of the heart by means of inspection, palpation, percussion and auscultation requires a degree of clinical skill which the dental student is not expected to acquire. He should appreciate, however, that by means of these techniques the doctor can obtain

valuable information regarding the heart size, the quality of the heart sounds, and the presence of heart murmurs.

Mention may be made of the apex beat which is normally produced by the apex of the left ventricle impinging against the chest wall during systole. It lies in the fifth left interspace within a line drawn vertically from the midpoint of the clavicle and its position is, in the absence of mediastinal displacement, a good guide to the heart size.

Radiology
The size of the heart and individual chambers may be more accurately determined by means of X-ray studies while information regarding cardiac function may be obtained from direct viewing of the heart movements under the X-ray screen (screening of the heart). Radio-opaque material may be injected into the aorta, heart or coronary arteries enabling their precise delineation.

Electrocardiography
The changes in electrical potential which occur when the heart muscle contracts and relaxes may be recorded by means of electrocardiography. This method of investigation is widely used in the study of coronary artery disease and it also yields valuable information in the arrhythmias.

Cardiac catheterisation
The pressure in the great vessels and heart chambers, and the oxygen saturation of the blood, can be measured via a cardiac catheter inserted via a peripheral vein.

CAUSES OF HEART DISEASE

A simple outline of the main causes of heart disease is set out in

Table 1. The cause of heart disease

Type	Frequency	Maximum age incidence
Rheumatic heart disease	COMMON	Children to middle age
Coronary artery disease		Middle age onwards
Hypertension		Middle age onwards
Pulmonary heart disease*		Middle age onwards
Thyroid heart disease	UNCOMMON	Middle age
Congenital heart disease		Infancy to early adult life
Syphilitic heart disease		Middle age

* Especially in industrial areas.

Table 1. The great majority of cases seen in ordinary clinical practice are accounted for by the first four causes listed—rheumatic heart disease, coronary artery disease, hypertension and, in industrial areas, pulmonary heart disease.

COMMON SYMPTOMS AND SIGNS

Dyspnoea

Dyspnoea literally means difficult or disordered breathing. It is an extremely important symptom of cardiac disease as it is often the earliest indication that cardiac function is impaired. Dyspnoea also occurs in various lung disorders, in anaemia, and where there is abdominal enlargement.

Cardiac causes

Cardiac dyspnoea may take one of two forms.

1. The breathlessness may be felt only on exertion and be relieved by rest. Thus it is common to obtain a history in cardiac patients that they are breathless on hurrying and on climbing hills or stairs and that it disappears in a relatively short time once they rest. As cardiac decompensation becomes more severe the degree of effort required to provoke dyspnoea becomes less until eventually the patient is breathless even at rest. At this stage he is invariably more comfortable in a propped-up or sitting position (orthopnoea) as the heart has less work to do in this posture.

2. The second variety of cardiac dyspnoea, which is termed paroxysmal nocturnal dyspnoea, occurs in cases of acute left ventricular failure (e.g. in hypertension or in coronary artery disease) and in cases of mitral stenosis with severe pulmonary hypertension; it is due to acute pulmonary oedema. The patient is wakened from sleep with a sense of suffocation or choking, the respirations are extremely laboured, he becomes cyanosed, is intensely distressed, and he coughs up frothy sputum which may be tinged with blood.

Lung disorders

Pulmonary causes of dyspnoea will be discussed in the chapter on respiratory diseases.

Anaemia

A substantial fall in the haemoglobin level causes impaired oxygenation of the tissues and resultant dyspnoea even when there is no intrinsic cardiac or pulmonary disorder. Dyspnoea is more likely to occur if the anaemia has developed quickly as compensatory mechanisms develop in anaemias of gradual onset.

Abdominal enlargement

Considerable abdominal swelling, e.g. from ascites, late stages of pregnancy, large cysts or tumours, causes elevation of the diaphragm with resultant pulmonary embarrassment and dyspnoea.

Cardiac pain

The most important variety of cardiac pain is that resulting from myocardial ischaemia which is usually a consequence of coronary artery disease. The symptom is a dramatic one and may take one of two forms.

1. Angina pectoris is the term given to the sensation of tightness or pain experienced behind the sternum when there is transient myocardial ischaemia. It tends to radiate across the chest and into the shoulders and arms. It is typically brought on by exertion, relieved by rest, and usually lasts not more than a few minutes.

2. The pain associated with myocardial infarction has the same pattern of distribution but it is usually much more intense and of considerably greater duration. Its onset is not determined by exertion and it is not relieved by rest.

Mention must be made of the chest pain complained of by the nervous, introspective individual who fears that he has cardiac disease. The pain is commonly described as sharp or stabbing in nature, it is located principally below the left breast, and it bears a poor relation to effort. In all these respects it is different from the pain of myocardial ischaemia.

Palpitation

Palpitation means an awareness of the heart's action. Some individuals describe the symptom as a 'thumping', others as a 'fluttering' in the chest. In the majority of instances there is no serious condition present.

Palpitation is experienced by normal individuals when the heart is acting forcibly as a result of exertion or emotional upset. Some nervous individuals, particularly women, experience the symptom after trivial exertion or emotional upset and it may be interpreted by them as an indication of heart disease. In some of these cases the cardiac rhythm is regular while in others there may be occasional extrasystoles. Once it is ascertained that no cardiac disease is present these individuals can be safely reassured.

Palpitation may occasionally be the presenting symptom of a significant cardiac disorder, e.g. the palpitation associated with an un-controlled atrial fibrillation or paroxysmal tachycardia.

Oedema

Oedema is the term given to the accumulation of an excessive amount of fluid in the tissues of the body. It occurs in congestive cardiac failure, in some forms of renal and hepatic disease, in beri-beri, in starvation, and as a local phenomenon in certain circum-stances.

Cardiac oedema

In congestive cardiac failure the site of the oedema is largely deter-mined by gravity, being most evident in the legs, particularly around the ankles, in cardiac patients who are ambulant, and in the lumbosacral region in patients who have been in bed for a period of time. In gross congestive cardiac failure fluid may also accumulate in the serous cavities of the body giving rise to ascites and pleural effusion; this is termed anasarca.

The oedema fluid, which is slightly yellowish in colour and re-latively low in protein, is formed as a passive transudate from the blood vessels. It was previously considered that the main cause was increased hydrostatic pressure (Fig. 6.5) but a more important fac-tor is decreased sodium excretion and consequent fluid retention.

The earliest indication of oedema is an increase in weight which, in an average adult, must rise by about 4·5 kg (10 lb) before visible changes occur. When swelling of the legs or of the lumbosacral region does develop it may be demonstrated to be due to fluid by the simple clinical test of producing pitting by pressure with the ball of the thumb or finger.

Renal oedema

In acute nephritis a slight or moderate degree of oedema is com-monly present; the earliest indication is often a puffiness of the face

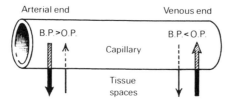

Fig. 6.5 Simplified representation of the relationship between the hydrostatic pressure (B.P.) and the osmotic pressure (O.P.) in a capillary.
Arterial end—fluid passes from vessel.
Venous end—fluid passes to vessel.

especially in the mornings. Gross oedema is a characteristic feature of the nephrotic syndrome (p. 204) where the sequence of events is protein loss in the urine—fall of plasma proteins—fall in plasma osmotic pressure (Fig. 6.5).

Starvation oedema
This is rarely seen in Western countries except under such grossly abnormal conditions as prevailed in concentration camps. It is not uncommon in many underdeveloped countries. Dietary deficiency leads to low plasma protein levels and thus to a fall in the plasma osmotic pressure.

Local oedema
Oedema is seen as a local phenomenon in inflammatory states and the dentist will frequently encounter examples of this in the buccal cavity. Obstruction to venous or lymphatic drainage will also produce oedema. Examples of this are the oedema seen in deep venous thrombosis, most commonly of the calf, and in lymphatic obstruction by malignant growths.

Cyanosis
Cyanosis is the term given to a bluish discoloration of the skin and mucous membranes due in most cases to the presence of an excessive amount of haemoglobin in the reduced or deoxygenated form (at least 5 g per 100 ml of reduced haemoglobin must be present before cyanosis is clinically apparent) and, less commonly, to the presence of certain abnormal haemoglobin derivatives.

Consideration of the causes given below will show that in many cases of cyanosis due to cardiac disease two factors are responsible, namely the central one of impaired pulmonary oxygenation and the peripheral one of increased conversion of oxyhaemoglobin to reduced haemoglobin.

Inadequate pulmonary oxygenation
This may result from pulmonary congestion due to congestive cardiac failure, mitral stenosis of long standing, left ventricular failure, or extensive lung disease

Increased peripheral deoxygenation
The conversion of oxyhaemoglobin to reduced haemoglobin may be increased peripherally because of general or local slowing of circulation. Examples are congestive cardiac failure, peripheral circulatory failure, Raynaud's phenomenon, and local venous obstruction.

Cardiovascular shunts

In certain forms of congenital heart disease some deoxygenated blood may pass directly from the right to the left side of the heart without traversing the pulmonary circulation.

Abnormal blood pigments

Cyanosis may be caused by the presence of sulphaemoglobin, or methaemoglobin, this usually being a toxic effect of certain drugs. Perhaps the commonest offender is phenacetin, present in some compound analgesic preparations.

DISTURBANCES OF CARDIAC RATE

The average cardiac rate in the healthy resting adult is about 70 per minute but it should be appreciated that there are considerable individual variations. The cardiac rate of the child is faster, in infancy being about 120 beats per minute and at the age of 10 about 90 per minute.

Tachycardia

When the cardiac rate in the adult is above the arbitrary level of 100 per minute tachycardia is said to be present. Tachycardia occurs physiologically after exertion and emotional upset. It is also seen as a normal reaction to fever, shock, haemorrhage, administration of adrenaline, and it is a characteristic feature of thyrotoxicosis. Tachycardia occurring in a person with organic heart disease is usually an indication that cardiac function is decreasing.

Paroxysmal tachycardia

This is a relatively uncommon condition characterized by the sudden development of tachycardia (e.g. 160 per minute) which may last from a few minutes to several hours and then as suddenly cease. The individual usually seeks advice because of the associated palpitation. In some cases the attack may be terminated by vagal stimulation, e.g. pressure on the carotid sinus or eyeballs.

Bradycardia

When the cardiac rate falls to 60 per minute or less bradycardia is said to be present. It is seen physiologically in certain athletes particularly highly trained distance runners. It is a typical feature of myxoedema, it occurs in association with jaundice and increased intracranial pressure, and it is one of the manifestations of excessive dosage with digoxin. Its occurrence otherwise should suggest the presence of heart block (*vide infra*).

DISTURBANCES OF CARDIAC RHYTHM

The cardiac rhythm is normally regular due to the activity of the sinoatrial node or pacemaker.

Sinus arrhythmia

This, the simplest form of cardiac arrhythmias, is seen physiologically in children and in many young adults. It consists of a quickening of the cardiac rate during inspiration and a slowing during expiration, and it is thought to be caused by alterations in vagal tone. Many students may personally demonstrate the condition by feeling their pulse during deep breathing. The condition does not produce any symptoms.

Extrasystoles

An extrasystole is a beat of the heart which is initiated in a focus of abnormal excitation outwith the sinoatrial node. Depending on the site of origin they may be classified as atrial, ventricular, or nodal (atrioventricular node); the distinction is made on electrocardiographic evidence.

The individual who has extrasytoles may experience no symptoms or he may have palpitation. On feeling the pulse the basically regular rhythm is interrupted from time to time by the occurrence of a premature beat which is weaker than normal and is followed by a longer pause (Fig. 6.6). Extra-systoles may be infrequent or so numerous as to mimic atrial fibrillation. Occasionally a premature beat occurs regularly after each normal beat producing coupling of the pulse (pulsus bigeminus); this is most often due to digoxin overdosage.

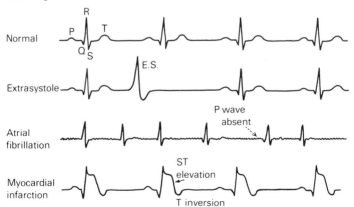

Fig. 6.6 Electrocardiograms showing the normal pattern, extrasystole (E.S.), atrial fibrillation, and early myocardial infarction. P represents the wave of excitation through the atria, Q R S and T the changes in the ventricles.

In most instances the presence of extrasystoles does not signify organic heart disease. Thus nervous instability, or overindulgence in tobacco, coffee or tea, may be responsible and all that is required is correction of the faulty habit and reassurance. Extrasystoles may also result from organic heart disease or from digoxin overdosage.

Atrial fibrillation

In atrial fibrillation the sinoatrial node no longer controls the heart rhythm. The atria beat very rapidly (about 400 per minute), and irregularly, by a process of excitation arising in the atria, the precise details of which are not fully understood. The atrioventricular node can transmit to the ventricle only about 140 to 160 of these irregular impulses per minute.

The most important causes of atrial fibrillation are rheumatic heart disease (particularly mitral stenosis), thyrotoxicosis, and myocardial ischaemia.

The pulse is completely irregular and, in the absence of treatment, usually rapid. At this stage palpitation is commonly experienced. The heart rate, determined by auscultation, is often considerably greater than the radial pulse rate because many of the ventricular beats are too feeble to produce a radial pulse; this phenomenon is known as a pulse deficit and it may number 20 or 30 beats per minute. The electrocardiographic pattern is characteristic (Fig. 6.6).

Atrial fibrillation throws an added strain on an already damaged heart and, in addition, embolization may occur. Clots tend to form in the atria because they are not emptying completely and a portion of clot may become dislodged and cause blockage, e.g. of a cerebral vessel producing paralysis, or of a limb vessel leading to gangrene.

Treatment consists in the use of digoxin to reduce the ventricular rate to the normal range (it does not produce a return to normal rhythm) and the management of the basic cause whether it be a cardiac lesion or thyrotoxicosis.

Atrial flutter

Artrial flutter is closely related to atrial fibrillation but the atrial rhythm, although very rapid, is regular. The atrioventricular node transmits every second, third or possibly fourth atrial impulse so that the ventricular rate will be one-half, one-third, or one-quarter that of the atrial rate (2 to 1, 3 to 1, or 4 to 1, atrial flutter). The pulse is therefore regular, although rapid.

Heart block

Interference with the transmission of the impulse from the atria to the ventricles may be caused in younger individuals by rheumatic fever, in older individuals by ischaemic changes in the conducting mechanism, or it may result from digoxin overdosage at any age.

Heart block may be potential, partial, or complete. The potential variety is detectable only be electrocardiography. In partial heart block some atrial impulses do not produce a ventricular response and the pulse is irregular due to 'dropped beats'. In complete heart block no impulses from the atria reach the ventricles and death occurs if idioventricular rhythm is not initiated within a few seconds. During these critical few seconds the individual usually loses consciousness, his colour becomes deathly pale and then cyanosed, and he is pulseless; this is termed an Adams-Stokes seizure.

CONGENITAL HEART DISEASE

In early foetal life the heart is represented by a simple tubelike structure which, by an extremely complicated process, evolves into the delicately regulated four-chambered structure that we know as the human heart. It is not surprising that sometimes this process is not completely flawless and a form of congenital heart disease results. An aetiological factor in certain cases is infection of the mother, in the early weeks of pregnancy, with the virus responsible for rubella.

Congenital heart disease may be classified according to whether cyanosis is present or not. In the cyanotic group (the 'blue babies') there is flow of some venous blood from the right side directly to the left side of the heart without traversing the pulmonary circuit. In general, the cyanotic forms have a graver prognosis.

Congenital heart disease is of importance to the dentist in two ways. Firstly, these patients may be high risks for dental anaesthesia or dental surgical procedures because of impaired cardiac function; secondly, they may develop subacute bacterial endocarditis after dental extractions unless appropriate phophylactic measures are taken.

Until relatively recent years no basic treatment was possible for any of the forms of congenital heart disease, but advances in thoracic surgery and anaesthesia now permit a striking benefit to be achieved in certain carefully selected cases.

Acyanotic congenital heart disease
Some of the less rare anomalies merit a brief description.

A defect may exist in the atrial or ventricular septum and if it is the sole abnormality and is small, may cause relatively little upset of cardiac function. In other instances the *septal defect* is associated with other anomalies, as in Fallot's tetralogy.

The ductus arteriosus, which is foetal life allows blood to pass from the pulmonary trunk to the aorta without traversing the lungs, may remain patent after birth permitting a flow of blood from aorta to pulmonary trunk which produces a very characteristic murmur at the base of the heart. Ligation of a *patent ductus arteriosus is* relatively speaking, one of the simpler operations that the thoracic surgeon may be asked to perform.

In *coarctation of aorta* the thoracic aorta is narrowed, causing a decreased blood supply to the lower part of the body associated with hypertension, which is a compensatory phenomenon, in the upper part. The arteries of the intercostal region become enlarged and tortuous in an attempt to provide a collateral circulation to the lower part of the body. From the dental point of view an increase in size of the mandibular arteries and the arteries leading to the individual teeth has been reported and, in consequence, there is a tendency to haemorrhage after dental extraction.

In *dextrocardia* the heart lies on the right side of the thorax. No symptoms are produced if dextrocardia is the sole defect and the condition may remain undetected until the individual undergoes some routine medical examination or has a chest X-ray.

Cyanotic congenital heart disease

The majority of infants with cyanotic congenital heart disease who survive the early months of life suffer from *Fallot's tetralogy* which comprises pulmonary stenosis, right ventricular hypertrophy, ventricular septal defect and dextroposition of the aorta. The presence of these defects permits the passage of unoxygenated blood from the right to the left side of the heart and the individuals affected show marked cyanosis, finger clubbing, dyspnoea, and retarded development. The buccal mucosa is often intensely cyanosed and has been likened to the colour of a ripe Victorian plum. There is delayed eruption of both deciduous and permanent teeth. An increase in the number of red cells occurs (polycythaemia), as a compensatory mechanism to offset the poor oxygenation of the blood. Cardiac surgery is used to correct the defect in a considerable portion of these unfortunate children and even very severe defects are now amenable to operation.

RHEUMATIC FEVER

Incidence

Rheumatic fever has its highest incidence in the autumn and winter months in countries with damp, temperate climates. The disease is now less common than it was but in Britain it is still the most important cause of heart disease in children and young adults. The maximum age incidence is 5 to 15 years.

Aetiology
Rheumatic fever is an immunological response to infection with the haemolytic streptococcus. The infection is usually in the throat and a history of an upper respiratory infection, or of scarlet fever, some 10 to 21 days before the onset of rheumatic fever is often present.

Pathology
The inflammatory reaction affects the connective tissues of the heart, the joints, and the subcutaneous tissues. The pathological changes are of greatest importance in the heart where the valves (endocarditis), the myocardium (myocarditis), and the pericardium (pericarditis), may be affected in greater or lesser degree. The valves are swollen and small, firmly adherent vegetations develop along the lines of contact of the cusps. After the acute stage has settled fibrous tissue reaction may produce permanent deformity and impaired function of the heart valves and also impaired efficiency of the myocardium. The mitral valve is most frequently affected, the aortic valve comes next in frequency, while the valves on the right side of the heart are rarely involved.

Clinical picture
The patient is usually a child or a young adult in whom it is often possible to obtain a history of an upper respiratory tract infection some two or three weeks before. The onset of the rheumatic fever is usually manifested by the development of arthritis which causes flitting pains particularly in the larger joints. The affected joints are tender to touch, painful, hot, swollen and red. The temperature is elevated, the pulse rapid, and the skin hot and sweating. The throat may still be inflamed from the previous streptococcal infection.

When the heart is seriously involved, cardiac enlargement occurs, the heart sounds are softer than normal and murmurs develop. Active pericarditis causes pericardial friction followed by pericardial effusion.

The blood sedimentation rate is accelerated and the level does not usually return to normal until the rheumatic process is quiescent (normal level is up to 12 mm in one hour by the Westergren method). Electrocardiography may yield evidence of potential heart block.

Diagnosis

In a typical case, such as described above, there is no diagnostic problem, but in some instances pain is much more prominent in one limb suggesting, for a time, a diagnosis of local inflammatory lesion or again joint pains are slight or absent, the picture being that of a child who is vaguely unwell, has a poor appetite and abdominal discomfort. Sometimes the symptoms are so mild that the child never comes under medical care.

Prognosis

Death in the acute stages of rheumatic fever due to cardiac failure is fortunately now rare. Many patients make a complete recovery and are left with no clinical evidence of any cardiac lesion. A substantial number, including some of the atypical or 'missed' cases, suffer permanent cardiac damage and this group will be discussed further in the section dealing with mitral and aortic valve disease.

Treatment

The individual with rheumatic fever is confined to bed until the process is deemed inactive by the absence of symptoms, and a return of pulse, temperature and blood sedimentation rate to normal levels. The duration of bed rest is, on an average, about six weeks. Salicylates are given in full dosage either as sodium salicylate or as aspirin. Salicylate therapy leads to a fall in the temperature (antipyretic effect), relief of joint pains (analgesic effect), and is generally believed to reduce the incidence and severity of permanent cardiac damage.

Steroid therapy, although it has a marked anti-inflammatory effect, does not lessen the incidence of permanent cardiac damage.

The after-care of the patient who has had rheumatic fever is important. The individual should take common sense precautions to avoid as far as possible the development of upper respiratory infections. As a prophylactic against further throat infections many favour long-term sulphonamide or penicillin therapy. In this respect mention must also be made of tonsillectomy; if the tonsils are diseased and the individual is having frequent sore throats he may benefit considerably from tonsillectomy, but healthy tonsils should never be removed in the hope of preventing further sore throats.

Chorea (Sydenham's chorea)

This is a less common manifestation of acute rheumatism. The maximum incidence is in children. It is characterized by oedema and focal changes in the brain especially the basal ganglia.

The main clinical features are involuntary jerky, purposeless movements of the limbs, facial grimacing, and 'jack-in-the-box' movements of the tongue. The risks of cardiac damage are as in rheumatic fever.

VALVULAR DISEASE OF THE HEART

For practical purposes we need consider only the mitral and aortic valve since the tricuspid and pulmonic valves are rarely affected. In the case of the mitral valve, rheumatism is the only aetiological factor, but with aortic valve lesions consideration must also be given to the possible role of syphilis and degenerative changes.

If the valve is deformed in such a way that its aperture is narrowed, the term stenosis is used, while if the deformity results in incomplete closure of the valve we used the term incompetence.

Pathological effects of valvular lesions

In mitral stenosis the valve cannot open properly, causing obstruction to the flow of blood from the left atrium to the left ventricle. The pressure in the left atrium rises, the left atrium enlarges and hypertrophies, pressure increases in pulmonary circuit producing pulmonary congestion, and the right ventricle hypertrophies.

In mitral incompetence the valve cannot close properly and when the left ventricle contracts some blood passes back through the mitral valve to the left atrium instead of all passing into the aorta. The left ventricle attempts to pass into the systemic circulation a normal quantity of blood and consequently hypertrophies.

In aortic stenosis the valve cusps become fused together so that the valve cannot open fully and there is obstruction to the free passage of blood from the left ventricle to the aorta; left ventricular hypertrophy results.

In aortic incompetence the valve does not close properly at the end of ventricular systole and there is a reflux of blood from the aorta to the left ventricle leading to left ventricular hypertrophy.

Clinical features

The majority of cases are seen in young adults. A past history of rheumatic fever, scarlet fever, or chorea is obtained in about 50 per cent. In the case of aortic lesions consideration must also be given to a past history of syphilis (aortic incompetence) and to the question of degenerative changes.

At first there are no symptoms, but later, when cardiac decompensation occurs, the individual experiences breathlessness on effort which becomes progressively worse. Palpitation may also be noted. Haemoptysis secondary to pulmonary engorgement is a feature in mitral stenosis and the patient may also have attacks of paroxysmal nocturnal dyspnoea.

The presence of mitral stenosis may be suspected by a malar flush due to cyanosis of the cheeks. In aortic incompetence the diastolic blood pressure is lowered as a result of reflux of blood to the left ventricle while the systolic pressure is often elevated because of more forcible left ventricular action, e.g. a blood pressure of 140/40 mm of mercury in common. The high pulse pressure produces the characteristic collapsing pulse of aortic incompetence. The pulse meets the examining fingers abruptly and forcefully but the impact is of very short duration as the pressure falls away quickly (Fig. 6.7).

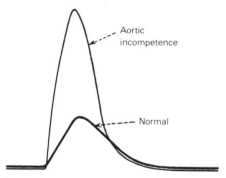

Fig. 6.7 Comparison between the normal pulse wave and that in aortic incompetence; the latter is sharply rising, sharply peaked, and sharply falling.

Clinical examination of the heart may reveal enlargement of one or more chambers and also the presence of various heart murmurs which, from their time, site and quality, indicate which form of valvular lesion is present.

Combination of valve lesions
In many cases more than one valve lesion is present, e.g. both mitral stenosis and incompetence, or both aortic stenosis and incompetence, or again a combination of mitral and aortic lesions. Double or multiple valve lesions obviously throw a greater strain on the heart.

Complications of valvular disease
The individual with rheumatic valvular disease of the heart may suffer three main complications and, as a result, the majority do

not survive beyond middle age unless surgical correction of the valvular lesion is possible.

1. Atrial fibrillation is particularly common if mitral stenosis is present. Fibrillation brings with it the danger of embolism.

2. Congestive cardiac failure is likely to occur if the valve deformity is producing considerable interference with cardiac function.

3. Subacute bacterial endocarditis may develop at any time.

Treatment

Until recently it was in effect the treatment of complications using digoxin for the control of atrial fibrillation, digoxin and other methods to relieve congestive cardiac failure and penicillin for the prophylaxis and treatment of subacute bacterial endocarditis. However, surgical treatment has now advanced considerably. Mitral stenosis can be treated by mitral valvotomy but other valvular disease is managed by open heart surgical methods using a temporary heart/lung bypass machine and valves may be repaired or replaced either by prostheses or by grafting techniques.

BACTERIAL ENDOCARDITIS

Bacterial endocarditis may be either acute or subacute. In the former, which is now very uncommon, virulent organisms such as haemolytic streptococci attack heart valves which were previously normal; it is a rare complication of virulent infections elsewhere in the body and as it has no specific dental importance, will not be discussed further. Subacute bacterial endocarditis, on the other hand, is of considerable importance to the dentist.

Aetiology and bacteriology

Subacute bacterial endocarditis is a bacterial infection of heart valves which are damaged or abnormal as a consequence of rheumatic disease or some congenital anomaly. The term 'locus resistentiae minoris' is sometimes used to describe the primary abnormality.

The infecting organism is, in the great majority of cases, the *Streptococcus viridans* which is a normal inhabitant of the buccal cavity. After many dental procedures, but especially extractions, there is a transient bacteraemia which in the healthy person is of no consequence but in a patient with damaged endocardium the organisms may gain a foothold on the damaged area resulting in bacterial endocarditis. All cases of subacute bacterial endocarditis are not the consequence of dental procedures. In some instances other operative procedures in the mouth or throat (e.g. tonsillectomy) or upper respiratory infections may be responsible, but in other cases the infection of the heart valves manifests itself insidiously in the absence of any apparent predisposing factor.

Pathology

Vegetations, which are composed of blood platelets, round cells, bacterial, and fibrin, are formed on the heart valves. These outgrowths are, in contrast to the vegetations of rheumatic fever, friable and small fragments may become detached and pass in the circulation to produce embolic phenomena in many parts of the body.

Clinical features

The condition may occur at any age but is most frequently seen in children or young adults. The presence of the underlying rheumatic or congenital heart disease may or may not have been known previously. A history of dental treatment, which may not necessarily include extractions, may be obtained. When subacute bacterial endocarditis does follow some dental procedure there is usually a latent period before symptoms and signs develop. The principal features are depicted in Figure 6.8.

The patient complains of loss of energy, loss of appetite, possibly of undue sweating, and he may have noted that he has become paler than normal. The skin and mucous membranes are pale and in advanced cases the skin has a light brownish tint sometimes described as an earthy pallor or a *cafe-au-lait* colour. The temperature becomes elevated but the degree of fever is usually slight and the fever is not constant; thus a single normal temperature recording by no means rules out the diagnosis. Finger clubbing develops but it is seldom gross and thus requires to be looked for carefully. Small petechial haemorrhages may be seen in the skin, the buccal mucosa, the conjunctivae and the nail bed. These are due to toxaemia which causes rupture of the small blood vessel walls. Enlargement of the spleen, again of slight or moderate degree, is a common finding, this being part of the body's defence mechanism against infection. Examination of the blood confirms the presence of anaemia and reveals also a leucocytosis and elevation of the blood sedimentation rate. The blood culture is not constantly positive and several cultures may have to be made before the *Streptococcus viridans* is isolated.

Examination of the cardiovascular system reveals tachycardia and

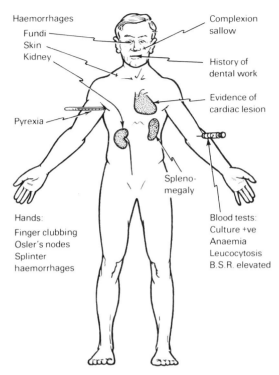

Haemorrhages
Fundi
Skin
Kidney

Complexion
sallow

History of
dental work

Evidence of
cardiac lesion

Pyrexia

Spleno-
megaly

Hands:

Finger clubbing
Osler's nodes
Splinter
haemorrhages

Blood tests:
Culture +ve
Anaemia
Leucocytosis
B.S.R. elevated

Fig. 6.8 The principal features in subacute bacterial endocarditis.

the doctor may note alterations in existing heart murmurs due to increasing deformity of already damaged valves.

The effects of embolism can be very diverse but the organ most frequently affected is the kidney. Slight degrees of haemuturia, detectable only be careful microscopy of the urine, are common, while occasionally there is frank haematuria and pain in the loin. Painful little swellings in the pulps of the fingers or toes (Osler's nodes) may result from impaction of portions of the vegetations in the digital vessels. Obstruction of larger limb vessels is much less frequent. Embolic phenomena may also affect the brain leading to various forms of paralysis.

Diagnosis
Subacute bacterial endocarditis should be suspected when any patient known to have rheumatic or congenital heart disease suffers deterioration in health. Careful enquiry regarding the symptoms outlined above should be made, followed by a detailed clinical examination, and examination of the blood and urine. Sometimes

there is difficulty in distinguishing between a recurrence of rheumatic activity and the early stages of subacute bacterial endocarditis and careful observation is necessary. It must be remembered also that patients with heart disease may develop infections other than subacute bacterial endocarditis, e.g. of the lungs or urinary tract.

Prognosis

Until the introduction of penicillin the prognosis in cases of subacute baterial endocarditis was hopeless. The outlook is now favourable provided the case is diagnosed reasonably early, the heart is not too badly damaged, and the organism is sensitive to penicillin or to an alternative antibiotic.

Prophylaxis

All patients with rheumatic or congenital heart disease, and those with prosthetic valves, are given a parenteral injection of an appropriate bactericidal antibiotic approximately 30 minutes (and not more than 60 minutes) before dental extraction to eradicate transient bacteraemia and thus prevent endocarditis. Provided that the patient has no history of penicillin sensitivity or of recent penicillin treatment he may be given either

1. benzyl penicillin in a dose of 600 mg (1 million units) intramuscularly followed by phenoxymethylpenicillin (Penicillin V) 500 mg four times daily by mouth for 48 hours.
2. a single 2 ml dose of Penicillin Triple Injection (Triplopen) which is a preparation containing a mixture of benethamine penicillin (500,000 units), procaine penicillin (250,000 units) and benzylpenicillin (500,000 units). This gives adequate cover for three days.

If the patient has received penicillin recently or if he is suspected of having penicillin allergy, lincomycin or cephaloridine can be used.

Since endocarditis due to *Streptococcus viridans* is much less common in edentulous patients, some authorities consider a recurrence of subacute bacterial endocarditis as an indication for a dental clearance in spite of an apparently satisfactory dental state.

Close cooperation between the dentist and the doctor is essential in these cases. The doctor should warn his patients with heart disease that they should always mention that they have a cardiac condition when they go to see a dentist; the dentist should be on the lookout for anyone who has cyanosis, breathlessness or some other feature suggesting heart disease and should, if necessary, defer treatment until a medical opinion has been obtained.

Treatment

Treatment consists in the administration of penicillin in high dosage for a period of several weeks (e.g. two million units daily for six weeks). Careful follow-up of cases has shown that this long period of treatment with a high dosage of penicillin is necessary to ensure complete control of the infection. If bacteriological studies indicate that the organism is not sensitive to penicillin other antibiotics will be required.

HYPERTENSION

Hypertension is said to be present when the blood pressure is clearly outwith the normal range. In healthy young and middle aged adults the systolic blood pressure should not, at rest, be higher than 140 mm and the diastolic pressure greater than 90 mm of mercury. The upper limits of normal are rather higher in older people, e.g. 150/100 mm of mercury or even possibly more. Since considerable increases of blood pressure may result from emotional upset or exercise, these factors should be excluded before a person is considered to be hypertensive.

In most cases of hypertension both the systolic and diastolic pressures are high. The systolic pressure alone may be elevated in elderly people with inelastic arterial walls; this is a less serious condition than diastolic hypertension.

Causes of hypertension

1. In the great majority of cases the hypertension appears to exist as a primary disorder and this variety is termed essential hypertension.

2. Hypertension results from bilateral renal disease such as glomerulonephritis or pyelonephritis and it also may follow unilateral affections of the kidney. It is important that the unilateral renal lesions are not overlooked as surgical treatment of the renal abnormality leads in some cases to cure of the hypertension.

3. Less common causes of hypertension include endocrine abnormalities such as phaeochromocytoma, Conn's syndrome and Cushing's disease and these also may be cured by surgical means. Coarctation of the aorta is a further rare cause of hypertension which is amenable to surgical therapy.

Essential hypertension

Incidence

Essential hypertension is a very common condition in people of middle age and over. Men are affected rather more than women. It is popularly believed to occur more frequently in people who have a forceful, driving personality and in physique are thickset and possibly a little overweight, but this association is far from constant.

Aetiology

Despite much experimental work the basic causation of essential hypertension is still unknown. There appears to be increased tone in the small blood vessels which causes an increased peripheral resistance, but the basic abnormality producing this deviation from normal has not yet been elucidated.

Pathology

Once hypertension has been present for some time it produces characteristic changes in the blood vessels, the heart, and the kidneys. The walls of the arteries become thicker and harder due to hypertrophy of the middle coat, while the lumen becomes narrower due to changes in the intima. These arterial changes are of greatest pathological import in the heart, the brain, and the kidney. The left ventricle enlarges and hypertrophies because it has to pump blood against a higher pressure but the arterial changes noted above lead to diminished blood supply to the myocardium and in time result in cardiac decompensation. The changes in the small blood vessels of the kidney produce ischaemia which in turn aggravates the already existing hypertension; a vicious circle of hypertension—arterial change—renal ischaemia—further hypertension is thus set up. The changes in the brain predispose to cerebral haemorrhage.

Clinical picture

In the early stages there may be no symptoms, the elevation of the blood pressure being discovered incidently during some routine examination, e.g. for insurance purposes. When symptoms do occur they include headache, which may be throbbing in character, breathlessness on exertion, chest tightness or pain on exertion, deterioration in visual acuity and epistaxis. Troublesome bleeding after dental extractions is not a common complication. Attacks of paroxysmal nocturnal dyspnoea due to acute left ventricular failure occur in severe cases. Congestive cardiac failure develops late in the course of the illness.

Blood pressure readings around 200/120 mm of mercury are common while much higher levels are seen not infrequently. The arterial changes may be noted in the radial vessel at the wrist, in the brachial vessel in the upper arm, and in the arteries of the retina by use of the ophthalmoscope. Haemorrhages, exudates, and swelling of the optic nerve head (papilloedema) may also be noted in the retina in advanced cases. The simplest clinical indication of left ventricular enlargement is displacement of the apex impulse downwards and to the left from the normal position; it may thus come to be felt in the sixth left interspace as far out as the anterior axillary line.

Prognosis
Many patients with quite marked degrees of hypertension live useful, active lives for several years after the condition has been detected. Death, when it does come, is most frequently from heart failure or a cerebrovascular catastrophe and less commonly from renal failure.

Treatment
Certain general measures are applicable in all cases and, if the hypertension is mild, may be all that is required. The individual is advised to conduct all his activities at a moderate tempo and to avoid, as far as far as possible, stress and anxiety. The provision of a mild sedative may make this advice more acceptable. If obesity is present it should be corrected. Alcohol should be taken only in moderation and tobacco is best avoided.

If the blood pressure remains elevated antihypertensive drugs are employed. In many patients effective control of the hypertension can be achieved by the use of a thiazide diuretic or a beta-adrenergic receptor blocking drug, either alone or in combination. In more severe cases additional drugs may be required; some of these act centrally, others produce a peripheral reduction in arteriolar tone.

Malignant hypertension
This term is used when the hypertension is very marked (e.g. diastolic blood pressure 130–140 mmHg) and is associated with severe fundal changes and rapid deterioration in renal function. It necessitates vigorous antihypertensive therapy.

CORONARY ARTERY DISEASE

Incidence
Coronary artery disease is a very common disorder which appears

to be increasing in incidence although this may be partly due to improved diagnosis. It is commoner in males. Those of middle age and over are mainly affected although cases in younger individuals, especially men, are not infrequent. Hypertension, diabetes mellitus and myxoedema are predisposing factors. Occupational surveys suggest that the incidence is higher in those engaged in sedentary work.

Aetiology
The reasons for the high incidence of coronary artery disease are obscure. Considerable attention has been paid to the possible role of the animal fat content of the diet, to the sugar content of the diet, and to the hardness of the water supply but there is no general agreement on these factors. Cigarette smoking is now firmly accepted as an important and preventable factor in the aetiology of coronary artery disease and obesity is also a significant factor.

Whatever the precise cause of it, the discernible pathological lesion is atheroma of the coronary arteries, which causes narrowing and irregularity of the lumen of the vessel and leads to fibrous tissue replacement of the medial coat. The blood supply to the myocardium is reduced by the arterial narrowing and thrombus formation may develop suddenly on atheromatous patches. These changes are seldom confined to the coronary vessels and involvement of the arteries of the limbs, the brain, and the kidney may materially affect the ultimate course of the disorder.

Coronary artery disease may become manifest by angina pectoris, myocardial infarction, or atrial fibrillation and cardiac failure secondary to fibrotic changes in the conducting mechanism and myocardium.

Angina pectoris
Angina pectoris, which literally means pain in the chest, is caused by transient myocardial ischaemia.

Clinical features.
The characteristic story is that the individual feels a retrosternal tightness or pain which tends to spread across the chest and to the shoulders and arms especially on the left side. Breathlessness is commonly associated. Angina pectoris is experienced when the heart is given extra work to do as on exertion, emotional excitement, after a meal, or after exposure to cold. An attack may be precipitated by the emotional reaction to a dental procedure. The pain is gripping in nature and may be severe. With rest it decreases

in intensity and passes off within a few minutes. The symptom has been graphically described as 'the cry of the heart for oxygen'.

Treatment
The patient should be advised to rest when the pain comes on. Prompt symptomatic relief follows the sublingual administration of a tablet of trinitrin which quickly dilates the coronary blood vessels, thus relieving myocardial ischaemia. The tablet should be allowed to dissolve under the tongue as absorption from the buccal mucosa is very rapid. Longer-acting coronary vasodilators are available but their action is less certain. If obesity is present it should be corrected. The patient is advised to avoid as far as possible activities known to produce angina and to stop smoking.

In recent years surgical treatment has become possible for stenosis of the coronary arteries. The methods include revascularization of the myocardium by implantation of the nearby internal mammary artery or direct reconstructive or bypass procedures on the coronary arteries themselves. This is usually done by carrying a bypass graft (using a segment of vein) from the aorta to the coronary artery beyond the block. Early results are encouraging particularly in relief of symptoms although it is not yet known whether the procedure improves prognosis in terms of life expectancy.

Myocardial infarction
Myocardial infarction results when an area of the myocardium has its blood supply markedly and suddenly reduced. It commonly follows thrombus formation on an atheromatous patch in a coronary vessel, haemorrhage into such a patch, and it may also result from obliteration of the lumen without actual thrombus formation. The

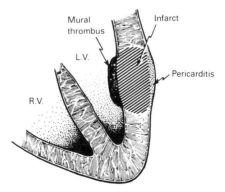

Fig. 6.9 Diagrammatic representation of a section through the wall of the left ventricle in a case of myocardial infarction.

descending branch of the left coronary artery is a common site for thrombosis to develop (Fig. 6.3). A mural thrombus may form on the endocardium underlying the zone of infarction in the heart wall and pericarditis may develop overlying it (Fig. 6.9).

Myocardial infarction may occur in a patient known to have had angina pectoris for some time or it may be the first indication of coronary artery disease.

Clinical features

In its most characteristic form there is a sudden onset of severe, crushing chest pain. The pain is felt behind the sternum and tends to radiate across the chest into the shoulders and into the arms. The onset is not determined by effort. The pain may last for hours unless relieved by morphine and is usually associated with evidence of shock. The patient frequently collapses and may lose consciousness for a period. The skin is cold, clammy and pale, the lips and fingers cyanosed, the breathing shallow, the pulse of poor quality, the blood pressure low, and vomiting is common. The heart sounds are faint and, after a day or two, pericardial friction may be audible.

The picture is not always so typical. Pain may be slight or absent or it may be felt largely in the abdomen raising the question of an acute abdominal emergency. In other cases there is more or less instantaneous death without time to indicate whether pain was present or not. Some patients who sustain a sudden cardiac arrest following myocardial infarction may be successfully resuscitated (see also p. 111).

Diagnosis

As a reaction to the tissue necrosis there is commonly slight pyrexia, leucocytosis, elevation of the sedimentation rate, and increase in the level of certain enzymes in the blood; these changes are often of diagnostic help. The diagnosis may be further substantiated by the characteristic changes in the electrocardiogram (Fig. 6.6), this being of particular value where the clinical features are not straightforward.

Course and prognosis

About one-quarter of patients die following myocardial infarction and most of these deaths occur in the first few days from uncontrollable shock, left ventricular failure, or a serious cardiac arrhythmia. Other hazards are embolism from the mural thrombus or from peripheral deep vein thrombosis. Congestive cardiac failure may also supervene.

In patients who recover from the initial attack of myocardial infarction the average expectation of life is about five to eight years but it is extremely difficult to judge prognosis in individual cases.

Treatment

The first essential is relief of pain and morphia has no equal in this respect. Bed rest is required usually for a period of about two weeks. Anticoagulants, given in the hope of reducing the tendency to further thrombosis in the coronary vessels and to minimize thromboembolic complications, used to be standard practice in myocardial infarction but they now tend to be used only in selected cases. The usual procedure is to give heparin intravenously at first, followed by an oral preparation such as phenindione or warfarin. Careful supervision, with periodic estimations of the prothrombin level of the blood, is necessary.

In view of the awareness of the frequency of sudden arrhythmias, some of which can be reversed by drugs, electrical stimulation or external cardiac massage, there is a growing tendency to look after the more severe cases of myocardial infarction in special *coronary care units* where continuous monitoring of cardiac rhythm and blood pressure can be carried out.

After recovery from the acute stages of a myocardial infarction the patient should have a period of convalescence followed by a gradual increase in activities but preferably stopping somewhat short of the previous level. Long-term anticoagulant therapy is used in carefully selected cases. Cigarette smoking should be stopped.

PULMONARY HEART DISEASE

Interference with the flow of blood through the lungs most commonly results from chronic bronchitis and emphysema. Right ventricular hypertrophy occurs and cardiac failure may ensue. This form of heart disease is commonly termed cor pulmonale. It may also result from the pneumoconioses or dust diseases.

The clinical picture is partly determined by the underlying lung disease and partly by the secondary cardiac failure. The individual will likely give a history of cough and spit associated with exertional dyspnoea. When cardiac failure supervenes, dyspnoea is increased, cyanosis intensified, and oedema develops.

Treatment of the cardiac failure is often only partially successful because the underlying lung disease is irreversible.

THYROID HEART DISEASE

Thyrotoxicosis in young individuals is seldom associated with any evidence of cardiac failure, but when the disorder occurs in middle-aged or elderly individuals cardiac complications are not uncommon. Extrasystoles or atrial fibrillation may occur and, in severe cases, congestive cardiac failure may follow. The diagnosis of thyrotoxicosis is not infrequently overlooked in such instances because eye signs and thyroid gland enlargement may be slight or absent. The cardiac failure will respond poorly to treatment until the thyrotoxicosis is controlled.

There is an increased incidence of coronary artery disease and of myocardial ischaemia in myxoedema. For this reason, when thyroxine is given the initial dose should be small and the dosage should be increased gradually.

CARDIAC FAILURE

The commonest causes of cardiac failure are rheumatic heart disease, hypertension, and coronary artery disease. The condition is usually considered under the headings of left heart failure and right heart failure, but pure examples of either variety are less common than combinations of the two types.

Left heart failure is seen most often in hypertension and coronary artery disease. It is characterized by paroxysmal dyspnoea, often nocturnal, due to acute pulmonary oedema. The administration of a diuretic along with a small dose of morphine usually produce quick symptomatic relief. Inhalations of oxygen are commonly given; digoxin may be required.

Congestive cardiac failure
This is commonly seen in cases of rheumatic heart disease particularly once atrial fibrillation is established. Not infrequently it develops subsequent to left ventricular failure. The dominant feature of the condition is accumulation of blood on the venous side of the circulation.

Clinical features
The main symptom is breathlessness. At first this is experienced only on exertion but in severe cases it is present at rest and the

individual cannot lie flat without acute distress. Oedema is most prominent around the feet and ankles of the ambulant patient, especially in the evenings. In the patient who has been confined to bed for some time it should be looked for in the lumbosacral region. Cyanosis of the lips, cheeks, ears and fingers is present and becomes more marked if the patient is exercised. The neck veins are engorged (see Fig. 6.4) and they may be made even more prominent by pressure over the liver (hepatojugular reflux), which is enlarged and tender because of its increased content of venous blood. Ascites develops in severe cases. The lungs are congested especially at the bases and in severe cases pleural effusion develops. The urinary output is low, the urine is concentrated and commonly contains albumin. The findings in the cardiovascular system depend on the basic cause but frequently the heart is enlarged and the rhythm irregular.

Treatment
The patient invariably finds it easier to be nursed in a propped-up position as this lessens dyspnoea. After the acute stage has passed he may with advantage sit in a comfortable chair for part of the day. Inhalations of oxygen may be required in severe cases.

Digoxin, which is prepared from the leaves of the foxglove plant, is an extremely valuable drug in cases of cardiac failure. It is usually given by mouth but is also available in an intravenous form for emergencies. Digoxin acts on the conducting system of the heart, slowing the cardiac rate and also has a direct action on the myocardium whereby the force of cardiac contraction is increased. Dosage has to be determined individually, and if too much is given there is nausea, vomiting, undue slowing of the pulse, extrasystoles.

The oedema may be quickly reduced by repeated administration of a diuretic such as one of the thiazide drugs or frusemide.

SYNCOPE

Syncope means transient loss of consciousness due to insufficient blood supply to the brain. The cerebral ischaemia may result from a simple fainting attack, from postural hypotension, from severe blood loss, or from a cardiac disorder such as heart block or myocardial infarction.

Simple fainting attack
This is the commonest form of syncope. The medical term for the condition is a vasovagal attack since it is due to the combined effects

of increased vagal tone which leads to slowing of the heart, and vasodilation, which leads to lowering of the blood pressure; these changes produce cerebral ischaemia.

Fainting attacks may be precipitated by prolonged standing or by some emotional shock which, in susceptible individuals, may be relatively slight. Examples are hearing bad news, witnessing an accident, seeing blood, or going through some form of medical or dental treatment particularly if pain is experienced or anticipated. The individual feels lightheaded, giddy, nauseated, and then loses consciousness. If this happens quickly he may fall to the ground and sustain injury. The skin is cold, pale, and clammy because of the profuse sweating which occurs. The pulse is slow (e.g. 40–50 per minute), weak, and the blood pressure is low. The pupils are dilated and the breathing is shallow. The duration of the attack is commonly a few minutes but it may last up to half an hour or so.

If consciousness is lost the individual should be laid flat on the floor or on a couch since a low position of the head improves cerebral blood flow; should a fainting attack affect a patient in a dental chair the chair should be tilted so that the head is as low as possible. Any tight clothing around the neck should be loosened and it should be ascertained that the airway is patent. Adequate ventilation around the individual should be ensured. Smelling salts may be administered; the sharp stimulus to the nasal mucosa restores the individual to consciousness a little sooner than would otherwise occur. Once consciousness is regained, a cup of tea is usually found to be beneficial. Alcohol should not be administered.

Postural hypotension

Most people have experienced the cerebral effects of postural hypotension in a minor form. A feeling of giddiness or lightheadedness is experienced on suddenly assuming the erect posture after sitting or lying flat for a period of time. In severe cases transient unconsciousness may occur. In the recumbent position blood tends to pool in the abdominal vessels and it is redistributed, by a reflex mechanism, on standing; before the redistribution is complete there may be temporary cerebral ischaemia.

Postural hypotension may be seen in patients who are receiving antihypertensive drugs which produce peripheral vasodilation.

Severe blood loss

It results in the reduction in blood volume leading to oligaemic shock. Consciousness may be lost as a result of cerebral ischaemia but in contrast to vasovagal attacks the pulse is usually rapid in this variety of syncope.

CARDIAC ARREST AND RESUSCITATION

Cardiac arrest describes the situation where there is no spontaneous cardiac output. It can be due to either cardiac standstill (asystole) or ventricular fibrillation. Both have the same presentation, and differentiation between them requires electrocardiography. Cardiac arrest can be due to:

1. Primary cardiac causes such as acute myocardial infarction.
2. Pulmonary embolism.
3. Sensitivity to drugs such as adrenalin or to local and general anaesthetics.
4. Respiratory obstruction due to inhalation of vomitus or the tongue falling back to occlude the airway.

Clinical features
The patient is unconscious, pulseless and cyanosed. To begin with respiration is stertorous but soon spontaneous respiration ceases and the pupils become dilated.

Management
It is essential to establish effective first-aid measures at once since irreversable brain damage due to hypoxia may occur as little as three minutes after cardiac arrest. The following measures are recommended.

1. Summon help. Note the time and summon help immediately. It is possible for one person to undertake mouth-to-mouth breathing and external cardiac massage but it easier when another person is there to help

2. Institute mouth-to-mouth ventilation (Fig. 6.10). Lay the patient down on a flat surface and clear the airway. Extend the neck to open the nasopharynx and help the tongue forward. Pinch the

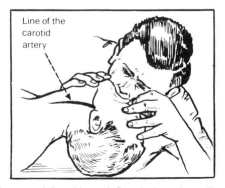

Fig. 6.10 Mouth-to-mouth breathing to inflate the lungs in cardiac arrest.

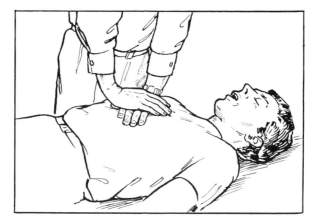

Fig. 6.11 External cardiac compression in management of cardiac arrest.

patient's nostrils shut and blow into the mouth. Make sure that the chest wall moves with the force of expiration. Repeat this 12 times per minute. It is recommended that a simple airway be available in the dental surgery for insertion over the tongue.

3. Initiate external cardiac massage (Fig. 6.11). A vigorous blow on the front of the chest may produce spontaneous cardiac activity. If this is not immediately effective, do not delay starting external cardiac massage. The heels of the hands should be placed on the lower sternum and sharp downward presses administered. These should be sufficiently forceful to depress the sternum by one to one and a half inches. The heart is compressed between sternum and spine and adequate cardiac massage will produce a palpable carotid or femoral artery pulse. External massage should be done approximately 60 times per minute. The ratio of four massages to one ventilation should produce an adequate circulation of oxygenated blood until hospital facilities are available.

PRACTICAL DENTAL CONSIDERATIONS

The following points summarize the main practical considerations which the dentist should bear in mind when dealing with cardiac patients:

1. Patients with cardiac disease should be considered as poor risks for any major surgical procedure. If multiple extractions or removal of a dental cyst or tumour is required prior consultation with a doctor is desirable. Multiple extractions should take place in several stages.

2. A local anaesthetic is usually preferable to a general in these patients but if general anaesthesia is required it should be undertaken by a fully trained anaesthetist.

3. Particular care should be taken to minimize emotional stress prior to any dental procedure and pain during it if the patient has coronary artery disease otherwise angina may be induced. Mild sedation for a day or two before the dental procedure may be helpful in severe cases.

4. In patients with rheumatic or congenital heart disease it is imperative that prophylactic measures be taken to prevent subacute bacterial endocarditis.

5. Rarely a patient with coronary artery disease may present initially as a dental problem because he experiences atypical angina felt only in the jaws and teeth. The relationship of the discomfort to exertion and emotional upset is important.

6. The dentist should be capable of carrying out first aid measures for cardiac arrest (p. 111) and should have in the surgery a simple airway to facilitate mouth-to-mouth respiration.

DISORDERS OF THE PERIPHERAL ARTERIES

Raynaud's disease

This is a disorder of the peripheral circulation which mainly affects young women. A family history is often present. There is paroxysmal vasoconstriction of the digital arteries associated with vasodilatation of the skin capillaries the blood in which is stationary and cyanosed. The fingers, which are cold, may be white for a short period at the beginning of an attack but they quickly become blue. Attacks usually follow exposure to cold or emotional upset. As the vascoconstriction wears off the fingers tingle and throb and regain their normal colour.

Cases of moderate severity are often controlled by avoidance of cold and abstinence from tobacco. Cervical sympathectomy may be of considerable value in severe cases but the effect of surgery does not always last for a long period.

Buerger's disease

This is a disorder of the peripheral circulation mainly affecting young men and always associated with tobacco smoking. It consists of a vasculitis affecting the hands and feet with peripheral ischaemia. Eventually gangrene of the digits results and amputation often becomes necessary; in severe cases the patient may lose a limb or limbs.

Treatment is by abstinence from smoking, by the use of cervical and lumbar sympathectomy in the earlier stages and later by appropriate amputation.

Peripheral arterial sclerosis

Arterial sclerosis of the peripheral vessels, especially those of the legs, is a common feature of elderly people and if marked, causes a decreased blood supply to the tissues hence the term obliterative or occlusive vascular disease. Hypertension, smoking and diabetes mellitus are predisposing factors. Similar changes are frequently present in the arteries of the brain, the heart and the kidneys.

The main complaints are of cold feet plus a cramping discomfort or pain in the calf muscles when walking with relief on rest. The latter symptom is termed intermittent claudication and is a direct result of muscle ischaemia. Examination reveals the feet to be cold and the skin smooth with loss of hair. The peripheral arterial pulses are weak or absent.

In severe cases the impairment of blood supply is sufficient to cause pain in the muscles even when the patient is at rest and especially at night. This condition of night pain at rest is important as it is a sign of impending gangrene which occurs when the blood supply is sufficiently impaired to cause death of tissues. Such gangrene is initially confined to a toe or toes but later the foot or even the leg may become involved. As gangrene sets in pain becomes extremely severe and the affected parts become cold, blue and then finally black. If the limb remains dry when the tissue becomes desiccated and a line of separation develops at the point where the healthy tissues have enough blood supply to maintain viability this condition is known as dry gangrene. However, if infection supervenes then the gangrene tends to spread. This is a dangerous condition known as wet gangrene.

Considerable improvements may occur in the early stages if the patient wears warm footwear, avoids injury and direct contact of the skin with heat. Abstinence from tobacco is important. Vasodilator drugs have been tried but it is extremely doubtful if they have much action on organically narrowed blood vessels.

Lumbar sympathectomy often improves the blood supply of the superficial tissues and is still a very important surgical measure. However, the effect on muscle blood supply is poor and although skin nutrition is frequently improved intermittent claudication is seldom alleviated for long periods.

Sympathectomy may be performed either by injection of the lumbar sympathetic chain with phenol or by surgical methods. Surgical reconstruction of the blood vessels by removal of the diseased core of tissue (disobliteration) or by bypass using autogenous vein or artificial materials is widely used with considerable success in selected cases. Even the aorta and iliac vessel may be replaced by such means.

The carotid artery may be affected by obliterative vascular disease resulting in cerebral effects and sometimes in unilateral blindness. In the early stages such narrowing can also be treated surgically.

Arterial aneurysms

Damage to the wall of the major blood vessels by arteriosclerosis can lead to weakening so that the arterial wall expands to form a saccular or fusiform distension known as aneurysm. This becomes partly filled with thrombus but the area is weak and the end result of such aneurysms is rupture. Large vessels are often involved (for example, the aorta and the iliac vessels) and death is not an infrequent outcome. However, surgical treatment for such aneurysms can be highly successful especially if they are treated before rupture. The aneurysm wall is removed and replaced by a synthetic prosthesis.

VENOUS THROMBOSIS

Superficial thrombophlebitis

In this disorder the superficial veins, particularly of the legs, become inflamed and thrombosed. The affected vein is red, tender, painful and hot. Varicose veins predispose to thrombophlebitis and the condition sometimes follows an infection such as a sore throat. Superficial thrombophlebitis is unpleasant but seldom dangerous.

Treatment consists of rest and the administration of antibiotics if there is an infective basis. Anticoagulants are usually given if the thrombosis is extensive or if extension to the deep veins is suspected.

A frequent cause of superficial thrombophlebitis, particularly in the arms, is the use of intravenous therapy. Treatment is simple and consists of removal of the intravenous infusion at that site.

Deep vein thrombosis

Thrombosis in the veins which lie deep in the calf and thigh muscles, is liable to occur in surgical patients after operation (see Chapter 3), in medical patients on strict bed rest and in obstetric patients after confinement. Details of the presentation of deep vein thrombosis and its management are discussed with postoperative complications (Chapter 3).

Cavernous sinus thrombosis

This is a special variety of venous thrombosis of direct dental interest. It usually arises from spread of infection from the face and the buccal cavity and a dental condition particularly dangerous in this respect is sepsis in the region of the third upper molars. Infection is likely to spread via the pterygoid plexus to the cavernous sinus if some surgical procedure such as extraction is performed when the infection is acute.

In a fully developed case the patient is extremely ill with a swinging temperature, oedema of the eyelids and the conjunctivae, prominence of the eyeballs (exophthalmos), severe headache, vomiting and leucocytosis. The infection and thrombosis may spread to the other intracranial sinuses and veins. Treatment consists of intensive antibiotic therapy plus the administration of anticoagulants.

7

Disorders of the respiratory system

ANATOMICAL AND PHYSIOLOGICAL CONSIDERATIONS

Anatomy

The principal anatomical components of the respiratory system are depicted in Figure 7.1 which is largely self-explanatory. The nose, air sinuses, pharynx, and larynx are usually termed the upper respiratory tract while the lower respiratory tract comprises the trachea, the bronchial tree, and the lung tissue.

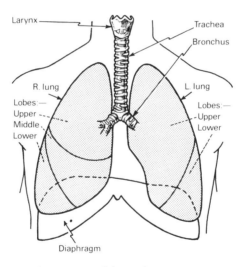

Fig. 7.1 The principal components of the respiratory system.

The trachea can normally be readily palpated in the suprasternal notch in the midline; if deviated it indicates mediastinal displacement. At the level of the second costal cartilage the trachea divides into the right and left main bronchi which soon subdivide into a bronchus for each lung lobe and thereafter subdivide again and again until very small bronchioles, each ending in a cluster of thin-

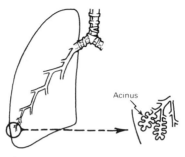

Acinus

Fig. 7.2 The division of the bronchial tree into the terminal air spaces.

walled air spaces or alveoli, are formed (Fig. 7.2). The right lung has three lobes (upper, middle and lower) while the left lung has only two lobes (upper and lower).

The pleura, or covering membrane, of the lungs is in two parts—the visceral pleura which is closely applied to the surface of the lungs, and the parietal pleura which lines the chest wall, diaphragm and mediastinum. Between the two layers is a thin film of fluid.

Chest movements

The lungs are kept expanded in the thoracic cavity by the difference between the positive pressure in the respiratory passages and alveoli (atmospheric pressure) and the negative pressure present between the pleural layers.

During inspiration the chest wall moves outwards and upwards (the ribs are hinged at the vertebrae), the diaphragm moves downwards, the negative pleural pressure increases and, in consequence, the lungs expand further. Expiration is largely a passive process depending on the elastic recoil of the lungs.

The amount of air which can be expired from the lungs by maximum expiration after maximum inspiration (vital capacity) varies from about 3½ to 5½ litres but, under ordinary conditions, only ½ litre is breathed in and out with each respiration; this illustrates the large reserve of respiratory tissue which exists for use in emergency.

Functions of the lungs

The prime function of the lungs is to provide the circulating blood with oxygen and to remove from it carbon dioxide. The alveolar walls, which are only one cell thick, have a very large surface area and they are covered with a rich network of thin-walled capillary blood vessels so that conditions are ideal for the rapid diffusion of oxygen and carbon dioxide. The air which is drawn into the alveoli with each inspiration is rich in oxygen (approximately 20 per cent) and low in carbon dioxide while the expired air contains a lower percentage of oxygen and a higher percentage of carbon dioxide. The respiratory rate rises from the normal level of 16–18 per minute when there is an increased demand for oxygen, as on exertion, or when some of the lung tissue is out of action, e.g. in lobar pneumonia.

The excretion of carbon dioxide by the lungs is an extremely important factor in the control of the acid-base balance of the body. When there is an increase of carbon dioxide (as carbonic acid) in the blood the respiratory centre in the medulla is stimulated and the breathing becomes deeper, quicker, and may have a hissing quality (Kussmaul respiration); this is a characteristic feature of uraemia.

The lungs play a part in the fluid balance of the body. In temperate climates about 500 ml of water are lost from the lungs each day by the process of insensible evaporation.

Defences of the air passages
We inhale many thousand litres of far from sterile air each day and yet only relatively rarely does infection of the respiratory passages or lung tissue arise. This is because the lungs have a very efficient protective mechanism which is constantly on guard.

1. In the nose, air sinuses and nasopharynx, dust particles and microbes are trapped on a sticky 'fly-paper' of ciliated epithelium and are the propelled towards the exterior by the movement of the cilia. The efficiency of this barrier is apparent if we examine the material blown from the nose on a foggy day.

2. A further defence is provided by the larynx, which closes reflexly if it is irritated.

3. The cough reflex, initiated by irritation of the respiratory mucosa, helps to keep the bronchial tree clear.

4. Infected material from the nasopharynx is often swallowed and rendered harmless by the powerful bactericidal activity of the gastric juice.

5. Organisms which penetrate the above defenses do not necessarily cause lung disease as many of them are dealt with by the local defences of the lung (macrophages and polymorphs).

INVESTIGATION OF RESPIRATORY DISORDERS

History
In addition to a full account of the patient's immediate symptoms specific enquiry must always be made regarding cough, spit,

haemoptysis, chest pain, dyspnoea, weight loss, occupation, and family history. The commoner symptoms are discussed in the next section.

Examination

On general examination we should look for cyanosis, dyspnoea, and finger clubbing; no special skill is required for their detection.

Examination of the chest by means of inspection, palpation, percussion and auscultation is a matter for the doctor but perhaps as an illustrative example one may mention the characteristic physical signs of an extensive pleural effusion. On the affected side there is impaired movement, a dull percussion note and absence of breath sounds; the effusion displaces the mediastinal contents to the opposite side shown by deviation of the trachea (felt in the suprasternal notch) and of the apex beat.

Sputum

Examination of the sputum is an important step in investigation of respiratory disorders. The presence of pus or blood is usually obvious on naked-eye examination. A very large volume of purulent sputum should always raise the suspicion of bronchiectasis. Microscopic examination of a stained smear is of value in defining the bacteria present; if tuberculosis is suspected the Ziehl-Neelsen staining technique is employed and several specimens must be examined before a firm negative answer is given. Culture of the organisms present and determination of their sensitivity to antibiotics is a valuable guide to treatment. Cytological examination of the sputum for malignant cells is a very important investigation if bronchogenic neoplasm is suspected.

Radiology

Radiological examination of the lungs is an essential step as it detects many cases of tuberculosis and carcinoma at a stage when clinical examination is quite negative, and it also gives much more precise information than physical examination in following the progress of lesions. Special techniques such as bronchography may be required, e.g. in bronchiectasis.

Bronchoscopy

Direct visualization of the mucosa of the upper part of the bronchial tree through a bronchoscope is of great importance in the diagnosis of bronchogenic carcinoma. A biopsy may be taken at the time of the examination.

COMMON SYMPTOMS AND SIGNS

Epistaxis

The vast majority of nose bleeds results from erosion of the vascular plexus in the anterior nasal septral mucosa. This is usually easily controlled by sustained pressure. However, should the bleeding become persistent or recurrent local electrocautery or chemical cautery under topical anaesthesia may be required.

Bleeding from the posterior part of the nose is much less common and may be more severe and difficult to control. Nasal packing may be necessary if the precise bleeding point cannot be identified and dealt with.

Cough

A cough is a defensive reflex set up by irritation of the mucosa lining the respiratory tract; it protects against the entrance of foreign material into, and expels secretion from, the respiratory tract. The term dry cough is used when no spit is produced and loose, or productive, cough when there is sputum.

Cough is a very common symptom of respiratory disease. A dry, irritating cough occurs in simple upper respiratory tract infections while if there is a more marked inflammatory reaction purulent sputum is produced. The commonest cause of chronic cough in this country is undoubtedly chronic bronchitis; characteristically the cough is worse in winter months. Cough is an important symptom of penumonia and is usually associated with pleuritic chest pain. Pulmonary tuberculosis is seldom forgotten as a cause of cough but it should be remembered that many early cases of the disease have no respiratory symptoms. In bronchiectasis the cough, and associated sputum, is most marked in the morning on rising. Carcinoma of the bronchus is a serious cause of cough in those of middle age and over.

Haemoptysis

Haemoptysis, which means the coughing up of blood from the respiratory tract, is a symptom which usually causes the patient great alarm and leads him to seek medical advice. The blood is commonly frothy and bright red in colour (oxygenated) due to admixture with air but, if the blood is small in amount, the sputum may be rusty in colour as in pneumonia, while if bleeding is copious, clots may be produced. The main causes of haemoptysis are:

   1. Pulmonary tuberculosis either in the early exudative stages,

or in the late stages due to erosion of a blood vessel in a cavity.

2. Lobar pneumonia—characteristic rusty sputum.
3. Bronchial carcinoma.
4. Bronchiectasis.
5. Pulmonary infarction, e.g. from peripheral vein thrombosis.
6. Heart disease
   a. mitral stenosis where the haemoptysis is due to pulmonary hypertension;
   b. acute left ventricular failure.
7. Haemorrhagic disorders.

Dyspnoea

Dyspnoea, which is more fully discussed in the chapter on cardiac disorders (p. 84) may arise from any pulmonary disorder which is extensive enough to cause impaired oxygenation of the blood passing through the lungs. Common examples are chronic bronchitis and emphysema, pneumonia, asthma, lung collapse, and pleural effusion.

Chest pain

The pain associated with cardiac disease has already been described (p. 85). Pain arises from respiratory disorders when the pleura is involved, as for example over an area of pneumonia, or if there is pressure on bony structures by tumour growth. Pleuritic pain is characteristically increased by coughing or deep breathing.

Hoarseness

The main causes of hoarseness of the voice are:

1. Laryngitis secondary to the common cold.
2. Chronic laryngitis due to excessive smoking or excessive shouting (e.g. newsvendors).
3. Tuberculous laryngitis—this is always secondary to pulmonary tuberculosis.
4. Syphilitic laryngitis—now rarely seen.
5. Neoplasm of the vocal cords, either papilloma or carcinoma.
6. Paralysis of the recurrent laryngeal nerve which supplies all the intrinsic muscles of the larynx with the exception of the cricothyroid.

On the right side the nerve arises from the vagus in the root of the neck but on the left it arises from the vagus in the upper part of the thorax and is closely related to the arch of the aorta and the left main bronchus in its ascent to the larynx. The left recurrent laryngeal may be compressed in the mediastinum by secondary carcinomatous lymph nodes or aortic aneurysm, while either nerve may be compressed at the root of the neck by enlarged lymph nodes or suffer damage at thyroidectomy.

7. Myxoedema causes hoarseness and should always be borne in mind when there is no apparent local cause.

Cyanosis
Cyanosis is dealt with in the section on cardiac disorders (p. 87); it may result from any pulmonary condition which interferes sufficiently with oxygenation of the blood.

Finger clubbing
The term finger clubbing is used to describe an enlargement of the ends of the finger which occurs in certain disease processes. A typical example of finger clubbing is shown in Fig. 7.3. The first change is an increase in the soft tissues of the nail bed so that the angle between the base of the nail and the skin is lost. Later there is a diffuse increase in the soft tissues of the finger end which becomes thickened both anteroposteriorly and laterally. The precise mechanism of finger clubbing is not fully understood, but the main factor is probably alteration in the oxygenation of the peripheral tissues. In marked cases the toes may also be involved.

1. *Pulmonary causes.* Suppuration in the lungs as in cases of bronchiectasis, lung abscess, and empyema usually produces finger

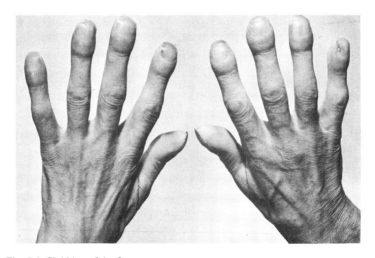

Fig. 7.3 Clubbing of the fingers.

clubbing which may be of a marked degree. Carcinoma of the lung is an increasingly important cause.

2. Cardiac causes. The cyanotic group of congenital heart disease is associated with finger clubbing which is often marked. Subacute bacterial endocarditis often causes finger clubbing, but the degree is usually slight.

3. Cirrhosis of the liver is a less common cause of finger clubbing.

Halitosis

The causes of halitosis, or foul breath, may conveniently be described in four main groups.

1. Sepsis or putrefaction in mouth and nasal sinuses. The dentist will encounter many examples of halitosis due to carious teeth, pyorrhoea, sepsis under crowns, etc. Other causes to be mentioned include Vincent's infection, septic tonsillar infection, neoplasm of nasal sinuses or nasopharynx, and syphilitic or tuberculous ulceration. Careful local examination will usually yield the diagnosis in these cases.

2. Sepsis or putrefaction in lungs. The most important causes are lung abscess, bronchiectasis, and tuberculous cavitation with secondary infection. In most of these cases the patient will give a history of cough and spit and examination of the fingers may show clubbing.

3. Drugs and foods. Excess tobacco smoking is a well-known cause of halitosis while onions and garlic are notorious for their effect on the breath. Paraldehyde is a drug which is used as a hypnotic in restless patients and its excretion in the breath gives a characteristic odour which may be smelt at some distance.

4. Other causes. In advanced renal failure the breath may have an unpleasant ammoniacal odour. In many alimentary disorders, ranging from simple gastric upsets to conditions like typhoid fever or peritonitis, the breath becomes foul.

Chest shapes

The principal medical terms for the common abnormalities of chest shape are as follows.

Kyphosis is the term used to describe increased curvature of the spine in the anteroposterior direction. This is seen commonly in the thoracic region giving rise to a hump-back. It occurs, in slight degree, as a more or less normal feature of ageing. It is seen in many cases of chronic bronchitis and emphysema. In some instances it is due to disease of the vertebrae, most often tuberculosis; this is the usual cause in severe hunch-back deformity.

Scoliosis signifies lateral curvature of the spine. Slight degrees are not uncommon and are usually due to faulty posture and development in childhood. Poliomyelitis may cause scoliosis if the vertebral muscles are unequally involved. Severe unilateral lung disease (e.g. tuberculosis, empyema) is an important cause of thoracic scoliosis. Unilateral hip joint disease frequently leads to lumbar scoliosis.

The term *barrel chest* is used where the anteroposterior diameter is greatly increased; there is increased curvature of the thoracic spine, the ribs are held more horizontally, and the sternum is usually more prominent (Fig. 7.4). Barrel chest is seen in some cases of chronic bronchitis and emphysema but its association with this form of lung disease is by no means constant. In chronic asthmatics barrel chest may develop but again the relationship is not constant. It is sometimes present in people with apparently healthy lungs.

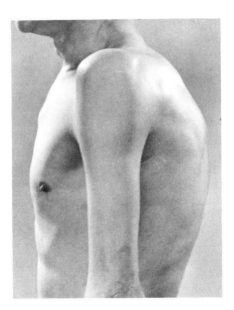

Fig. 7.4 Barrel-shaped chest.

CORYZA

Coryza, or the common cold, is an extremely frequent infection particularly in the winter months. The virus responsible has a high infectivity and, unfortunately, the immunity resulting from an attack is short lived. The incubation period is short, in the majority of cases being two to three days.

Clinical features
These are so well known from personal experience that a description is hardly necessary. The individual has symptoms of a mild or moderate toxaemia which is followed by catarrhal inflammation of the nasal passages, i.e. rhinitis.

Treatment
No specific treatment is available. Rest, warmth, hot drinks and aspirin usually alleviate symptoms but it is doubtful if they shorten the course of the illness. Instillation of nasal drops containing a vasoconstrictor substance such as ephedrine may be employed to relieve nasal congestion.

Complications
Complications of the common cold are very frequent and are due to secondary bacterial infection, e.g. with staphylococci, streptococci, pneumococci and *Haemophilus influenzae*. There is an increase of general malaise, commonly with mild or moderate fever, and symptoms are indicated below.

1. Sinusitis—frontal headache or a dull ache over the maxillary sinus. In a severe case of maxillary or frontal sinusitis appropriate irrigation may be necessary in addition to antibiotic therapy.

2. Pharyngitis—sore throat, dry irritating cough.

3. Laryngitis—sore throat, hoarse voice and cough.

4. Tracheitis—soreness or rawness behind the upper sternum increased by cough.

5. Bronchitis—cough and purulent sputum.

6. Bronchopneumonia—see details below.

7. Otitis media—Eustachian tube catarrh leads to deafness and when the middle ear is involved there is in addition, pain in the ear.

Acute otitis media is almost exclusively a problem of childhood. It is often associated with infected lymphoid tissue of the nasopharynx and adenoid hypertrophy. This may be associated with nasal obstruction and mouth breathing. Adenoidectomy may minimise nasal difficulty and reduce the chances of chronic infection.

The most common bacteria involved in otitis media are streptococcus pneumonia and haemophilus influenzae. Symptoms consist of early stuffiness of the ear followed by severe pain. If the tympanic membrane ruptures a serous or purulent discharge may present at the external ear. Treatment consists of systemic antibiotics continued for at least 10 days. If the infection does not respond readily an alternative drug (one of the broader spectrum antibiotics) should be substituted. Nasal and auditory tube decongestants in the form of nose drops or sprays may help. When the pain is especially severe and associated with bulging of the tympanic membrane, then incision of the tympanic membrane (myringotomy) should be considered. This gives immediate and dramatic relief of pain.

Complications of acute suppurative otitis media are meningitis, facial paralysis, mastoiditis and subdural or brain abscess.

Chronic otitis media characterised by persistent perforation of the tympanic membrane may necessitate mastoidectomy.

INFLUENZA

Aetiology
Three related viruses, termed A, B and C, may cause influenza. Virus A is responsible for most of the epidemics, virus B tends to cause more limited outbreaks, while infection with virus C is rare. If the infection becomes particularly widespread the term pandemic is used—in the great pandemic of 1918–19 it is estimated that approximately twenty million people died, the majority of them from secondary bacterial pneumonia.

Clinical features
The incubation period is short, in most cases being one to three days. Unfortunately the immunity after the attack lasts only a few months so that it has usually disappeared before the next mild epidemic occurs.

The onset is abrupt with headache, aches and pains in the limbs and in the trunk, sweating, fever, and often vomiting. There is usually an associated catarrhal inflammation of the upper respiratory passages.

In most cases recovery takes place after a few days. In some, secondary bacterial infection leads to bronchitis or bronchopneumonia while in others, fortunately a minority of those infected, the illness takes an extremely rapid and fatal course.

Treatment
Bed rest, warmth, hot drinks and aspirin are sufficient to control symptoms in the majority of cases while the disease runs its course. Antibiotics should be given in full dosage if there is suspicion of secondary bacterial infection especially in the old, the very young,

or the frail. Influenza virus vaccines, which give relatively short-lived protection, may be given annually or at times of epidemics.

ACUTE BRONCHITIS

Aetiology
Acute bronchitis is most often the sequel to a severe or neglected attack of the common cold; the common bacterial invaders are streptococci and pneumococci.

It should be remembered that when a child has an attack of what appears to be acute bronchitis he may be in the prodromal stages of one of the common infectious diseases such as measles or whooping cough.

Pathology
The bronchial mucosa is red and congested and covered with an exudate which is first thin and later purulent.

Clinical features
There is evidence of the constitutional upset which is usually associated with any bacterial infection—malaise, shivering, sweating, fever, tachycardia, and leucocytosis. The respiratory symptoms comprise cough and spit. The spit may be small in amount at first but later becomes purulent. Auscultation of the chest reveals abnormal sounds (rhonchi) produced by the secretion in the bronchi.

Prognosis
The prognosis is very good in otherwise healthy people but in infancy, old age, and in association with other illnesses, acute bronchitis can be a serious problem and may be followed by bronchopneumonia.

Treatment
The general measures used for the treatment of an infection, namely rest, warmth, and a light diet, are employed. Antibiotics are usually reserved for severe infections or at the extremes of life.

CHRONIC BRONCHITIS

Aetiology
Chronic bronchitis is an extremely common condition in this country, especially in industrial districts. The most important aetiol-

ogical factors are the contamination of the atmosphere in large towns with products from open fires and industrial processes ('smog'), the prevalence of cigarette smoking, and the unfavourable atmospheric conditions associated with certain occupations such as foundry workers and miners. Other factors that may be of importance in individual cases are faulty chest development, chronic foci of infection in the sinuses, and damage to the bronchial passages from repeated attacks of acute bronchitis. In many cases there is a combination of predisposing factors, e.g. a dusty occupation, excess cigarette smoking, and residence in an area where 'smog' is or has been common.

Clinical features

The individual has a history of chronic cough and spit which is characteristically worse in the winter months when atmospheric conditions deteriorate. The spit may be relatively clear at times but is purulent when exacerbations of the bronchitis occur. Breathlessness on exertion occurs and may be very marked. In the majority of cases emphysema develops and this may be followed by right heart failure. There may be attacks of asthma superimposed particularly when the bronchitis undergoes an acute exacerbation.

Finger clubbing is not usually present unless there is a marked degree of suppuration in the bronchial tree; in such instances one should consider the presence of underlying bronchiectasis.

Treatment

In the majority of cases it is impossible to produce a cure but treatment may lead to considerable improvement. The principal measures are:

1. Reduction in cigarette consumption.

2. Antibiotic therapy when there is active infection present and, in some cases, over the winter months.

3. Instruction in breathing exercises.

4. Change of occupation if this is an aetiological factor.

The public have a great faith in cough mixtures but it is certain that many of them have little action other than a psychological one. A sedative cough mixture such as syrup of codeine phosphate is useful at night, however, while if there is bronchospasm this may be relieved by a bronchodilator.

Patients suffering from chronic bronchitis tolerate anaesthesia badly and have a marked tendency to develop a postoperative bronchopneumonia. Patients should where possible be stopped from smoking for at least one week before operation and it has been shown that prophylactic antibiotics reduce the incidence of postoperative chest infection, especially for operations in the upper abdomen and involving the chest wall.

CHRONIC SINUSITIS

Recurrent or chronic attacks of sinusitis despite adequate antibiotic therapy should suggest some underlying disease such as dental infection, scarring from previous trauma with inadequate drainage or perhaps diabetes. Medical or surgical attention to these underlying problems is essential in order to eliminate secondary infection.

The condition is important to the dentist and indeed pain in maxillary teeth with tenderness to percussion is not infrequent. Furthermore, the condition may be associated with meningitis, orbital cellulitis and abscess, or even with brain abscess. Surgical drainage procedures may be necessary as part of the treatment.

EMPHYSEMA

Emphysema is most commonly seen as a sequel to chronic bronchitis. Prolonged overdistension of the alveoli by the strain of repeated coughing leads to weakening and rupture of the alveolar walls with the formation of larger air-containing spaces or bullae. The lungs occupy a greater volume and usually cover the anterior surface of the heart. Emphysema has two important effects:

1. There is a reduction in the total alveolar surface available for gaseous exchange so that there is impaired oxygenation of the blood and a tendency to carbon dioxide retention.

2. There is interference with the blood flow through the lungs leading to hypertrophy of the right ventricle.

Clinical features
Breathlessness on exertion is the dominant symptom. Physical examination is a notoriously poor guide to the presence of emphysema and it is now appreciated that the erstwhile textbook picture of a barrel-chested individual with increased resonance on percussion is by no means constant. Poor chest expansion is almost always present and the vital capacity is reduced. Cyanosis may be evident.

Chest X-ray usually shows the increased volume and increased translucency of the lungs.

If right heart failure supervenes, dyspnoea and cyanosis are intensified and oedema, hepatic engorgement, etc., develop.

Treatment

The measures outlined for chronic bronchitis are required in the majority of cases. Digoxin and diuretics are used when cardiac failure develops.

LOBAR PNEUMONIA

Lobar pneumonia usually attacks young, previously healthy adults. The incubation period is short, often two to three days. The organism responsible is most frequently the pneumococcus.

Pathology

As the name indicates, there is inflammation of part or all of a lobe or lobes of a lung. In the earliest stages the principal change is intense engorgement of the lung tissue which still contains air, but this is soon followed by the infected alveoli becoming packed with oedema fluid and cells and thus the lung tissue becomes airless or consolidated. Red cells predominate initially (the stage of red hepatization), and leucocytes and phagocytes later (the stage of grey hepatization). During the stage of resolution the alveolar contents are liquefied by proteolytic enzymes and debris is removed by phagocytosis and by coughing.

Clinical picture

There is a sudden onset often with a rigor. The temperature rises quickly and may reach 40°C (104°F) or higher. The individual is breathless and has pain over the affected lobe due to involvement of the overlying pleura; the pain is increased by deep breathing or coughing and, in consequence, he takes quick, shallow breaths and tends to place the hand over the affected area when coughing. The cough produces sputum which is tenacious, small in amount at first, and tinged with blood giving it a rusty colour. The pulse is rapid, cyanosis is present, and there is a leucocytosis. Herpes labialis is often a feature.

The doctor can detect the consolidated lobe by percussion and ausculation. X-ray of the chest confirms the diagnosis.

Course and prognosis

Before antibiotics were produced the course of the illness was determined by a battle between the infecting organism on the one hand and the patient's resistance on the other. The usual picture was of a very severe illness with a high fever for five to seven days, at the end of which time there was, in favourable cases, a rapid drop in temperature and a lessening of dyspnoea and other symptoms; this was termed the crisis. The aim of treatment was to sustain the patient's strength until by the production of antibodies he had overcome the infection.

The organisms were not always overcome in this favourable manner and peripheral circulatory failure (often fatal), spread of infection to the pleural cavity with suppuration (empyema), and lung abscess were important complications.

Treatment
Antibiotic treatment should be instituted promptly. Penicillin is the drug of choice in the majority of cases, but if the organisms are resistant other antibiotics will be required. Some guidance may be obtained from bacteriological examination of the sputum. Oxygen may be required initially. Pleuritic chest pain may require to be relieved by an analgesic.

Bronchopneumonia

Pathology and bacteriology
Bronchopneumonia, or lobular pneumonia, is characterized by a patchy infection of many lobules of lung tissue usually scattered through more than one lobe. The lung bases are most often involved. Normal, or relatively normal, areas of lung are seen between the airless, consolidated areas.

Bronchopneumonia is due to a descending infection from the upper respiratory passages by organisms which are often found normally in the respiratory tract, e.g. staphylococci, streptococci, *Haemophilus influenzae*, and pneumococci (group 4). It occurs as a complication of acute bronchitis, especially at the extremes of life, in measles, whooping cough, severe influenza, or following inhalation of infected material into the respiratory passages. Importantly, bronchopneumonia occurs as a complication following anaesthesia and operations and especially if there have been collapsed areas of lung (atelectasis).

Clinical features
There is usually evidence of the predisposing cause. The symptoms and signs of any bacterial infection develop namely malaise, fever, tachycardia and leucocytosis. Dyspnoea and cyanosis are present and may be of alarming degree in the infant. Cough and purulent spit may not be as prominent as in lobar pneumonia and this is particularly the case in young children who tend to swallow what

sputum is produced. Discomfort or actual pain in the chest, worse on breathing or coughing, may be experienced but again it is not usually as marked as in lobar pneumonia.

The areas involved are revealed by the presence of crepitations; dullness on percussion is less striking than in lobar pneumonia.

Course and prognosis

As in the case of lobar pneumonia the prognosis has been immeasurably improved by the use of antibiotics but bronchopneumonia is still a serious condition at the extremes of life and in the frail.

Treatment

The measures described for lobar pneumonia apply. In inhalation bronchopneumonia the inhaled material may have to be sucked out. Following operation the patient may be unable to cough effectively, so that to assist in clearing secretions tracheostomy (p. 46) with assisted ventilation and suction toilet of the bronchial tree may be necessary.

Hypostatic pneumonia

This is the term given to the pneumonic change which occurs in the congested and oedematous lung bases of the bed-ridden individual in whom it is a common terminal event.

LUNG COLLAPSE

Collapse of a lung, or a portion of a lung, most frequently results from obstruction of the related bronchus. The air in the portion of lung supplied by the bronchus becomes absorbed and the lung becomes much reduced in volume or collapsed; this is often termed absorption collapse. Bronchial obstruction may result from:

1. Inhalation of a foreign body. The dentist is particularly concerned with the possible inhalation of blood clot or portions of teeth in the anaesthetized patient. Children may inhale coins or other small objects placed in the mouth. If vomiting occurs in an unconscious patient there is considerable danger of the vomitus being inhaled into the respiratory passages.

2. Bronchogenic carcinoma.

3. External pressure on bronchus, e.g. by enlarged tuberculous or neoplastic lymph nodes.

4. Postoperative collapse due to blockage of a bronchus by tenacious mucus or secretions.

Of these various causes the most important from a dental viewpoint is, of course, inhalation of foreign bodies, and the remarks which follow apply to this variety of lung collapse.

Clinical features
Following the inhalation of a foreign body into the lungs there is sudden breathlessness and cyanosis. Absorption collapse occurs distal to the site where the bronchus is obstructed. The affected lung is smaller in volume and there is a compensatory shift of the mediastinum to that side; clinically this may be detected by noting alteration in the position of the trachea and the apex beat. The doctor will be able to detect dullness on percussion and reduced breath sounds over the affected area. Infection is likely to supervene (Figs. 3.1 and 3.2).

The inhalation of infected blood from a tooth socket or other operation site in the mouth or throat is more likely to result in a patchy bronchopneumonia rather than lung collapse.

The principal complications which may later develop as a consequence of inhalation of foreign material in the respiratory tract are lung abscess and bronchiectasis (Fig. 7.5).

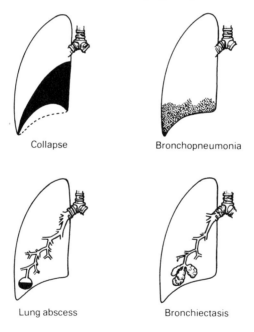

Collapse   Bronchopneumonia

Lung abscess   Bronchiectasis

Fig. 7.5 The complications which may follow inhalation of foreign material into the respiratory passages.

Treatment
Prophylaxis is extremely important. During any operation in the mouth or throat, precautions must be taken to guard against the possible entry of blood clot, etc., into the respiratory passages and this is particularly important in the anaesthetized patient. If a foreign body is inhaled then it is worth while, as a first-aid measure, leaning the patient forward and thumping him firmly on the back in the hope that this, plus coughing, will lead to the foreign body being dislodged. If this is not successful, or if there is any anxiety that there is any residual material in the lungs, then medical advice should be sought immediately; bronchoscopic removal of the material is indicated in view of the complications outlined above.

LUNG ABSCESS

Aetiology
Lung abscess is a less common occurrence since the introduction of antibiotics but it may still be seen in the following circumstances.

1. Inhalation of infected material into the bronchial passages after operations on the mouth and throat conducted under general anaesthesia unless proper care has been taken.
2. Sepsis distal to obstruction of the bronchus by carcinoma.
3. The sequel to a severe pneumonia caused by antibiotic-resistant organisms.

Pathology
The organisms responsible are most commonly streptococci, staphylococci, and pneumococci. The abscess cavity is filled with pus, has fibrous tissue walls which, in chronic cases, may be very thick, and is surrounded by a zone of lung inflammation. If the abscess is near the surface of the lung there is likely to be a pleural reaction with pleural effusion and possible empyema.

Clinical features
A history suggesting an aetiological factor is usually obtained. A swinging temperature, sweats, rigors, tachycardia, and leucocytosis indicate the presence of sepsis. Finger clubbing occurs. A cough and purulent sputum are present if the abscess is in communication with a bronchus. The signs in the chest are usually those of consolidation or effusion. It may be possible to see a fluid level in the abscess cavity on X-ray film.

Treatment
Prevention is important as emphasized in the preceding section of lung collapse. This is particularly so following inhalation of infected material into the respiratory passages. Bronchial obstruction due to carcinoma cannot always be relieved. Antibiotics are given preferably after determination of the sensitivity of the infecting organism. Drainage of the abscess cavity via the chest wall is sometimes necessary and if there is empyema then surgical drainage is mandatory.

BRONCHIECTASIS

Aetiology
In clinical practice there are two main types of onset. The commoner variety is that which dates from a severe childhood attack of measles or whooping cough complicated by bronchopneumonia and bronchial obstruction due to viscid plugs of mucus. The other variety, which is of direct dental interest, is that following bronchial obstruction by an inhaled foreign body. In both instances the bronchiectasis results from the combined effects of bronchial obstruction and infection. Obstruction leads to absorption collapse with outward tension on the bronchial walls while the infection weakens the walls.

Pathology
There is a dilation, which may be either saccular or cylindrical, of the terminal portions of the bronchi especially at the lung bases. Chronic sepsis develops in these dilated portions and may spread to adjacent lung tissue or even to distant parts via the blood stream, e.g. to produce brain abscess.

Clinical features
Cough and spit, worse in the mornings, are the dominant symptoms. The sputum is copious, purulent and sometimes blood-streaked. Halitosis is common and the dentist is likely to be made unpleasantly aware of this sign if he has a bronchiectatic patient. Clubbing of the fingers is a typical feature. If the degree of suppuration in the chest is marked then the general health will suffer and the individual is likely to be underweight and have a poor appetite.

On auscultation of the chest the doctor may be able to hear adventitious sounds at the lung bases. Confirmation of the diagnosis is usually obtained by means of a bronchogram. This comprises an

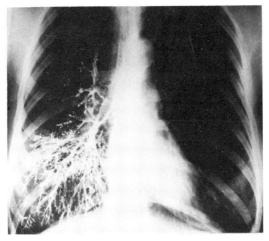

Fig. 7.6 Normal right lower lobe bronchogram.

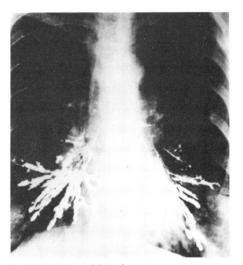

Fig. 7.7 Bilateral cylindrical bronchiectasis.

X-ray picture of the bronchial tree after it has been delineated by a radio-opaque material (Figs. 7.6, 7.7 and 7.8). The bronchiectatic areas are sometimes likened to a bunch of grapes.

Prognosis
The prognosis has been much improved by antibiotics. The infection can be more readily controlled so that the dangers of secondary pneumonia or metastatic abscess are lessened.

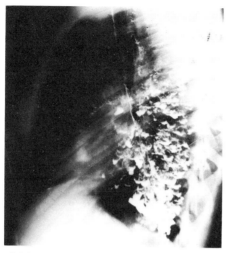

Fig. 7.8 Saccular left lower lobe bronchiectasis (lateral view).

Treatment

This may be either medical or surgical. The aim of medical treatment is to keep the dilated portions empty and free from infection
by the use of postural drainage and antibiotics. Successful postural
drainage necessitates careful localization of the affected areas so
that the optimum position for drainage may be adopted. The procedure must be carried out regularly.

Surgical treatment is possible only where the bronchiectasis is
localized to one lung and preferably to one lobe of that lung. In
such cases lobectomy may give a permanent cure.

MALIGNANCY OF THE RESPIRATORY SYSTEM

Laryngeal neoplasms

Cancer of the larynx is much more common in people who smoke
and drink heavily. As in the mouth, such neoplasms may arise
from areas of leukoplakia. Squamous cell carcinoma is the most
common tumour of the larynx. It has significantly different clinical
behaviour in different locations. Vocal cord cancers have a favourable prognosis because early presentation with hoarseness leads to
early detection and therapy. In addition the vocal cord is especially
devoid of lymphoid tissue and drainage and therefore cervical
spread does not generally occur early. Irradiation therapy is the
treatment of choice for early vocal cord cancer.

Cancer of the supraglottic and subglottic larynx on the other hand tends to metastasise early to the cervical lymph nodes because of the rich lymphatic drainage. Clinical presentation is generally later than in a case of vocal cord tumour. The most common early symptom is pain, particularly on swallowing with referred pain to the ear. Palpable lymph node metastases may also be one of the presenting signs. Since these tumours are generally more advanced when first detected, they are usually best treated with combination surgery and X-ray treatment.

Carcinoma of the maxillary antrum

A cancer may arise from the lining of the maxillary antrum. This may present as sinusitis, as unilateral facial swelling or may present with erosion into the oral cavity presenting with loosening of the upper teeth, or of a previously well fitting denture. The diagnosis is confirmed by appropriate biopsy. Treatment is by a combination of surgery which involves complete maxillectomy and radiotherapy. The resultant defect must be repaired and the dentist is often required to fix an appropriate obturator.

Bronchogenic carcinoma

Bronchogenic carcinoma is now probably the commonest variety of malignant tumour seen in the medical wards of hospitals. This is partly because of better diagnosis and partly because of a real increase in the incidence of the disorder (Fig. 1.1). It is seen more frequently in men and the majority of cases occur over the age of 40 years.

Aetiology

The basic cause of cancer remains unknown, but in the case of bronchogenic carcinoma there now appears to be incontrovertible evidence that a heavy cigarette consumption is associated with an increased incidence. Men who regularly smoke over 20 cigarettes a day are over 20 times more liable to develop carcinoma of the bronchus than non-smokers. Pipe smoking or cigar smoking is much less harmful in this respect. Atmospheric pollution may be an additional aetiological factor in large towns.

Pathology

The growth starts in the wall of a bronchus usually near the lung hilum although a few are peripheral and a few apical. There are three histological types—the round cell tumour which is most malignant, the columnar cell adenocarcinoma which is intermediate in malignancy, and squamous cell adenocarcinoma which has the slowest rate of growth.

The tumour spreads to the lymphatic glands in the mediastinum and neck, to the pleura, and by the blood stream to bones, brain and liver.

Clinical features

Bronchogenic carcinoma may present in many ways and a high level of clinical skill is necessary if the diagnosis is to be made at a time when surgical treatment is possible. Cough and haemoptysis may occur early or late; their presence is always an indication for a detailed examination of the lungs. When the growth is large enough to cause bronchial obstruction infection in the retained secretions distal to the block is likely to occur and the patient may develop a febrile illness which is taken for pneumonia; only when the 'pneumonia' does not clear up may the underlying neoplasm be suspected. Spread of the tumour to the pleura results in chest pain, which is worse on breathing, and a blood-stained pleural effusion develops. Spread of the growth to the glands in the mediastinum is likely to produce congestion of the neck veins, fullness of the neck, and hoarseness due to pressure on the recurrent largyngeal nerve. In some patients the first indication of the presence of the tumour is symptoms arising from secondary deposits in the bones, brain, or liver. Loss of appetite, energy, and weight, which are features common to the cachexia of any malignant neoplasm, may occur before, or along with, any of the above symptoms.

Diagnosis

It is important that the doctor thinks of bronchogenic carcinoma if an adult presents with any of the symptoms or signs mentioned above. Chest X-ray is a very important aid to diagnosis while bronchoscopy is a further valuable step as it enables visualization of the tumour and biopsy.

Treatment

The only curative treatment possible is surgical removal of the growth by lobectomy or pneumonectomy but, unfortunately, this is not a feasible step in the great majority of patients as, by the time symptoms bring them for medical attention, the condition is too far advanced. Deep X-ray therapy may slow the progress of the disorder and relieve, to some extent, troublesome symptoms. Morphia is the most useful drug in the latter stages of the disease.

Other tumours of the respiratory system

Adenoma of the bronchus is an infrequent cause of cough and haemoptysis. Bronchoscopy and biopsy are required in diagnosis.

Secondary deposits in the lung occur commonly; the most important primary sites are the breast, the alimentary tract, bones, the prostate, and the kidney.

LUNG DISEASE DUE TO DUST

Those lung diseases which are caused by the inhalation of dust are known collectively as the pneumoconioses. There are many varieties, but *silicosis* will be taken as an illustrative example.

Aetiology

The disease is due to the inhalation over long periods of fine particles of silica; this is an occupational hazard of miners, stone masons, sand blasters, etc. The tiny particles of silica pass to the alveoli, where they are taken up by macrophages and deposited in lymph nodes throughout the lungs. The silica slowly goes into solution and sets up an irritative fibrotic reaction.

Clinical features

The individual will give a history of having been in an occupation involving exposure to silica dust for many years. A latent period of several years is usually present before symptoms arise. The main symptoms are cough, spit, and dyspnoea which is progressive and eventually incapacitating. The diagnosis may be confirmed by chest X-ray.

Complications

Patients with silicosis have a greatly increased liability to develop pulmonary tuberculosis. The other main complication is right heart failure secondary to the fibrotic changes in the lungs.

Treatment

There is no curative treatment for the condition and preventive measures are all-important. The dust in the atmosphere should be kept down as far as possible by various mechanical means, and if this is not sufficient respirators should be worn. Those at risk should be examined at regular intervals and at the earliest sign of the disease should be removed from that occupation. Silicosis is one of the diseases covered by the Workmen's Compensation Act.

PNEUMOTHORAX

Aetiology
Pneumothorax, which means air in the pleural space, may be due
to a penetrating wound of the chest wall, rupture of a tuberculous
focus near the surface of a lung, escape of air through a weakened
portion of the visceral pleura (the spontaneous variety), or it may
be induced as a therapeutic measure in tuberculosis.

Features of spontaneous pneumothorax
The patient is usually a young adult who suddenly develops pain in
the affected side of the chest and becomes breathless and cyanosed.
Examination shows that the mediastinum is shifted to the opposite
side and the percussion note on the affected side is more resonant
than usual (Fig. 7.9). Chest X-ray shows the air-containing pleural
space and the collapsed lung.

In most cases there is no continued leak, the air in the pleural
cavity is absorbed in two or three weeks, and the lung re-expands.
All that is required is sedation to relieve the initial pain and a
period of rest. In the valvular type air passes into the pleural cavity
with inspiration but none escapes during expiration; in such cases
the tension in the chest must be relieved via a needle passed
through an intercostal space. The pneumothorax which follows
penetrating wounds is often accompanied by bleeding into the
pleural cavity (haemo-pneumothorax). There is frequently a valvular mechanism with a build-up of air in the pleural cavity (tension
pneumothorax). In such cases the air must be relieved by the passage of one or more large intercostal drains connected to an under-
water drainage system and suction may be necessary to keep the

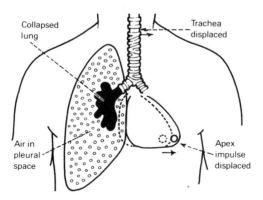

Fig. 7.9 The changes in a right sided pneumothorax.

lung expanded. Continuing leakage of air or bleeding may necessitate operation on the chest (thoracotomy) to seal the air leak and control bleeding.

In some cases of pneumothorax air may escape from a punctured lung via the pleural cavity into the muscle planes and subcutaneous tissues (surgical emphysema). This is usually a harmless condition and is diagnosed by a subcutaneous crackling on palpation. Occasionally large quantities of air escape and track upwards into the neck where they may cause respiratory embarrassment.

PLEURISY

Aetiology

The principal causes of pleurisy and pleural effusion are as follows:

1. Tuberculosis, either as a reaction to the primary infection, or secondary to well-established tuberculosis of the lungs.

2. Other lung infections, especially pneumonia.

3. Bronchogenic carcinoma or secondary tumour deposits in the lungs.

Pathology

The term 'dry pleurisy' is often used to describe the early stages when the pleura is inflamed but there is little in the way of exudate. When fluid accumulates in the pleural cavity we use the terms wet pleurisy or pleural effusion.

The nature of the effusion varies with the cause. In the primary tuberculous variety it is straw coloured, contains lymphocytes, is sterile on culture, and tubercle bacilli are usually demonstrable only after guinea-pig inoculation; in pleurisy following pneumonia pus cells are present in the fluid and one may have all stages from a slightly hazy fluid to a frank empyema; pleural effusion due to carcinoma is usually blood stained.

Clinical features

Pleuritic chest pain, which is characteristically sharp and increased by breathing or coughing, is most likely to be present before effusion develops. At this stage also the doctor may hear with the stethoscope pleural friction caused by the movement of the inflamed pleural layers. Breathlessness becomes progressively more marked as fluid accumulates in the pleural cavity. The effusion produces impaired movement, dullness of percussion note, impaired or absent breath sounds on the affected side, and a shift of

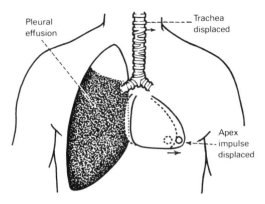

Fig. 7.10 The changes in a right sided pleural effusion

the mediastinum to the opposite side (Fig. 7.10). Chest X-ray shows an opacity due to the fluid.

It is relatively simple matter to remove the fluid, either for diagnostic purposes or for relief of breathlessness, through a hollow needle passed under local anaesthesia through an intercostal space. Treatment depends upon the basic cause.

EMPYEMA

The term empyema is employed where there is pus formation in the pleural cavity. It used to be a relatively complication of severe pneumonia or lung abscess but is now uncommon.

The patient shows all the features of a severe bacterial infection with a swinging temperature, rigors, leucocytosis, etc., while examination of the chest shows evidence of fluid in the pleural cavity. Diagnosis is confirmed by paracentesis of the chest.

The main points in treatment are the intensive use of antibiotics and the aspiration of pus from the pleural cavity. Formal surgical drainage with a removal of a rib to gain access may be necessary.

SMOKING AND HEALTH

The annual Report of the Chief Medical Officer of the Ministry of Health for the year 1967 contains the following statement: '. . . the abolition of cigarette smoking would be the greatest single contribution to the improvement of the public health still open to us'.

The principal reasons for such a view may be summarized as follows:

1. Deaths from cancer of the lung continue to increase and there

is a greatly increased incidence in those who are heavy cigarette smokers.

2. Chronic bronchitis is a widespread condition, with a considerable morbidity and significant mortality, and it is very much more common in heavy cigarette smokers.

3. Morbidity and mortality from coronary heart disease and from peripheral vascular disease (e.g. of the lower limb) continue to rise and are greater in the heavy cigarette smoker.

In addition to these major causes of morbidity and mortality it should be remembered that the heavy cigarette smoker is usually a greater anaesthetic risk.

Abolition of cigarettes appears an impracticable dream but health education in regard to the hazards of cigarette smoking should nevertheless be pursued. Young people should be advised to stop, to reduce, or to change to a pipe or cigars.

8

Disorders of the alimentary tract

THE BUCCAL CAVITY

General considerations

The buccal cavity is referred to by Sir William Osler as a mirror of the rest of the body and it is essential that the dentist should have a clear understanding of the oral changes produced by systemic disorders. He should also appreciate the possible effects of dental abnormalities on the body generally.

1. For the efficient mastication of food, it is necessary that a sufficient number of teeth are present and that the soft tissues of the mouth be healthy. Thorough mastication of food is a very important first step in the complex process of digestion. While it is probably true that no specific alimentary disease is actually due to inadequate mastication, it must be accepted that insufficient teeth, extensive dental caries and poor oral hygiene are wholly undesirable in any person and that they may well have a positively adverse influence in those with gastritis, peptic ulceration or disordered bowel function. Lack of teeth is likely to be more important in older people in whom the digestive powers of the stomach may be decreased.

2. A patient suffering from an illness of medical nature may initially consult his dentist because of a prominence of oral symptoms. As an example of this, we may recall the bleeding gums of acute leukaemia. One of the authors well remembers a case of acute monocytic leukaemia occurring in a middle-aged man in whom the bleeding gums led him to seek dental advice. Unfortunately, the dentist's suspicions were not aroused by the obvious pallor and ill-health of the man and he proceeded to extract several teeth in the mistaken belief that he was dealing with an advanced case of periodontal disease.

Similarly, in underdeveloped areas of the world, scurvy due to vitamin C deficiency may present with bleeding gums.

3. In other instances, the dentist may observe during the course

of routine work, some oral abnormality which gives a clue to the fact that a general medical disorder is developing. In this connection, one may note that the dentist is often seeing his patients at regular intervals for a 'check-up' on the state of the teeth, whereas the doctor is seldom consulted until the patient feels positively ill. The classically quoted, but seldom seen, buccal pigmentation of Addison's disease is an example of an early oral manifestation of systemic disease. Similarly, infectious mononucleosis may present with oral signs of oedema of the fauces, enlarged cervical lymph nodes and occasionally with oral petechial haemorrhages seen in the palate.

4. The dentist should have an awareness of the various systemic infections which may produce local lesions in the mouth. This is partly for reasons of his own safety as in syphilis but also that he may not continue with local measures alone in circumstances where general measures are urgently required. Perhaps the most striking example of this is the folly of attempting to deal locally with the oral lesions of syphilis or tuberculosis.

5. There has been much speculation regarding the role of dental sepsis in the aetiology of disorders of the alimentary tract. At one time some held that the swallowing of septic material from diseased periodontal tissues migh predispose to peptic ulceration but support for this view is now very scanty. Haemotogenous spread of organisms from the buccal cavity to the gall-bladder to produce cholecystitis is, however, still actively considered by some to be of importance.

Dental sepsis has also been considered as playing a part in the causation of rheumatoid arthritis, but the evidence for this theory is far from convincing. The great majority of patients with dental sepsis do not develop rheumatoid arthritis and, conversely, rheumatoid arthritis may be present in those with healthy teeth or with dentures.

6. In subacute bacterial endocarditis there is no doubt that the buccal cavity is the source of infection in the majority of cases.

Examination of the buccal cavity

A dentist, by the nature of his training and profession, should be extremely proficient at examining the buccal cavity, but there may be a tendency, particularly if he has a very full schedule, for him to devote his attention to the teeth and gums to the exclusion of the other structures in the mouth. This is obviously undesirable and when one considers the number of disorders which may have local manifestations in the buccal cavity it is apparent that the dentist should include even a brief examination of all the structures in the mouth in his initial appraisal of the patient.

The essentials for a proper examination are good illumination, a comfortable relaxed patient, and a well practised routine on the part of the dentist. It does not matter in what order the various structures are examined provided they are all included. The lips, the gums, the mucosal lining of the cheeks, the palate, the tongue and the throat should all be inspected. Regarding the tongue, it may be noted that while it is seldom examined nowadays with the detail and reverence accorded it by the physicians of Victorian times, nevertheless it is an important mirror of disease and it should never be ignored. The dorsum of the tongue, the sides and the under surface should all be inspected and this should be followed by observations of the movements of the tongue and soft palate. Palpation of the tongue is necessary to detect any lesion or abnormality within the substance of the organ such as a lingual thyroid. In health, the tongue is moist, pinkish in colour, has a slight fur on the surface, and the papillae are easily seen.

THE LIPS

Colour
Cyanosis is often most evident in the lips; it is more prominent after exertion or in cold weather. Pallor of the lips may be due to shock (e.g. after haemorrhage or myocardial infarction) or due to anaemia. With regard to pallor of the lips it must be remembered that examination of the skin and mucous membranes affords only a rough guide to the haemoglobin level. Furthermore, the true colour of the lips is more often than not a matter for conjecture in women.

Herpes and other viral infections
Many viruses can affect the oral tissues but the herpes virus especially seems to result in significant oral disease. Primary herpetic gingivostomatitis is common as the result of infection with the herpes simplex virus. The infection is characterised by small painful blisters or vesicles situated near the mucocutaneous junction of the lips. These may enlarge and coalesce and cervical lymph node enlargement is not uncommon. The lesions may become severe in eczema herpeticum or in immunologically suppressed hosts. The virus is probably a normal inhabitant of the buccal cavity, capable of producing inflammatory changes only when the resistance is

lowered (e.g. during an attack of coryza, influenza or pneumonia).

Recurrent herpes simplex infections are common and a recurrence may be precipitated by a minor cause such as exposure to sunlight or menstruation. Most recurrences are manifest on the lips (herpes labiales). Herpes zoster of the maxillary or mandibular division of the trigeminal nerve produces a unilateral facial rash limited to the affected dermatome and in association with unilateral oral ulceration. The pain is severe and may simulate toothache and this is important since the pain may precede the appearance of the characteristic rash. In some rare cases the facial nerve is affected, causing a unilateral lower motorneurone facial nerve palsy in association with skin lesions in the external ear and oral ulcers on the palate (Ramsay Hunt syndrome). Once the rash has disappeared there may be post-herpetic neuralgic pain.

Accidental infection with the vaccinia virus may occur from a vaccination site to the lip or tongue and may cause marked swelling and oedema with vesicle formation that progress to pustules. In infection due to measles, spots resembling grains of salt on a red erythematous mucosa may develop in the buccal cavity (Koplik's spots). The oropharynx is also inflamed and the characteristic macular skin rash appears soon after.

Other abnormalities
The effects of vitamin deficiency and of syphilis on the lips are considered later in this chapter along with the effects of these disorders on the buccal cavity generally. Carcinoma of the lip is discussed with other tumours in Chapter 4.

CLEFT LIP AND PALATE

Approximately 1 in 800 babies is born with either a cleft lip, a cleft palate or both. The deformity is a major challenge to plastic surgeons and requires in addition the help of a speech therapist and frequently other specialist care, including expert counselling of the parents.

The condition is classified as to whether the primary palate (that is, the lip and alveolar ridge) or the secondary palate (that is, the hard and soft palate) or both are involved. Clefts of the lip may be minor but may extend well up into the nostril and the condition may be bilateral, extending back through the primary palate on both sides and involving the central area of the secondary palate.

Management of the condition is best undertaken by early consultation between the surgeon and orthodontist. The case is evaluated and it may be advisable to insert a dental obturator very early on in the neonatal period in order to prevent later arch deformity.

Surgical repair is carried out for cleft lip at an early stage, usually the first three months of life, but in cleft palate surgical treatment is best delayed for some time, but should be performed somewhere between one year and eighteen months of birth.

GINGIVAL HYPERTROPHY

Hypertrophy of the gingival tissues is most frequently the result of local causes (e.g. chronic sepsis and irritation) and the dentist, who will be familiar with such conditions, should always consider such local aetiological factors before turning to the less common systemic causes of gum hypertrophy described below.

1. In scurvy the gums are swollen and haemorrhagic.

2. In acute leukaemia, especially the monocytic variety, bleeding swollen gums are often present.

3. The drug phenytoin (Epanutin or Dilantin), which is used in the control of epilepsy, may lead to gingival hyperplasia. In severe cases alternative anticonvulsant therapy may have to be employed.

4. Gum hypertrophy develops in some women during pregnancy and may be sufficiently marked as to cause prominent gingival swellings or 'pregnancy tumours'. Similar, but less prominent, changes may be seen at menstruation. In many of these cases the gum changes are probably hormonally induced exaggerations of pre-existing minor gingival hypertrophy caused by local infection.

STOMATITIS AND GINGIVITIS

Stomatitis simply means inflammation of the mouth and gingivitis a more localised inflammation of the gums adjacent to the teeth. The changes may occur on the tongue or on the buccal mucosa.

A generalised form of stomatitis may be found within the mouth and may occur in infants where the hygiene is poor, or in any ill person where care of the mouth is neglected. It may be seen after excess smoking or alcohol consumption or, in some cases, after the prolonged use of penicillin or other antibiotic lozenges. The mucosa of the mouth is red and dry, the tongue swollen and covered with a brownish fur, and the breath foul. Care of the mouth is extremely important in any severe or prolonged illness and in hospitals it is standard practice to pay very careful attention to maintaining a healthy state of the buccal cavity. Mouth washes, e.g. with hydrogen peroxide, followed by swabbing of the tongue with a preparation such as Compound Glycerin of Thymol is carried out at frequent intervals.

Aphthous stomatitis

Aphthous stomatitis is characterized by the appearance of small, painful, superficial ulcers in the mouth (dyspeptic ulcers). Excess salivation is usually associated. Sometimes these ulcers occur for no particular reason while in other instances they occur following some gastrointestinal upset or a febrile illness. Mild cases often clear up spontaneously although recurrence is common. Mouth washes containing hydrogen peroxide, or the local application of a 1 per cent solution of gentian violet or of a paste containing triamcinolone acetonide (a steroid preparation) are often helpful.

Fungal infections

Stomatitis due to infection of the buccal cavity with fungi is not uncommon. The most frequent cause in this country is by the yeast-like fungus *Candida albicans*. This is known as thrush. Many normal people harbour candida albicans in the oral cavity but infection becomes clinically apparent when the resistance is lowered. Candidiasis thus provides a reflection of health and tends to become rampant where there is general debility and especially after the use of broad spectrum antibiotics in the treatment of general infection.

It tends to manifest at the extremes of age, and is common in bottle-fed infants if hygiene is imperfect. It is frequent also in the elderly, especially where there is associated generalised debility. A variety of immunological disorders predispose to candidiasis and it is not uncommon is diabetes mellitus, and also occurs in pregnancy. It is a frequent finding in the dehydrated ill patient. White or yellow patches appear in the buccal mucosa and on the throat and may lead to considerable discomfort and interference with eating. The disorder frequently responds to the local application of 1 per cent aqueous solution of gentian violet but a more efficacious form of treatment is with the antibiotic known as nystatin and this is usually given by topical and oral administration. In some patients a form of chronic candidiasis develops in association with the wearing of dentures (denture stomatitis). This affects the palate only but is sometimes associated with cracks and inflammation at the corners of the mouth (angular cheilitis).

Ulceromembranous stomatitis

Ulceromembranous stomatitis (Trench mouth, or Vincent's infection) is due to the combined effects of a fusiform bacillus and an anaerobic spirochete. A healthy mouth has a considerable degree of natural resistance to these organisms, but again this may be lessened by systemic illness, fatigue, or local factors.

The infection usually commences and is most severe at the gum margins and in the interdental papillae which are quickly affected, but it also may spread to the rest of the buccal cavity and to the throat. Vincent's infection is very rare in the edentulous mouth. The charateristic lesion is a superficial ulcer of a rather irregulat shape. It is usually covered with a greyish membrane. The adjacent mucosa is markedly inflamed. Excess salivation is present and the breath is offensive with a characteristic odour. The submandibular lymph nodes are usually tender and enlarged.

The drug of choice is metronidazole and mouthwashes containing hydrogen peroxide often lead to rapid improvement. It is important to ensure that the infection has been completely eradicated, especially from the interdental areas. In chronic or recurrent cases, attention must be paid to the general health of the individual and a search made for local factors which may predispose to persistence of the infection.

Diabetes mellitus

Patients with diabetes mellitus are prone to infection and the oral cavity is no exception. It should be noted that the forms of stomatitis referred to above are more likely to develop in the diabetic and meticulous dental care and careful stabilisation of diabetes are indicated.

Gangrenous stomatitis

Gangrenous stomatitis, noma, or cancrum oris is now uncommon. It used to be seen as a complication of severe illnesses in debilitated children with very poor resistance. The gangrenous changes were usually maximal in the tissues of the cheeks and sometimes caused penetration to the exterior.

DRUGS AND THE BUCCAL CAVITY

Several drugs may produce symptomatic or objective changes in the buccal cavity and it is important that the dentist has an awareness of them. Some of these are mentioned in other chapters but it will be of value to summarize them here. Mouth washes and other local remedies are not included.

Iron
Fluid preparations of iron, used in the treatment of hypochromic anaemia, produce blackening of the tongue and teeth unless taken through a straw. The same effect, though usually in lesser degree, will be observed with iron tablets if the patient does not swallow them promptly.

Liquorice
Mixtures containing liquorice produce blackening of the tongue; their use is now much less common.

Phenytoin
Gum hypertrophy may follow the use of the anticonvulsant drug phenytoin (Epanutin).

Atropine
Dryness of the mouth is an important side effect of treatment with atropine-containing remedies used for some alimentary disorders.

Hypotensive drugs
Dryness of the mouth occurs as a complication of treatment of hypertension with ganglion-blocking drugs.

Heavy metals
The long continued administration of bismuth, lead, and mercury leads to a blue line on the gum margin around the natural teeth due to a deposit of the sulphide salt of the metal in the presence of local infection. Stomatitis, excess salivation, and foul breath are usually also present. These heavy metals used to be in common use for the treatment of syphilis but they have been almost completely superseded by penicillin. Lead poisoning may also occur as an industrial disease or be due to contaminated drinking water.

Antibiotics
Stomatitis may occur as a complication of antibiotic therapy due to alterations in the bowel flora causing deficient synthesis of the vitamin B complex. A brownish-yellow discolouration of the teeth may result from prolonged administration of tetracycline in childhood.

Drug allergy

Oedema of the throat and glottis may occur as an allergic response to certain drugs in susceptible individuals. Some patients develop stomatitis, excess salivation, rhinitis and conjunctivitis if they are given iodides or bromides (iodism, bromism); a skin eruption may also be present.

Aspirin burn

Painful burns are seen not uncommonly in the buccal cavity due to the local irritative effect of an aspirin tablet held in the mucobuccal fold near a painful tooth in the mistaken belief that proximity to the site of pain enhances the analgesic effect of the drug.

THE BUCCAL CAVITY AND SYSTEMIC DISORDERS

The principal systemic disorders which may produce changes in the buccal cavity are summarized below. The student is referred to the appropriate chapter for an account of the various diseases.

Blood diseases

The principal changes to be remembered are the glossitis of hypochromic anaemia and pernicious anaemia, and the tendency to haemorrhage and infection in acute leukaemia, thrombocytopenia, and agranulocytosis.

Vitamin deficiency

The gum changes of scurvy, the tongue and lip changes of vitamin B deficiency, and the dental consequences of vitamin D deficiency are the important oral manifestations.

Endocrine disorders

The pigmentation of Addison's disease, the tongue enlargement of cretinism, and the enlargement of the jaw and tongue of acromegaly are the main points to be remembered.

Infectious diseases

The principal buccal changes to recall in the common infectious disorders of childhood are the Koplik's spots of measles, the vesicles of chickenpox, the difficulty in mastication and swelling of the parotid duct orifice in mumps, the tongue changes in scarlet fever, and ulceration of the fraenum of the tongue in whooping cough. Buccal lesions may occur in congenital, primary, secondary and tertiary syphilis. Superficial ulceration may be present in chronic pulmonary tuberculosis. In the United States actinomycosis, blastomycosis, histoplasmosis, and coccidioidomycosis are important causes of chronic, indurated, suppurative lesions of the buccal cavity and jaws.

Neurological disorders
The main changes are the paralysis of tongue associated with bulbar and pseudobulbar palsy, hypoglossal paralysis, scars of the tongue in epilepsy, tremors of the tongue in general paralysis of the insane, and the jack-in-the-box movements in chorea.

Gastrointestinal disorders
Halitosis, whilst often a symptom of oral disease or dental caries, also occurs in association with fungating infected carcinomata of the stomach or oesophagus. Crohn's disease, a chronic inflammatory disease of the bowel, may also present with oral ulceration, mucous tags or areas of induration within the oral cavity. Peutz-Jeughers syndrome consists of intestinal polyposis affecting predominantly the small bowel. This disease often presents with small bowel obstruction due to intussusception and is associated with pigmented areas on the lips within the buccal cavity and on the dorsum of the hand.

MISCELLANEOUS CHANGES IN THE TONGUE

Leukoplakia
This is an uncommon condition, the causation of which is poorly understood. The main aetiological factors usually considered are irritation of the tongue from roughened edges of teeth or dentures, irritation from chronic smoking, and from syphilis. It should be noted that dysplastic degeneration of the mucous membranes occurs most commonly in those who smoke and drink alcohol to excess.

White, firm, smooth patches develop on the surface of the tongue particularly on the lateral aspects, and also on the undersurface of the tongue and the adjacent floor of the mouth. This area is often overlooked in routine oral and pharyngeal examination and should be given special attention. In chronic cases, fissures appear and may cause considerable pain and discomfort. In severe cases, the process may also involve other parts. The Wassermann reaction should always be performed in cases of leukoplakia and, if found to be positive, anti-syphilitic treatment must be given. Good oral hygiene is essential and any possible aetiological factors such as carious or roughened teeth should be dealt with.

Leukoplakia is a pre-cancerous condition and because of this patients with leukoplakia should be kept under careful observation. The development of nodules or ulcers indicates that a biopsy should be performed but it should not be deferred if any suspicion exists. If the histological changes reveal incipient neoplasia then excision of the affected mucosa with skin-grafting can be performed. If frank neoplastic change is confirmed, then surgical resection and radiotherapy are employed as described in Chapter 4.

Lichen planus
This is a skin disorder which may produce lesions in the mouth resembling leukoplakia to some extent. It never, however, produces a uniform white patch but rather a framework of whitish lines, often radiating from a central area. It may also present as a silvery or violaceous patch on a mucosal surface and this may be associated with some burning pain. Topical corticosteroids may be helpful in some cases.

Dryness of the tongue
Dryness of the tongue occurs in people who habitually breathe through the mouth as a result of nasal obstruction; this may be caused by hypertrophy of adenoidal tissue or be due to deviation of the nasal septum. Dryness of the tongue is an important manifestation of dehydration (e.g. in diabetic coma) and is a useful clinical guide in assessing the fluid balance of the patient. Dryness of the mouth due to drugs is discussed on page 153. Deficient secretion from the parotid glands results in dryness of the mouth; this is considered on page 159.

Furring on the tongue
Some individuals become very alarmed if they notice that the tongue is furred and they may seek medical advice regarding this. The majority of them believe that fur on the tongue is a sign of disorder of the bowels or stomach, but in many instances it does not have any serious significance. It is seen after excess smoking, on 'the morning after the night before', after milk drinking if the hygiene of the mouth is poor, and in any febrile illness. It also occurs in many alimentary disorders ranging from simple gastric upsets to serious conditions like peritonitis and typhoid fever. In severe renal

failure a brownish fur on the tongue is common, especially if the hygiene of the mouth has been neglected. The characteristic fur on the tongue in scarlet fever has already been noted. Lastly it should be noted that some apparently perfectly healthy individuals have a rather prominent fur on the tongue.

Fissured or scrotal tongue

In this condition the fissures on the tongue are abnormally deep. The fissures may run longitudinally, transversely, irregularly, or radiate out in a herringbone pattern from the centre. The disorder is congenital in origin and does not signify any disease.

Geographical tongue

Geographical tongue, or wandering rash of the tongue, is the descriptive term employed for a condition characterized by patchy desquamation of the superficial epithelium after initial local overgrowth. The patch is slightly raised and has a yellowish-white or greyish colour; where desquamation has occurred there is a red, raw looking area. The patches gradually change in shape, often forming circles which may touch. Healing occurs slowly but fresh patches may form over several months until the condition finally clears up. Pain is not usually present but the disorder often produces considerable anxiety to the patient until he is reassured that it is not of serious import. The cause of the disorder is unknown. There is no specific treatment but it is worth while trying the effect of simple mouth washes.

Black hairy tongue

This is an unusual condition which usually occasions considerable alarm on the part of the sufferer. It is due to infection with a fungus which produces a dark pigment and causes proliferation of the filiform papillae. The infection may occur without apparent antecedent cause or it may follow systemic or local antibiotic therapy due to an upset of the normal mouth or bowel flora. The disorder improves following the use of hydrogen peroxide mouth washes or alternatively, the use of 10 per cent salicylic acid.

The burning tongue

Sometimes the dentist will be consulted by patients whose principal symptom is a burning sensation in the tongue and in whom examination of the organ is either negative or reveals nothing more than a little redness. The symptom is usually more pronounced after taking hot, wellseasoned, or rough items of food and drink.

In these circumstances the main considerations which the dentist should bear in mind are set out below. It will be readily seen that in many cases both dental and medical advice may be necessary.

1. Is there any occult source of irritation in the mouth such as rough edges of teeth, ill-fitting dentures, etc.?

2. Sometimes a burning tongue may be associated with denture stomatitis (see above) and in such cases a stainless steel denture which does not cover a wide area of the palate is a useful alternative.

3. Are there dental fillings of different metallic composition which when in contact produce a minor electric current in the buccal cavity?

4. Is the patient anaemic?

5. Is there deficiency of the vitamin B complex?

6. Has the patient been taking any medicines which could directly irritate the mucous membranes of the mouth (e.g. too strong mouth washes) or upset the normal buccal or bowel flora (e.g. antibiotics)?

7. Is there coronary artery disease present? The pain of myocardial ischaemia is usually experienced in the chest and may be referred to the shoulders, arms, and jaws and gums; occasionally it may be maximal in one of the referred sites.

8. In some instances the symptom occurs in women at the time of the menopause and it is generally believed that hormonal imbalance is responsible, although the mechanism is obscure. A chronic desquamative gingivitis may also be seen at the menopause.

9. Traumatic ulcer of the tongue. Chronic ulceration of the tongue which can be difficult to differentiate from carcinoma may develop as a result of chronic trauma from a roughened tooth or dental appliance. Such ulcers heal rapidly after elimination of the cause of irritation and failure to do so is an indication for biopsy.

Oral antral fistula
Occasionally an oral antral fistula will develop following extraction of an upper molar tooth, the roots of which often protrude into the maxillary sinus. Such a fistula is easily closed by rotating a small flap of oral mucosa across the defect. Oral antral fistulae may also develop as a result of tumours, but this is a much more rare event and if suspected biopsy is essential.

THE SALIVARY GLANDS

The principal diseases of the salivary glands are considered below but epidemic parotitis or mumps is described on page 5.

Ptyalism

Excess secretion of saliva is a distressing symptom. It may occur in any irritative or inflammatory lesion of the buccal cavity, in Parkinsonism (page 322), as a result of the administration of iodides or heavy metals, and in anxiety states. Ptyalism may also occur in some instances of carcinoma of the oesophagus. Management consists in correction of any causal factor and the symptomatic use of atropine preparations such as belladonna.

Xerostomia

The term means a dry mouth. It occurs in habitual mouth breathers and where there is a deficient secretion of saliva. The latter occurs in dehydration from any cause, in Sjögren's syndrome, and from excessive use of atropine preparations.

Inflammatory parotitis

Associated with salivary calculus

Calculus formation is common in the submandibular gland, unusual in the parotid gland and unknown in the sublingual gland. The submandibular gland secretes a highly mucous saliva and the duct has a long course. The calculi are composed of calcium phosphate and carbonates. Their clinical features consist of swelling below the angle of the jaw which develops at meal times and accompanied by mild discomfort and sometimes severe pain. There is oedema and swelling of the floor of the mouth and frequently a discharge of purulent saliva from the duct. There is sometimes an unpleasant taste present. In a proportion of patients the stone can be palpated bimanually and X-ray shows the calculi. If the stones are in the floor of the mouth they can be removed through an intraoral incision but if in the submandibular gland then the gland itself must be removed since it is fibrosed and chronically damaged. Calculi within the parotid gland or duct are uncommon, the stones being usually translucent and seen as filling defects on a sialogram.

Acute suppurative parotitis

Suppurative parotitis (Fig. 8.1) is seen as a complication of debilitating illness or in postoperative patients in whom the hygiene of the mouth has been neglected; dehydration is an important predisposing factor. There is a spread of bacteria, usually staphylococci or streptococci up the duct of the gland. The gland becomes swollen, very tender, and pus may be seen extruding from the ductal

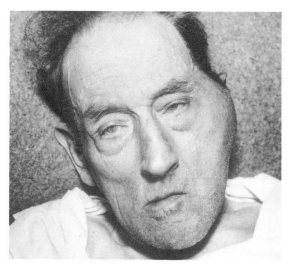

Fig. 8.1 Acute parotitis. Affected left parotid gland in a debilitated patient. Appearance of mixed parotid tumour is very similar.

orifice within the mouth. Pyrexia and leucocytosis, together with generalized illness develop. Prevention by strict oral hygiene is very important. In established cases antibiotics are employed and surgical drainage may be required in staphylococcal infection.

Chronic recurrent (non calculus) parotitis
In a minority of cases this condition may be due to main duct obstruction, e.g. stenosing papillitis as a result of operative trauma or ill-fitting dentures. In such cases dilation may be successful. The remainder of patients have no such stricture, the disease being of unknown aetiology. It is frequently seen in children, the individuals suffering from periodic pain and swelling of one or both parotid glands, often for many years. Radiological studies may show sialectasis (dilatation of the duct system). Treatment is by the establishment of drainage, by massage of the gland and sialagogues and parotidectomy may be required in severe cases. Division of the auriculo-temporal nerve in the middle ear has been successfully employed.

Mikulicz's syndrome
The term Mikulicz's disease should be reserved for cases of benign enlargement of the salivary and lacrimal glands of unknown cause. Histological examination shows atrophy of the gland acini and an

increase of lymphoid tissue. When the glandular enlargement is due to some recognizable pathological process such as Hodgkin's disease, lymphatic leukaemia or lymphosarcoma the term Mikulicz's syndrome is used.

Sjögren's syndrome

Comprises an affection of the salivary and lacrimal glands producing troublesome xerostomia and a sense of grittiness in the eyes. The majority of patients are women and they may also suffer from rheumatoid arthritis. It is thought to be due to an auto-immune process.

Uveoparotitis (Heerfordt's syndrome)

This is a local expression of sarcoidosis which is an uncommon disorder characterized by histological changes similar to those seen in tuberculosis except that caseation does not occur and tubercle bacilli are not present. The Mantoux reaction is negative. There is a concomitant swelling of the parotid glands and inflammatory changes in the uveal tract of the eyes. Other manifestations of sarcoidosis may be extremely varied and include enlargement of the mediastinal lymph nodes, lesions of the lung tissue, enlargement of the spleen and skin lesions.

Salivary tumours

Simple adenomata and cysts of the salivary gland may occur but are extremely uncommon. Similarly lipomata and neurofibromata of the facial nerve may present as swellings within the parotid gland and bony tumours such as adamantinoma of the mandible may be mistaken for true lesions arising within the parotid.

Mixed salivary tumour (pleomorphic adenoma)

This is a slow growing tumour usually found in patients over 30 years old. 90 per cent occur in the parotid gland and 5 per cent in the submandibular gland and the remainder are found in the palate, cheek or lip. The tumour is lobulated and has a false capsule. On cutting it has a translucent appearance and histologically is composed of cellular elements which are epithelial and a myxomatous matrix which may have the consistency of cartilage. Treatment is by removal of the tumour with the surrounding parotid gland (superficial parotidectomy) and care must be taken to preserve the facial nerve. In the submandibular gland and in other areas such as the lip or palate complete excision is practiced.

Adenocarcinoma

This presents as a hard, ill-defined swelling steadily enlarging and infiltrating the surrounding skin. If involving the parotid gland there is, unlike the pleomorphic adenoma, involvement of the facial nerve with facial palsy and subsequently, as the base of the skull is involved, other cranial nerves become affected. Glandular metastases may occur in the neck and more rarely distant metastases in liver or lung. Treatment is by wide excision and skin grafting and by deep X-ray therapy.

Adenoid cystic carcinoma (cylindroma)

This is a malignant tumour arising usually in the submandibular gland or in the palate. It metastasizes along nerve sheaths or tissue planes rather than to regional nodes. The tumour is radioresistant and requires very wide excision.

Adenolymphoma (Warthin's tumour)

This accounts for approximately 10 per cent of all parotid swellings. It is a round or ovoid cystic tumour with a smooth surface and is filled with brownish material. Histologically it consists of columnar epithelium with lymphoid stroma probably arising from salivary duct epithelium and lymphoid tissue within the gland. Local enucleation is curative.

SORE THROAT

Sore throat is a very common complaint. The majority of cases are due to simple upper respiratory tract infections, which are self-limiting, but it is important to remember that there are more serious causes.

1. Soreness of the throat due to local infection. The more important of the local infections of the throat are the pharyngitis of the common cold, streptococcal sore throat, Vincent's infection spreading from the buccal cavity, and extension of thrush from the buccal cavity. There is seldom any diagnostic problem in these cases but, in cases of doubt, the diagnosis can be quickly established by microscopic examination of a stained smear from the throat.

2. Soreness of throat in association with the infectious fevers. The infectious fevers are discussed elsewhere, but it may be recalled here that sore throat is a feature of the early stages of measles, cerebrospinal fever, and poliomyelitis, and is a cardinal part of the clinical picture of diphtheria and scarlet fever.

3. Secondary syphilis. Soreness of the throat may be present in secondary syphilis if the mucosal lesions, which are characterisitc of this stage of the infection, spread from the buccal cavity to the throat.

4. Sore throat associated with blood disorders. The principal disorders of the blood which may be associated with sore throat are acute leukaemia, agranulocytosis, and infectious mononucleosis.

Investigation of sore throat

A careful history will often reveal helpful information, e.g. contact with cases of infectious disease, presence of a recent tendency to haemorrhage, or skin rashes. On general examination attention should be paid to the presence of pallor, skin rashes, enlarged lymph glands, enlarged spleen, evidence of bruising, and purpura. The appearance of the mouth and throat may give diagnostic help (e.g. the difference between the streptococcal throat and the throat of diphtheria, or the presence of Koplik's spots). A swab of the throat for bacteriological study will yield diagnostic information in many instances and, in addition, will give valuable therapeutic help by indicating the sensitivity of the organisms to the various antibiotics. Examination of the blood is necessary to establish the diagnosis in cases of leukaemia, agranulocytosis and infectious mononucleosis. Two serological tests may be of value—the Wassermann or Kahn reaction in cases of syphilis, and the Paul-Bunnell reaction in cases of infectious mononucleosis.

DISORDERS OF THE OESOPHAGUS

Anatomical considerations

The oesophagus is a hollow tube, about 25 cm long, which extends from the lower border of the cricoid cartilage to the cardiac orifice of the stomach which is at the level of the eleventh thoracic vertebra. The distance from the incisor teeth to the lower end of the oesophagus is about 40 cm.

The oesophagus lies in a loose bed of areolar tissue in the posterior mediastinum. The principal relations are the trachea, the thyroid, the aortic arch, and the left main bronchus anteriorly, while the vertebral column lies posteriorly. The left recurrent laryngeal nerve lies between the aortic arch and the oesophagus.

The oesophagus has an outer longitudinal and an inner circular muscle layer with connective tissue containing nerves (Auerbach's plexus) and the blood vessels between. The mucous membrane consists of stratified squamous epithelium which changes abruptly to gastric mucosa at the cardia.

The upper end of the oesophagus is kept closed, except on swallowing, by a sphincter formed by the cricopharyngeus muscle. Reflux of gastric contents into the lower end of the oesophagus is prevented by the cardiac sphincter of the stomach, the muscles of the diaphragm around the oesophageal opening and the difference between the thoracic and intra-abdominal pressure. Ordinarily it takes above five seconds for a bolus of food to traverse the oesophagus. The parasympathetic fibres to the oesophagus are carried in the vagus nerves. Should oesophageal obstruction exist then the level of obstruction can often be precisely located by the patient. Oesophageal pain is felt in the retrosternal area and at the root of the neck.

Dysphagia

The commonest symptom in disorders of the oesophagus is difficulty in swallowing, or dysphagia, and a description of the main causes of dysphagia will, in fact, be an account of the principal oesophageal lesions. In addition it should be remembered that dys-

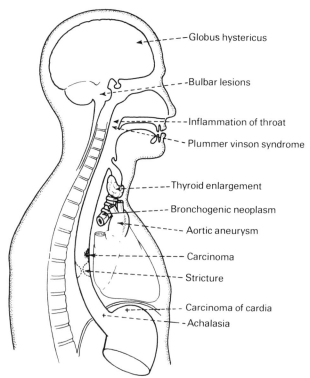

Fig. 8.2 The causes of dysphagia.

phagia may result from painful conditions of the throat which have already been described. The causes of dysphagia are shown diagrammatically in Figure 8.2.

Dysphagia may result from lesions in the posterior one-third of the tongue or in the oral or the laryngo-pharynx but it more commonly results from disorders affecting the oesophagus.

Dysphagia due to pressure on the oesophagus

1. Enlarged lymph glands in the mediastinum are a not uncommon cause of dysphagia. The enlargement may be due to Hodgkin's disease, tuberculosis, lymphosarcoma or metastatic carcinoma particularly from the bronchi.

2. Thyroid enlargement must be of considerable degree before it causes difficulty in swallowing if the thyroid is in its usual position but, if the thyroid is retrosternal then relatively slight enlargement may be sufficient to cause dysphagia as the gland cannot readily be enlarged in an anterior direction. Dysphagia due to thyroid enlargement is usually accompanied by tracheal deviation and compression.

3. Bronchial carcinoma. Carcinoma of the bronchus near the carina or involving mediastinal glands close to the oesophagus may directly invade the oesophageal wall.

4. Abnormalities of the great vessels. Aneurysms of the aortic arch or of the great vessels at the root of the neck or abnormalities in their origin and anatomical course are rare causes of dysphagia.

5. A pharyngeal diverticulum may develop from a weak area between the inferior constrictors of the pharynx and the crico-pharyngeus. The dysphagia is accompanied by a gurgling in the neck when the diverticulum empties and there may be attacks of coughing and halitosis. An oesophageal diverticulum is more likely to result from traction on the oesophagus by a localized area of postinflammatory fibrosis, e.g. infected lymph glands. Either form may exert pressure on the oesophagus and cause dysphagia. Barium swallow is usually diagnostic.

Dysphagia due to intrinsic oesophageal lesions

1. Carcinoma of the oesophagus is a very important cause of dysphagia which progresses until the patient cannot swallow even his own saliva. The disease is discussed in detail in Chapter 4.

2. Simple fibrous stricture of the oesophagus may result from trauma caused by swallowing a foreign body, a corrosive substance or extremely hot fluids. The most common cause of stricture, however, results from longstanding oesophagitis consequent on reflux of acid gastric contents and bile into the oesophagus. This is usually accompanied by an hiatus hernia. The dysphagia which results may cause considerable loss of weight as a result of impaired nutrition but is not associated with the cachexia of malignant growth. The treatment in most cases is by periodic dilatation of the stricture by oesophageal bougies. If an hiatus hernia is present and reflux can be demonstrated then repair of the hernia and prevention of reflux can result in cure. Occasionally, it is necessary to resect a very tight stricture and reconstruct the defect by an oesophagogastric anastomosis.

3. *The dysphagia of the Plummer-Vinson or Kelly-Paterson syndrome* is due to degenerative changes occurring in the upper part of the alimentary canal, particularly the pharynx. In severe cases webs of tissue form in the pharynx and upper oesophagus. The syndrome comprises chronic iron deficiency anaemia, glossitis, dysphagia and koilonychia. The term 'sideropenic dysphagia' is sometimes employed.

Dysphagia due to neuromuscular or functional causes

1. Difficulty in swallowing is a common symptom in hysterical individuals. The usual description is of a constant lump in the throat as though something was lodged there. The main points of diagnostic value are the absence of evidence of any organic lesion and the personality of the patient. The condition is termed *globus hystericus.*

2. Difficulty in swallowing is an important feature of lesions of the lower brain-stem nuclei (*bulbar palsy*) or of the pyramidal fibres which supply these nuclei (*pseudobulbar palsy*). Vascular lesions and degenerative processes account for the majority of cases. Impaired function of the tongue and larynx causing difficulty in eating and speaking are associated symptoms.

3. Dysphagia may be due to disturbed function of the sphincter at the lower end of the oesophagus, which does not open in the usual reflex manner in response to swallowing. *Achalasia*, which means failure to relax, is a better term than cardiospasm which was used when it was thought that there was active spasm of the sphincter. It occurs more often in women and the aetiology is poorly understood.

The dysphagia is often intermittent at first. In severe cases there may be considerable weight loss because of impaired nutrition. An attempt may be made to improve the faulty mechanism of the cardiac sphincter by periodic dilation with an oesophageal bougie. This is sufficient in many cases but, if it fails to give relief, recourse may be made to surgical division of the muscle fibres at the lower end of the oesophagus (Heller's operation). In longstanding achalasia there is an increased risk of carcinoma of the oesophagus and this possibility should be borne in mind during investigation.

Investigation of a case of dysphagia

A careful history may reveal some causal factor such as swallowing a foreign body or a corrosive substance, or there may be associated symptoms of the cause such as cough or haemoptysis in bronchogenic carcinoma. It should be ascertained whether the dysphagia is progressive as in carcinoma or intermittent as in achalasia. Often the patient will indicate the level of obstruction accurately.

The clinical examination should pay particular attention to the presence of anaemia, koilonychia, weight loss, thyroid gland enlargement and cervical lymphadenopathy. In the mouth the tongue should be inspected carefully for glossitis and the throat should be thoroughly examined. Blood examination will be required if anaemia is suspected.

The next step in investigation is usually recourse to radiology. An X-ray of the chest will reveal evidence of most of the causes of external pressure on the oesophagus. An X-ray of the oesophagus, taken after the patient has swallowed a thick paste of barium, will reveal the level of hold-up and, in many cases, gives a clue to the nature of the obstruction. In carcinoma the characteristic finding is an irregular filling defect, in simple stricture the narrowing is usually symmetrical, while in achalasia there is smooth uniform enlargement of the lower part of the oesophagus above the closed sphincter.

A further diagnostic step is oesophagoscopy—this is essential and can be carried out either with a flexible or rigid oesophagoscope and is of particular value in differentiating carcinomata from benign strictures as one is able to visualize the growth and take a biopsy for histological examination.

Other oesophageal conditions

Oesophageal varices
Dilation of the veins at the lower end of the oesophagus results from a rise in pressure in the portal circulation most commonly as a consequence of cirrhosis of the liver. These oesophageal varices are prone to bleed, giving rise to copious haematemesis. They may be visualized as small filling defects on barium swallow X-ray examination.

Hiatus hernia

This is an important cause of indigestion and heart-burn, especially in women of middle age and over. Due to widening of the opening in the diaphragm through which the oesophagus passes, a portion of the upper part of the stomach passes through into the thorax (Fig. 8.3). This is associated with inefficiency of the cardiac

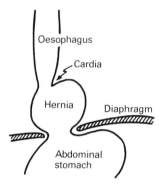

Fig. 8.3 Relationship of a hiatus hernia to the diaphragm.

sphincter and a reflux of acid gastric contents resulting in oesophagitis. The symptoms in hiatus hernia are characteristically worse on stooping or lying flat since in these positions oesophageal reflux is more likely to occur. Treatment is by weight-reducing diet and the avoidance of stooping. The patients are encouraged to sleep in a semi-upright position. Should these simple measures fail then surgery may be necessary for severe symptoms or for stricture.

DISORDERS OF THE STOMACH AND DUODENUM

Anatomical and physiological considerations

The shape and form of the stomach (Fig. 8.4) varies widely in different individuals and according to whether it is full or empty. The body of the stomach secretes most of the gastric juice which contains hydrochloric acid, pepsin, lipase, mucus and intrinsic factor. The secretion is initiated by a psychic flow produced by the taste, sight, smell or thought of food and completed by a reflex and humoral response to the presence of food, especially meat extracts, in the antrum of the stomach. The antrum mixes the food and propels it through the pylorus into the duodenum. The arterial blood supply which is derived from several vessels arising indirectly from the abdominal aorta is abundant.

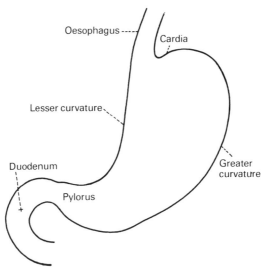

Fig. 8.4 The configuration of the normal stomach.

The stomach is not an essential part of the alimentary tract but it has the following important functions.

1. Motor. It acts as a reservoir for the food enabling us to take large meals relatively infrequently. The food mass lies initially in the body of the stomach where it is softened by admixture with the gastric juice. It then passes into the antrum where active peristaltic movements, plus gastric digestion, complete the transition of food to a semi-liquid consistency for delivery in small quantities to the duodenum over a period of two to six hours depending on the nature of the meal.

2. Digestive. In the presence of free hydrochloric acid, pepsin begins the digestion of proteins by breaking them down into proteoses and peptones, and fats are hydrolysed to a limited extent by lipase, but the main digestive processes do not take place until the semi-liquid food reaches the small intestine.

3. Protective. The stomach protects the more delicate small intestine in several ways. Very hot or very cold foods are brought to body temperature, chemical irritants such as alcohol are diluted, many bacteria are destroyed by hydrochloric acid, grossly irritant material is rejected by vomiting, and improperly masticated food is softened and broken up by gastric peristalsis and digestion.

4. Haemopoietic. The cells of the gastric mucosa secrete a substance called the intrinsic factor which is essential for the absorption of vitamin B_{12} (the extrinsic factor). Deficiency of vitamin B_{12} is a very important cause of anaemia (p. 219).

Investigation of gastric and duodenal disorders

A careful history is essential. Special tests include the employment of a barium meal examination and the performance of gastroduodenoscopy. This is carried out with the flexible fiberoptic instrument and allows confirmation of X-ray findings and biopsy of tissues for histological examination. Resting gastric juice or the secretion of gastric juice stimulated by the administration of a drug such as histamine or pentagastrin can be used to assess the acid peptic secreting ability of the stomach.

Other special investigations include the assessment of the speed of gastric emptying and of the integrity of its nerve supply.

It is important to realize that a proportion of barium meal X-ray examinations reveal no abnormality despite the presence of disease so that endoscopy is essential should symptoms continue.

Dyspepsia

One of the principal ways in which disorders of the stomach and duodenum may present is by indigestion, or dyspepsia. The main causes of this common symptom are as follows.

1. Simple or functional dyspepsia. This term is used to describe recurrent dyspepsia without any detectable lesion in the stomach or duodenum and in the absence of disordered function of other organs such as the liver and kidneys.

It is most often seen in nervous, tense people especially when they are overworked or otherwise keyed-up. The reason for the dyspepsia is not known with certainty, but hypermotility and spasm of the pylorus and duodenum are likely factors. Symptomatic relief is often obtained with alkalis and sedation.

2. Gastritis. Acute inflammatory change in the gastric mucosa is most often due to dietary and alcoholic indiscretion. Abdominal discomfort, nausea, and vomiting are present and there may be haematemesis in severe cases.

Atrophic and hypertrophic forms of chronic gastritis have been described largely on the basis of gastroscopic appearances. The aetiology of the condition is obscure. Dyspepsia, which does not usually have the periodicity characteristic of peptic ulceration, is the main symptom.

3. Peptic ulcer.

4. Carcinoma of stomach.

5. Hiatus hernia.

6. *Secondary dyspepsia.* Dyspepsia is frequently due to disordered function of the stomach secondary to defects of other organs or systems. Important examples are gallbladder disease, hepatic dysfunction (e.g. cirrhosis of liver), anaemia, congestive cardiac failure, and chronic renal disease.

Peptic ulceration

The term 'peptic ulcer' includes duodenal ulcer, gastric ulcer, and the less frequent ulcers which may occasionally be seen at the lower end of the oesophagus or at the junction of a gastroenterostomy (stomal ulcer). Duodenal ulcer is the commonest variety.

Incidence

Peptic ulceration is a common disorder which affects 10 per cent of all adults at some time during their life. Duodenal ulceration is commoner in men while the sex incidence of gastric ulcer is about equal. Duodenal ulcers usually start in early adult life whereas most gastric ulcers develop in middle age or later; either variety, however, may develop at practically any age. A family history of peptic ulceration is often present.

Aetiology

The causation of peptic ulceration is not fully understood although two facts seem reasonably clear:

1. The lesion occurs only in those parts of the alimentary canal in contact with the gastric juices, i.e. the stomach and duodenum, and the small intestine after short-circuit operations.

2. The actual ulceration is apparently caused by proteolysis of the mucosa and it is probable that pepsin and hydrochloric acid are the important constitutents of the gastric juice in this respect.

What is less well understood is why some people develop peptic ulceration whereas others do not. It is widely believed that peptic ulceration is commoner in the ambitious, self-driving, worrying type of person who leads a restless life taking inadequate time for meals, for rest and for leisure, e.g. many of those in executive positions and in the medical and dental professions. It must not be thought, however, that peptic ulceration is a prerogative of the intelligent, ambitious person, for it is seen quite commonly in the unskilled worker either clerical or manual. Two factors that probably are of great importance are irregular hurried meals and frustration; these may occur in many widely differing walks of life.

Many attempts have been made to define local predisposing factors in the upper alimentary tract. Inadequate blood supply to certain portions of the mucosa, deficiency of some protective enzyme rendering the mucosa vulnerable to the action of gastric juice, and focal sepsis causing mucosal damage have all been considered as possible aetiological factors but none has been proven.

Pathology

The majority of duodenal ulcers occur in the first part of the duodenum about one inch from the pylorus. The commonest site for a gastric ulcer is on the posterior wall of the lesser curvature. The ulcer is at first superficial, involving only the mucosa, but chronic ulcers may penetrate deeply into the wall of the stomach or duodenum and be surrounded by much fibrosis. Ulcers usually measure about quarter to half an inch in diameter but larger lesions may develop. In some cases more than one ulcer may be present. Malignancy may develop within the wall of a gastric ulcer.

Clinical features

The characteristic symptom of peptic ulceration is indigestion or dyspepsia. In a typical case of duodenal ulceration the patient usually states that about one to three hours after a meal, or just before a meal, he experiences discomfort in the upper part of the abdomen. This may be a vague, 'blown-up' feeling of distension, while at other times a gnawing pain may be experienced. The discomfort usually settles temporarily if food or an alkali is taken. Flatulence, a burning sensation behind the sternum (heartburn), and the eructation of mouthfuls of sour liquid (waterbrash), are often associated. When the dyspepsia is severe, vomiting is likely to be frequent. These symptoms may also waken the patient from sleep in the early hours of the morning.

In duodenal ulceration the dyspeptic symptoms are characteristically intermittent. A common pattern is dyspepsia for a few days to a few weeks, followed by a period of freedom from symptoms lasting for a few weeks or months. Recurrence of symptoms is frequently associated with worry or overwork. More severe symptoms include vomiting and the development of pain in the back.

The symptomatology in gastric ulceration is similar to that in duodenal ulceration with the exception that the discomfort usually comes on much sooner after meals and may be less intermittent.

Clinical examination of the patient is often not helpful in establishing the diagnosis. While it is true that many patients with peptic ulceration have a worried, lean face with deeply etched nasolabial folds (dyspeptic facies), this association is far from constant. Weight loss may occur if the ulcer is very active and vomiting is pronounced, but it is not a feature in uncomplicated cases. Examination of the abdomen may reveal tenderness in the epigastrium.

Investigations
Should barium meal X-ray examination reveal a duodenal ulcer then endoscopy is unnecessary. However, in cases of gastric ulceration endoscopy is essential to visualize the lesion, obtain biopsy and observe progress.

In duodenal ulceration there is characteristically a hypersecretion of acid gastric juice (hyperchlorhydria) although in gastric ulceration there is very seldom excess acid secretion.

Prognosis and course
An acute peptic ulcer may heal with or without treatment and remain healed. In many individuals, however, the lesion becomes chronic while, in others, the ulcer may heal but a further ulcer develops some time later. Many patients learn to 'live with their ulcer' and suffer only occasional discomfort. Others, however, find it a severe disability and economic handicap. Various complications (Fig. 8.5) may develop especially in the case of chronic ulcers.

1. Haemorrhage may occur from the ulcer producing haematemesis and/or melaena (See Ch. 4).

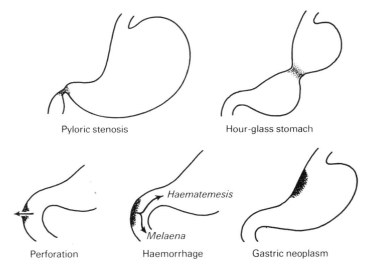

Pyloric stenosis

Hour-glass stomach

Perforation

Haematemesis

Melaena

Haemorrhage

Gastric neoplasm

Fig. 8.5 The complications of peptic ulceration. See text for discussion regarding gastric neoplasm.

2. The ulcer may penetrate through the wall of the stomach or duodenum leading to perforation and acute peritonitis.

3. Excessive fibrosis may develop around the ulcer which, if situated at the pylorus, produces pyloric stenosis. A less common site for fibrotic narrowing is in the body of the stomach producing hour-glass deformity.

4. Malignant change may be found in a segment of the wall of an otherwise simple gastric ulcer. This is most important to recognize. Although there has been some debate as to whether the neoplasm is in fact a complication of gastric ulceration the argument is of no great clinical importance.

Treatment

Rest is of undoubted value in the treatment of peptic ulcer. Most patients with chronic ulcers find that a few quiet days will often settle an exacerbation of symptoms, while a holiday away from business worries is almost invariably beneficial. The rest should be both physical and mental and, to attain the latter, mild sedation is helpful.

Certain broad principles about the diet may be stated. The meals should be taken at regular hours and the individual should have a midmeal snack such as a glass of milk and a biscuit. The food should be properly masticated and it is therefore important that the patient has an adequate number of teeth in good repair or is provided with efficient dentures. He should rest for a while after meals to permit digestion to occur in optimal circumstances. These broad principles are more important than the precise composition of the diet which should never be allowed to become an obsession with the patient, as may sometimes happen. In general, the diet should not contain foods which are liable to cause gastric irritation (e.g. highly seasoned foods), or which are very difficult to digest. Milk products, eggs, fish, chicken, and tripe are common items on the diet but soup, meat, vegetables, and fruit are all permissible, and in fact desirable, provided they are cooked in such a way as to render them easily digestible. The peptic ulcer patients may, unless care is taken with his diet, have a poor intake of vitamin C; this is very undesirable as vitamin C plays an important part in healing.

Tea and coffee should preferably be taken rather weak with plenty of milk and alcohol in moderation after meals. Tobacco smoking is best avoided altogether and it has been shown that abstinence from smoking may be associated with an increased incidence of healing of duodenal ulceration

Most patients find quick, albeit temporary, relief from dyspepsia with an alkali and in consequence of this there is a great variety of proprietary preparations available for self-medication. Sodium bicarbonate, or baking soda, is one of the most commonly used drugs but, although reasonably effective, it is far from ideal as it causes liberation of carbon dioxide in the stomach producing flatulence, stimulates further secretion of hydrochloric acid, and may lead to an upset in the acid-base balance of the body (alkalosis) because it is so readily absorbed. Two widely prescribed substances which are efficient and safe are aluminium hydroxide and magnesium trisilicate. The symptomatic benefit obtained from the use of alkali-drugs is without doubt but it is less certain that their long-term use promotes healing of the ulcer.

Recent years have seen remarkable changes in the management of peptic ulceration and in particular duodenal ulceration by the development of the drug cimetidine (Tagamet). This drug acts by inhibiting histamine receptors specific to the stomach and so inhibiting secretion of an acid gastric juice. The drug has been shown to heal peptic ulcers and may be taken for prolonged periods as a maintenance therapy to prevent relapse.

Indications for surgery in peptic ulcer

In gastric ulceration surgical treatment is clearly indicated in the presence of perforation or excessive fibrosis leading to hour-glass deformity. If there is doubt after observation as to the healing of a gastric ulcer or doubt as to whether an ulcer is simple or malignant, then surgery is likewise required.

In chronic duodenal ulceration where the symptoms are persistent and intolerable, surgery is likewise required as it is in cases of perforation and pyloric stenosis.

Many patients with peptic ulceration bleed (haematemesis and/or melaena) and surgery may be required where bleeding is persistent or recurrent.

The results of surgery for gastric ulcer and duodenal ulcer are in general good but cure cannot be guaranteed and especially in duodenal ulcer, recurrent ulceration or complications of operation develop in approximately 7–10 per cent of patients.

Carcinoma of stomach

The stomach, especially the pyloric region, is a common situation for cancer. The tumour is usually an adenocarcinoma. It may present as an ulcer and be difficult to distinguish from a simple peptic ulcer. Endoscopy and biopsy is essential in this differentiation.

Clinical features

The clinical features may be considered conveniently in three groups. Firstly, there may be symptoms specifically related to the stomach the most important being a vague form of indigestion occurring for the first time often in late middle life in an individual with a previously good appetite. Dyspepsia is progressive and not subject to relapses and remissions as in peptic ulceration and is poorly relieved by alkalis. Abdominal pain and vomiting usually develop later. Secondly, there are the symptoms which are common to many malignant neoplasms, namely loss of appetite, loss of energy and loss of weight and in addition there may be anaemia which often develops early and results from persistent slight bleeding. Thirdly, the tumour may present with secondary deposits in the liver, bones or abdominal lymph nodes and very occasionally there is a tumour deposit in the lymph nodes at the root of the neck, especially on the left side.

Diagnosis

Gastric neoplasm should be suspected in any middle-aged or elderly individual who loses his appetite and develops vague indigestion. Clinical examination in the early stages is often negative but later will show evidence of weight loss and an abdominal mass or an enlarged liver. A barium meal will usually show a filling defect while gastroscopy may permit visualization and biopsy of the growth. Specimens may be obtained for exfoliative cytology. The gastric juice commonly contains blood and has an offensive odour.

Treatment

The only curative treatment is surgical resection of the stomach (gastrectomy) but, unfortunately, the lesion is inoperable in many cases by the time a diagnosis is established.

Haematemesis and melaena

Causes

The main alimentary causes of haematemesis and melaena are acute erosive gastritis, acute or chronic peptic ulceration, ruptured oesophageal varices and rarely gastric neoplasm. Other causes include vomiting of swallowed blood, e.g. after epistaxis, and the haemorrhagic blood disorders. Aspirin, which is irritant to the gastric mucosa, may precipitate alimentary bleeding, especially in those with peptic ulceration. Excess alcohol intake is a common precipitating factor in many instances.

Clinical features

If much blood is lost the patient is shocked (Ch. 4). If the blood is vomited immediately after haemorrhage occurs it will be red in colour but more frequently it is retained in the stomach for some time and owing to the action of the gastric juice it becomes progressively darker and may come to resemble coffee grounds. The melaena stool is black, shiny and offensive in odour and is sometimes described as a tarry stool. In contrast to the appearance of the blood in haematemesis the blood in haemoptysis is usually bright red in colour and frothy due to admixture with air.

Treatment

The main points in treatment are rest, sedation and adequate blood transfusion in severe cases. Patients are managed by a physician and surgeon acting together and early diagnosis of the site of bleeding, particularly by endoscopy, is important. Recently, there have been some successful results by coagulation of bleeding points using a laser beam directed endoscopically. Surgery is indicated for persistent or recurrent bleeding.

After the emergency is over diagnostic measures are necessary to establish the source of bleeding and the patient should receive iron to enable him to replace the lost blood.

DISORDERS OF THE BOWEL

It is proposed to deal quite briefly with the various bowel disorders. In the majority of cases the main symptomatology is disordered bowel rhythm, i.e. diarrhoea and constipation. An account will be given of the principal causes of these two common symptoms, together with an explanatory note where desirable.

Diarrhoea

Diarrhoea may be defined as the abnormally rapid passage through the gut of the intestinal contents leading to frequent, loose stools. Colicky abdominal pain may occur. Considerable quantities of fluid and electrolytes may be lost in severe cases of diarrhoea and their replacement is an essential part of treatment (e.g. in bacillary dysentery, cholera, etc.). The presence of blood and mucus in the stools indicates ulceration of the colon.

1. Transient diarrhoea may result from many *simple causes*, e.g. the eating of indigestible food such as green apples, emotional upset, or a change in climate.

2. *Infection of the bowel* is very important cause of diarrhoea; in this group are bacterial food poisoning, bacillary dysentery, amoebic dysentery, typhoid, and paratyphoid fever, cholera, and tuberculosis of the intestine. Bacterial food poisoning is most frequently due to organisms of the Salmonella group. Other important agents are certain strains of staphylococci and *Clostridium botulinum* (botulism). The principal clinical features are an abrupt onset, nausea, vomiting, and diarrhoea.

3. *Malignant tumour* of the bowel is very common in the colon or rectum but much less so in the duodenum and small bowel. Adenocarcinoma is the common variety and this grows so as to form a circumferential lesion which causes stricturing and ulcerates. The symptoms are initially of intermittent diarrhoea alternating with constipation. For tumours on the left side of the colon or in the rectum bleeding is a common accompaniment whereas lesions in the ascending colon and in the caecum more often present with loss of weight, loss of appetite and loss of energy. There is often a palpable mass and in rectal lesions the tumour can be felt by digital examination. The liver may be palpable due to the presence of secondary deposits. In some patients the stricture becomes so tight so as to cause complete intestinal obstruction and the patient presents with a distended abdomen, colicky abdominal pain and vomiting.

Diagnosis is by means of barium enema X-ray examination and by sigmoidoscopy or fiberoptic colonoscopic examination and biopsy. The treatment is surgical and involves excision of the primary tumour with either end to end anastomosis or the formation of a colostomy. Should there be secondary deposits in the liver then usually a palliative resection is carried out or the tumour is bypassed so as to avoid the complication of obstruction.

4. *Crohn's disease.* This is a relatively uncommon non-specific chronic inflammatory condition of the bowel of unknown cause. The commonest area affected is the terminal ileum but the disease can affect any part of the gastrointestinal tract including the mouth. The presentation may be with pain in the right iliac fossa with diarrhoea, weight loss and anaemia and with loss of energy but occasionally a more acute onset with perforation of the bowel or fistula formation occurs.

Treatment is supportive by means of adequate nutrition and blood transfusion if anaemic. Surgical resection may prove necessary for obstruction, fistula formation or other complications. Unfortunately resection is followed by recurrence of the disease in up to 50 per cent or more of patients.

5. *Ulcerative colitis* is a relatively uncommon but very important

cause of diarrhoea. The condition, which is of uncertain aetiology, affects young adults and is commoner in females. The individual has recurrent bouts of diarrhoea, the stools containing blood and excess mucus. Progressive weight loss and anaemia occur. The disease is a serious one and may prove fatal. Some patients respond to a low residue diet, steroids and blood transfusion while in others surgery is necessary. It has been shown that the best results are obtained by total removal of the colon and rectum although some surgeons still practice partial colectomy. Removal of the colon and rectum (proctocolectomy) necessitates the creation of a permanent ileostomy.

It is important to know that longstanding ulcerative colitis involving the whole colon is a predisposing cause of cancer of the colon and this is an added reason to consider colectomy in severe disease.

6. Impaired absorption of fat from the small intestine leads to the passage of pale, bulky, offensive stools containing excess fat. The disorder is termed *steatorrhoea; coeliac disease* is the childhood variety. The absorption defect is seldom limited to fat, however, there is commonly associated a deficiency of iron, calcium and vitamins (especially D and B) so that anaemia, glossitis, and rickets or osteomalacia, are usually present in addition to loss of weight.

Many cases improve on a diet free from gluten, which is a constituent of ordinary flour.

7. Diarrhoea may also result from *poisoning* with various substances. In medicolegal circles the most important is arsenic.

8. Self-medication with *purgatives* is a common cause of intermittent diarrhoea in introspective individuals with a 'bowel complex'. This is discussed further in the section below.

Constipation

Constipation may arise either from delay in the passage of faeces through the intestine or delay in the evacuation of faeces from the rectum. From a practical viewpoint, patients with constipation may be divided into two main groups, namely those in whom there is no organic cause, and those in whom there is some underlying pathology. It should be emphasized that the first group is by far the larger.

1. No organic lesion. A very large number of individuals complain that they suffer from constipation. There are usually two main factors which have contributed to this state of affairs. The first is that in many there has been, in the early years of life, a tendency to neglect to empty the bowel when the reflex mechanism of the rectum has indicated that it is full, owing to social inconvenience or laziness. After a time there is blunting of the reflex mechanism and the individual, who now has a 'lazy bowel', begins to use purgatives at first intermittently but later regularly. The other factor is that many people have the erroneous idea that a variety of ill-defined diseases will overtake them if evacuation of the bowel is not frequent and regular. Advertisements in the press and elsewhere encourage this misconception and serve to focus still more the attention of the rather hypochondriacal individual on the bowel function. It should be realized that for some individuals it is perfectly natural for the bowels to move on alternate days or at even greater intervals. Furthermore, there is no convincing evidence that constipation causes 'poisoning of the system' or leads to disease in any other way.

Management of this group of patients is difficult and requires re-education of the patient to break the purgative habit, reassurance, advice to take as much exercise as possible, a diet containing natural roughage such as fruit and vegetables, and a high fluid intake.

2. Organic cause. The other group of patients with constipation is those in whom there is some organic cause. Among the simpler of these are painful haemorrhoids, and fissure and pregnancy. Among the more serious are carcinoma of the colon, as referred to above, and external pressure on the intestine from other varieties of abdominal growths (e.g. a large ovarian carcinoma pressing on the pelvic colon). It is obvious that the essential step in the management of patients in this group is detection and correction of the underlying lesion.

Hernia

Hernia is an extremely common abdominal condition. The term means the protrusion or herniation of a portion of the bowel (or other abdominal viscus through the abdominal wall). There are a large number of herniae described but the common varieties occur in the inguinal and femoral region. They are characterized by a swelling which has a cough impulse and can commonly be reduced. Apart from the discomfort they cause the importance of hernia lies in the fact that the loops of bowel they contain may become strangulated (cut off from their blood supply) and thus become gangrenous. This is a serious condition and threatens life. The treatment of hernia is to reduce the contents into the abdominal wall and remove the hernial sac (herniotomy) and then to repair the defect in the abdominal wall (herniorrhaphy). In case of strangulation the devitalized bowel must be removed and the continuity of the gastrointestinal tract repaired by end-to-end anastomosis. The hernia is then repaired.

Haemorrhoids

This is an extremely common condition in the Western world, the piles presenting either as bright red bleeding per anus or as a prolapse at the anal verge. Occasionally piles may strangulate with severe pain. Treatment is by the avoidance of constipation, by injection in the submucosa of the anal canal in early cases but haemorrhoidectomy is frequently necessary.

Diverticular disease

This is an extremely common condition particularly in obese middle-aged women. It is especially common in the Western world and is said to be associated with a lack of dietary fibre. Small pouches bulging from the colonic wall form mainly in the left side of the colon and in the sigmoid region especially.

The symptoms consist of aching pain in the left lower abdomen, often accompanied by constipation. Occasionally one of the diverticulae perforate causing a pericolic abscess or peritonitis. This is a very dangerous condition which frequently ends fatally. Very occasionally a diverticulum bleeds heavily and can lead to collapse and shock.

Diagnosis is by barium enema X-ray examination. In the late stages when fibrosis and scarring has occurred the differentiation from cancer can be difficult and sigmoidoscopy or colonoscopy is necessary.

Treatment is by adjustment to the diet and the consumption of a high fibre or bran diet is often beneficial. Occasionally surgical resection is needed for advanced cases and is always needed for the treatment of pericolic abscess or perforation.

Investigation of patients with bowel symptoms

In the clinical examination of the patient particular attention should be paid to the nutrition, temperature, the presence of anaemia, and the presence of masses in the abdomen. The spleen and the liver should be particularly sought for and enlargement noted. Digital examination of the lower part of the rectum must always be performed since it is not uncommon for a small rectal carcinoma to be detected even though the symptoms may not suggest such a lesion. Visual examination of the lower bowel by the use of a proctoscope and sigmoidoscope and more recently examination of the entire colon through a flexible fiberoptic colon-scope are also necessary and biopsy specimens may be removed for histological examination.

The stool should be examined by the naked eye (the appearances may be practically diagnostic as in steatorrhoea) for blood, and for pathogenic organisms, if there is any suspicion of an infective aetiology.

Radiological examination of the bowel after a barium enema is an extremely useful way of detecting structural changes and if air is introduced into the colon along with the barium then a more clearly defined picture is obtained. The characteristic changes in cancer are those of an irregular filling defect. Diverticulae can be seen as referred to above and in ulcerative colitis or Crohn's disease the bowel wall can be seen to be rigid and narrowed with loss of characteristic mucosal pattern.

INTESTINAL OBSTRUCTION

Obstruction of the gastrointestinal tract can occur at any level. Obstruction affecting the oesophagus and pyloric outlet of the stomach have already been described.

Obstruction of the small bowel is usually the result of impaction of small bowel within a hernial orifice, or due to twisting (volvulus) of the bowel upon itself or in relation to an intra-abdominal band or adhesions. If the blood supply to the bowel is also obstructed, gangrene of the affected length of the bowel wall results. Obstruction of the large bowel is usually due to tumours.

The cardinal features of intestinal obstruction are abdominal pain, vomiting, distension and constipation. The pain is colicky, often abrupt in onset, and becomes progressively more severe. In small bowel or proximal colon obstruction it is felt in the upper abdomen whereas the pain of distal colonic obstruction is subumbilical. Vomiting occurs early in obstruction of the small bowel but is often a late feature in colonic obstruction. It tends to be particularly early, profuse and frequent in proximal small bowel obstruction and leads to dehydration and loss of electrolytes. Abdominal distension occurs earlier and is much more marked in obstruction of the colon but may be less prominent in upper small bowel obstruction. Obstruction in the distal colon causes initial swelling and tenderness in the right iliac fossa but this is soon followed by small bowel distension once the pressure forces open the ileocaecal valve. Complete obstruction of the bowel is associated with absolute constipation (failure to pass flatus or faeces) although one or two small motions may be passed shortly after the onset of obstruction.

The features of intestinal obstruction may be accompanied by evidence suggesting the underlying cause, e.g., the presence of a tender, non-reducible hernia indicating probable small bowel involvement, a history of change in bowel habit and perhaps the passage of blood and mucus per rectum suggesting a colonic neoplasm, or the patient may already be known to be suffering from a disorder such as Crohn's disease which may predispose to small bowel obstruction.

The level of the obstruction may be confirmed by taking a straight X-ray of the abdomen in the erect and supine positions. Fluid levels are seen within the distended bowel and the pattern of the gas shadows and their distribution may be helpful in reaching a diagnosis.

The principles of treatment are the early relief of pain, the passage of a nasogastric tube to alleviate vomiting and allow aspiration of fluid from the stomach and small bowel, the correction of dehydration and electrolyte deficits, and surgical intervention to relieve the obstruction. The abdomen is opened and the small bowel, if entrapped, is relieved. Any gangrenous segments of bowel are excised and the continuity of the bowel is restored by anastomosis. In obstruction of the large bowel, a similar approach may be possible but very frequently it is necessary to decompress temporarily the bowel by means of a colostomy opening on to the body surface. Such a colostomy may be permanent if the obstruction has been caused by an inoperable distal tumour, but may be temporary, allowing the surgeon to return at a second operation for removal of a resectable cancer and reconstitution of the bowel.

9

Disorders of the liver, gall-bladder and pancreas

ANATOMICAL AND PHYSIOLOGICAL CONSIDERATIONS

The liver is a very large organ which plays an essential part in many of the body functions. It is situated in the right upper abdomen under the dome of the diaphragm. Venous blood from the alimentary tract is carried to the liver by the portal vein and arterial blood via the hepatic artery from a branch of the abdominal aorta. Bile is drained from the liver by the common hepatic duct and passes to the gallbladder where it is concentrated. From the gallbladder the bile passes to the duodenum by means of the common bile duct which, in its terminal portion, traverses the head of the pancreas.

The main functions of the liver may be considered under the following headings.

1. Protein metabolism. The liver plays a vital role in the breakdown of protein to a form which is suitable for energy use. It also plays a part in the synthesis of fibrinogen, albumin, globulin and prothrombin.

2. Carbohydrate metabolism. Glycogen is stored in the liver. It is derived partly from the carbohydrate of the food but, in addition, the liver is able to synthesize glycogen from protein and from fat.

3. Fat metabolism. The bile salts produced by the liver are essential for the emulsification and digestion of fat. Liver cells also play a part in lipid metabolism and fat oxidation.

4. Detoxicating function. Many toxic by-products of metabolism are disposed of by the liver, and also a great variety of drugs, some by direct excretion in the bile, some by oxidation (e.g. alcohol), some by conjugation with other chemical substances, and some by destruction.

5. Secretion of bile. One of the main functions of the hepatic cells is the extraction of bilirubin from the blood carried to the liver from the spleen and other parts of the reticulo-endothelial system and the active secretion of it into the bile passages where it forms bile pigment.

6. *Other functions.* The liver is an important storage organ for a variety of essential substances including vitamins A, D, K, B_{12}, iron and water. It also produces a number of factors concerned in blood coagulation amongst the most important of which are fibrinogen, prothrombin (factor VII) and factor V.

JAUNDICE

Jaundice or icterus, is a yellowish discolouration of the skin due to an increase in the pigment bilirubin in the blood and tissue fluids. When the increase is slight it is detectable only by chemical analysis of the blood but as the concentration of bilirubin rises a yellow tint appears in the sclera and is followed by yellow colouration of the skin and mucous membranes. In mild cases the yellowness is discernible only by careful examination in good light. In severe cases the yellow colour is intense and may assume a green hue.

The increase in pigment always occurs as a result of a disturbance in the normal metabolism of bilirubin and to understand the causation of jaundice it is necessary to have a simple appreciation of normal bile metabolism.

Normal bilirubin metabolism.

This may conveniently be considered to occur in the following stages (Fig. 9.1).

1. The red blood cells survive for about 100 days and are then broken down in the spleen and other parts of the reticuloendothelial system. The haemoglobin from the cells is broken into haem and globin and the haem is further divided into an iron-containing part, which is stored for further use, and an iron-free residue, which forms the bile pigment bilirubin.

2. Bilirubin is transported to the liver and in this prehepatic phase it is bound to plasma albumin and is said to be unconjugated. It is actively secreted by the hepatic cells into the tiny intrahepatic ducts of the biliary system and in its passage through the liver cells it becomes detached from albumin and conjugated with glucoronic acid. The unconjugated bilirubin is not soluble in water and cannot be filtered by the glomerulus of the kidney whereas the posthepatic or conjugated bilirubin can be filtered and hence can appear in the urine.

3. The biliary system drains the bile from the liver to the gallbladder where it is concentrated by the absorption of water. The bile then passes down the common bile duct, which traverses the head of the pancreas on its way to the duodenum; as will be seen

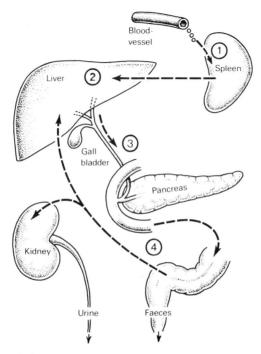

Fig. 9.1 The principal steps in normal bilirubin metabolism.

later, this is a very important relationship. Bile pigment, altered to urobilinogen in the alimentary canal, is responsible for the normal colour of the faeces.

4. A small amount of urobilinogen is reabsorbed from the alimentary tract and some of it is excreted in the urine as urobilinogen. Normal urine does not contain bilirubin (bile).

Many classifications of jaundice have been proposed. The following is perhaps the simplest.

Haemolytic jaundice.

This is due to excessive production of bilirubin resulting from abnormally rapid destruction of red blood corpuscles. The liver secretes much of this bilirubin which is subsequently converted in the gut into urobilinogen. The stools therefore contain larger amounts of urobilinogen than normal and are consequently dark orange in colour. The urobilinogen content of the urine is also increased. In many patients, however, the liver is unable to deal with all the excess bilurubin which accumulates in the plasma and this results in jaundice. This excess bilirubin is unconjugated and cannot pass through the kidney and hence cannot appear in the urine.

A well known example of this variety of icterus is congenital acholuric jaundice (congenital spherocytosis) which is discussed in the chapter on blood disorders. Other examples are the jaundice which accompanies diseases causing haemolysis of blood, such as malaria.

Obstructive (*cholestatic*) *jaundice*

Here there is no excessive production of bilirubin but there is an obstruction to the passage of bilirubin from the liver cells and it regurgitates into the blood stream causing jaundice. The bilirubin is conjugated after its passage through the liver cells and is therefore water soluble and appears in the urine where it can be readily detected by simple tests. On account of the obstruction the bilirubin reaching the intestine is reduced in amount or in complete obstruction, is entirely absent. Consequently the urobilinogen is diminished or absent resulting in pale or even white 'clay coloured' stools.

Obstructive jaundice may be grouped into intrahepatic and extrahepatic disorders.

Intrahepatic cholestasis

Obstruction to the small biliary canaliculi can occur as a result of drug toxicity and in association with some diseases which damage the liver cells with disorganization of its structure. Thus severe intrahepatic cholestasis can occur following ingestion of the drug chlorpromazine and can also occur as part of the disease picture in infective hepatitis.

Extrahepatic cholestasis

Extrahepatic jaundice is due to obstruction to the flow of bile through the extrahepatic bile ducts system. The commonest cause for this is the presence of gallstones within the common bile duct but carcinoma of the common bile duct or head of the pancreas are not infrequent. At first the obstruction is incomplete but progresses until no bile reaches the intestine at all and clay coloured stools result.

Hepatocellular (*hepatic*) *jaundice*

A number of diseases directly damage the liver cells so that they are unable to metabolize the bilirubin which is delivered to them. In most of these conditions there is also an element of intrahepatic cholestasis so that the picture is intermediate between that of haemolysis and frank extrahepatic obstruction. Viral hepatitis (which includes hepatitis due to virus A, virus B, and non A-non B hepatitis) is the commonest cause of jaundice due to hepatocellular damage in Western countries. Other important causes include alcohol excess and drug induced disease such as following overdosage with paracetamol.

Infective hepatitis

Aetiology
It is due to a virus (hepatitis A virus) ingested with the food and has an incubation period of about one month. Infective hepatitis has its maximal incidence in children and young adults; outbreaks are not uncommon in schools, institutions, and in the armed services. The infectivity is greatest before the onset of jaundice; thereafter there is little danger of those in contact with the patient contracting the infection.

Clinical features
The common sequence of events is that for a few days the patient feels out of sorts, depressed, has a very poor appetite and may vomit a few times. The diagnosis is made evident by the development of jaundice, first apparent in the eyes and later in the skin. The degree of jaundice varies from being very slight (perhaps detectable only by chemical analysis) to being very intense. The urine is darker than normal in colour and contains both bile and urobilinogen. The stools are usually only slightly pale in colour except in severe cases with gross intrahepatic obstruction. The liver is commonly slightly enlarged and tender. A haemorrhagic tendency, due to complex defects, is present in severe cases (p. 235).

Course and prognosis
The majority of patients make a complete recovery after an illness lasting for a few weeks. In a small proportion the infection is so virulent that fatal hepatic necrosis is caused. A further small proportion are left with chronic inflammatory changes in the liver and subsequently develop cirrhosis of the liver.

Treatment
There is no specific treatment for infective hepatitis. The usual measures employed are rest, a diet low in fat but high in carbohydrate

and complete abstinence from alcohol during the period of jaundice and for several months thereafter.

Hepatitis B virus (serum hepatitis)

Hepatitis B virus is transmitted by syringes or needles which have been imperfectly sterilized (hence the earlier term syringe hepatitis), by the transfusion of blood or plasma donated by an individual who is a carrier of the virus (hence the term serum jaundice) and it is now known that it is also propagated from person to person by close contacts. In the United Kingdom about 1:500 of the population are symptomless carriers of hepatitis B surface antigen (HBsAg) and in some geographic areas, e.g., the Middle East and the Far East, the prevalence of carriers is much higher. The prevalence of the carrier state is also higher in patients from institutes for the mentally handicapped, in patients with haemophilia and other blood disorders who receive multiple transfusions of blood or blood products, in drug addicts, and in patients attending renal dialysis units for long term treatment. Dental practitioners should be particularly alert regarding possible transmission of infection, including to themselves, from such patients.

Dentists and members of their staff who are antigen positive may constitute a risk of infection to patients. It is recommended that they should wear gloves when treating patients and that they should cover any cuts or abrasions so that blood cannot be transferred to the patient.

Sterilization of instruments by boiling is not sufficient to prevent this type of viral infection. Instruments should be autoclaved or, alternatively, disposable equipment used. This applies especially to syringes and needles.

The incubation period of type B hepatitis ranges from 30 to 180 days with the majority being between 60 and 110 days. In any patient with jaundice suspected of viral nature it is very important to make enquiry as to any injection, transfusions, or other treatment received at such times. The clinical features of the condition are indistinguishable from those of type A hepatitis. The prognosis and treatment likewise are similar.

Non A—non B hepatitis

Non A-Non B hepatitis is also caused by a virus, or viruses, and is probably spread by direct contact as well by percutaneous introduction. The incubation period may be as short as 10 days or up to 150 days. Our knowledge of the condition is still fragmentary.

Extrahepatic cholestasis

This variety of jaundice is often referred to as 'surgical' jaundice since it is amenable to cure or relief by surgical methods. It is important to realize that in operating for jaundice or (of importance to dentists) in the presence of jaundice, there is a haemorrhagic tendency (page 235) and prior to surgery injections to vitamin K must be given so that the level of prothrombin is restored to normal within the blood.

In this variety of jaundice the pigmentation may be very marked and may assume a greenish hue but it is important to realize that the obstruction may be incomplete as occurs when a gallstone intermittently obstructs the common bile duct. The stools are usually pale so that no bile pigment reaches the intestine and the urine contains large amounts of bile (bilirubin) and appears very concentrated and greenish-black in colour. In severe cases they may be bradycardia and pruritus, due to the retention of bile salts.

Although clinical evidence of the cause of obstruction is usually present this is not always so and it is always important to think of obstruction as a cause of jaundice. In the case of gallstones there is

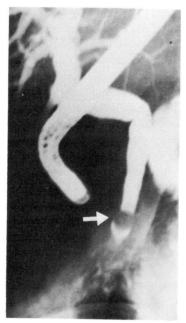

Fig. 9.2 Endoscopic retrograde cholangiogram showing a gallstone at the lower end of the bile duct (arrowed). The endoscope has been passed through the oesophagus and stomach to lie in the duodenum allowing the passage of a fine catheter into the bile duct from below

frequently a typical history of attacks of colicky pain in the right upper abdomen associated with intermittent attacks of jaundice. By contrast in cancer, either of the pancreas or of the common bile duct, the classical picture is of progressive jaundice associated with loss of energy and loss of weight and usually without pain. On the other hand there may be quite severe back pain in cancer of the pancreas. In extrahepatic obstruction the diagnosis may be established before operation by radiological methods (Fig. 9.2). Exploratory operation with intraoperative radiology is only rarely necessary. Stones within the common bile duct are always associated with stones in the gallbladder and treatment is by cholecystectomy and exploration of the common bile duct with removal of the stones. Occasionally a bypass operation between the common bile duct and the intestine is performed.

In cancer of the pancreas the prognosis is poor and indeed most tumours are inoperable by the time the patient comes to surgery. All that is possible in these situations is to bypass the flow of bile to the intestine and so relieve the jaundice. Radiotherapy and chemotherapy may be employed but no great success has attended either. In the few patients in whom a small operable pancreatic or common bile duct tumour is found an extensive operation removing the entire head of pancreas and loop of the duodenum (pancreatico-duodenectomy) is possible. The risk of the procedure is high and reconstruction of the integrity of the gastrointestinal tract difficult.

There are a variety of rarer conditions which can cause extrahepatic obstruction and amongst these are carcinoma of the ampulla of Vater or duodenum, a number of congenital cysts of the extrahepatic bile duct system, benign structure of the bile duct and chronic pancreatitis with fibrosis in the head of the pancreas.

Other hepatic disorders

Cirrhosis of the liver

Cirrhosis of the liver may be caused by the late effects of infective hepatitis, or overindulgence in alcohol for many years especially if the diet has been neglected. In many cases, however, neither of these factors is apparent and the cause is obscure.

The condition is characterised pathologically by a progressive replacement of liver cells by fibrous tissue. The fibrosis leads to deterioration in hepatic function with eventual liver failure (cholaemia) and also to interference with the flow of blood through the liver resulting in portal hypertension.

The main clinical features of liver failure are a poor appetite, a tendency to morning dyspepsia, a sallow complexion with a trace of jaundice, ascites and oedema. The liver is enlarged and firm in the early stages but later becomes small in size as the fibrous tissue contracts. Portal hypertension causes splenic enlargement and the development of oesophageal varices with the likelihood of recurrent alimentary haemorrhage. Small dilated blood vessels, descriptively termed spider naevi, may be seen on the face and on the upper part of the trunk. There may also be redness of the palms of the hands (palmar erythema). The course of the disorder is usually steadily progressive.

Surgical measures to reduce the portal hypertension by shunting portal blood to the low pressure systemic system are sometimes feasible but in many circumstances it is preferable to rely on medical treatment the main points being adherence to a suitable diet and the avoidance of alcohol, the use of blood transfusion to deal with haematemesis and the control of ascites by diuretics.

Tumours of the liver

Primary tumour of the liver is extremely rare in Britain but it is a common malignant neoplasm in Africa and South-East Asia. If the lesion is small, then partial resection of the liver can be curative but this is rarely so. The results of palliative therapy are poor and there is usually a rapid progression to death.

On the other hand, secondary tumours involving the liver are a very common development following primary cancer of the stomach, bowel, lung, and breast. Here again the outlook is poor but effective palliative treatment can be afforded by the skilled use of chemotherapy and surgical resection has an occasional use for localized solitary lesions.

Hepatic necrosis

Acute hepatic necrosis, or acute yellow atrophy, is fortunately uncommon. There is massive death of hepatic cells due to overwhelming infection (severe cases of infective hepatitis or Weil's disease), gross nutritional deficiency, or chemical poisoning. In many cases there is an associated acute renal failure. The prognosis is extremely grave but perfusion through charcoal columns and the skilled use of blood coagulation factors may allow a time for the liver to recover.

Liver transplantation

Transplantation of the liver has been used in some patients for the treatment of advanced cirrhosis, and liver tumours.

DISEASES OF THE GALLBLADDER

Cholecystitis

Inflammation of the gallbladder may be acute or chronic. The condition occurs most often in middle-aged people and it is commoner in women and more likely to develop in obese individuals. The disease is almost always accompanied by the presence of stones in the gallbladder and the infecting organism is most frequently *E. coli*. The patient may suffer attacks of repeated inflammation which should be distinguished from attacks of biliary colicky pain which occurs in association with the presence of the gallstones.

In the acute stages of the disorder the patient has severe right sided upper abdominal pain which has a tendency to pass through to the right shoulder blade. The temperature is elevated, vomiting is common, there is tenderness over the gallbladder and a trace of jaundice is frequently present. In association with this the urine may be rather dark for a short period due to the presence of bile although the stools seldom become pale. In severe cases the acutely inflamed gallbladder may become filled with pus (empyema of the gallbladder) and in very severe cases gangrene and perforation of the gallbladder may occur with consequent peritonitis. Acute cholecystitis usually settles following the use of an antibiotic and restriction to a fluid diet for a few days but the presence of a rising pulse rate, continued fever and spreading abdominal tenderness are an indication for surgery. After subsidence of the acute attack a low fat diet with a high carbohydrate content is prescribed but there is a considerable tendency for the infection to recur with the subsequent development of chronic cholecystitis.

Chronic cholecystitis is characterized by a flatulent dyspepsia plus recurrent bouts of right sided upper abdominal pain due to acute exacerbations. Attacks are often precipitated by the taking of fatty foods. Mild cases may remain largely free from symptoms provided they adhere to a low fat diet but, if the attacks are recurring frequently and are severe then removal of the gallbladder (cholecystectomy) is the treatment of choice. Indeed, provided the patient is otherwise well many surgeons recommend cholecystectomy for chronic cholecystitis with associated gallstones because recurrence is so frequent and because the complications can be dangerous.

Gallstones

Gallstones arise because of the precipitation of cholesterol and calcium bilirubinate from the bile. This occurs in association with alterations in the constituents of the bile, with stasis in the gallbladder with the presence of infection. Gallstones (cholelithiasis) are usually present in association with chronic cholecystitis. The attacks of pain are very similar to those experienced by the patient with acute cholecystitis but fever and constitutional illness are not present. If a stone passes into, and becomes lodged within the common bile duct obstructive jaundice results. This is a dangerous condition characterized by fever, rigor and jaundice and may be complicated by infection passing into the blood stream (bacteraemia). However, stones may remain within the common bile duct for many years and be quite symptom free and revealed only by X-ray study. Very occasionally the gallbladder may become adherent to the adjacent duodenum and a gallstone erode into the small bowel. If such a stone is large enough it may obstruct the small bowel.

The treatment of gallstones is cholecystectomy and this should be performed if the general condition of the patient permits. The patient with stones within the common bile duct is seldom well and indeed the condition is sufficiently dangerous to warrant exploration of the common bile duct and removal of the stone. At operation for removal of the gallbladder it is a good practice to X-ray the common bile duct at operation to ensure that stones within it are not missed.

PANCREATITIS

Inflammation of the pancreas may be acute, recurrent or chronic. The disease is commonly associated either with the presence of gallstones or in association with a high alcohol intake.

In acute pancreatitis the patient is suddenly stricken with upper abdominal pain and repeated vomiting. There is considerable associated shock with a high pulse rate and low blood pressure and not infrequently the patient experiences respiratory difficulty and is cyanosed. The serum amylase is grossly elevated. Treatment is by conservative means including the use of intravenous fluids and pethidine for the relief of pain. The bowel is rested by means of nasogastric suction and oral fluids are prescribed. If gallstones are present they are removed and the patient is instructed to abstain from alcohol and to remain on a low fat diet.

In the presence of gallstones, particularly in the common bile duct, attacks may become recurrent and chronic pancreatitis is particularly likely to develop in those patients who consume much alcohol. Chronic pancreatitis is an extremely difficult condition to treat. The patient must abstain from alcohol and any biliary pathology must be treated surgically. Occasionally, surgical removal of a portion of the pancreas (pancreatectomy) is effective. The fibrosis which occurs in the head of the pancreas with compression of the common bile duct and resulting in jaundice has been alluded to earlier.

10

Disorders of the renal system

PHYSIOLOGICAL CONSIDERATIONS

The kidneys, which are measure about 12 cm in length, are situated retroperitoneally in the posterior part of the abdomen. Each is covered with a firm capsule. If the kidney is divided longitudinally the appearances are as shown diagrammatically in Figure 10.1. At the hilum, the pelvis of the ureter, the renal artery, and the renal vein are in close proximity. The blood supply is very abundant; the renal artery is short and arises directly from the abdominal aorta.

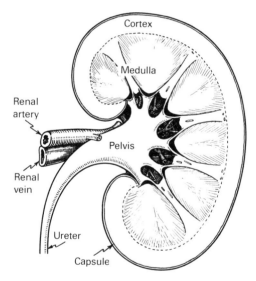

Fig. 10.1 The appearance of the kidney on section.

The nephron

The nephron, comprising the glomerular tuft, Bowman's capsule, and the tubule, is the essential functional unit of the kidney; each kidney contains approximately one million nephrons. The glomeru-

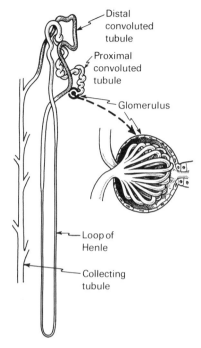

Distal convoluted tubule

Proximal convoluted tubule

Glomerulus

Loop of Henle

Collecting tubule

Fig. 10.2 The principal components of the nephron.

lus is a tuft of capillaries which invaginates Bowman's capsule, the expanded end of the renal tubule, as shown in Figure 10.2. The tubule comprises the proximal convoluted tubule, the loop of Henle, and the distal convoluted tubule. Collecting tubules carry the urine to the renal pelvis from where it passes to the ureters and the bladder.

Formation of urine

The main steps in the formation of urine are as follows:

1. A large volume of filtrate, similar in composition to plasma, except that it is free from protein and fat, is formed from blood flowing through the glomerular capillaries.

2. The filtrate is modified in its passage down the renal tubules in the following ways:

(a) The volume is greatly reduced by the absorption of water.

(b) Other substances which are of value to the body (e.g. glucose, electrolytes) are wholly or partly reabsorbed.

(c) Certain substances are excreted into the filtrate by the tubule cells (e.g. creatinine).

(d) The pH is adjusted according to the need to excrete excess acid or alkali.

Features of normal urine

The average 24-hour urinary volume in the healthy adult is 1,500 ml. Normally the night volumes is less than the day volume, a fact of considerable convenience.

Urine is a clear, straw-coloured fluid with a specific gravity which may vary from about 1·002 to about 1·030 depending upon the concentration of solutes. It does not normally contain sugar or protein (albumin).

Functions of the kidney

The main functions of the kidneys are the elimination of waste products of metabolism and the control of fluid and electrolyte balance.

1. The kidney is the most important route for the elimination of the waste products of metabolism particularly the end products of protein metabolism. A useful index of this function is the level of the blood urea (normal 15 to 40 mg per 100 ml or 2·5 to 7·0 mmol per 1).

2. The kidney plays a vital role in regulating the fluid balance of the body. Thus, if there is a high fluid intake the kidney compensates by excreting a large volume of dilute urine, while if there is a danger of dehydration (either from low fluid intake or from excess fluid loss by other channels as in diarrhoea and vomiting) the urinary volume is low.

3. Control of the pH of the blood within very narrow limits is essential for health and the kidney is one of the main instruments by which this is achieved. If there is a tendency for an increase in the acid radicals in the blood (acidosis), the kidney excretes a more acid urine and, conversely, if there is an increase in the alkali radicals (alkalosis) an alkaline urine is formed. The lungs also play an important part in controlling acid-base balance.

4. Many drugs used therapeutically, or toxic substances taken accidentally or suicidally, are excreted by the kidney either in their original form or as breakdown products.

It is important to realize that the kidneys have a great reserve of function. This is amply illustrated by the fact that an individual can lead a perfectly healthy life should one kidney have to be removed (nephrectomy) because of traumatic damage or unilateral renal disease.

INVESTIGATION OF RENAL DISORDERS

In the investigation of renal disorders the customary practice of taking a full history and performing a full clinical examination is adhered to and is followed by examination of the urine, assessment of renal function, and, in certain cases, by radiological or visual examination of the renal tract.

History
The main points about which specific enquiry must be made are past history of sore throats, the presence of oedema, the occurrence of painful micturition (dysuria), or frequency of micturition, and any alterations in the appearance of the urine.

Clinical examination
Attention is directed particularly to the presence of oedema, the blood pressure, the size of the left ventricle, the appearance of the optic fundi, the presence of enlargement or tenderness of the kidneys, the bladder size, and, in males, the size of the prostate gland (this is assessed by digital rectal examination).

Examination of urine
This entails determination of certain physical characteristics (especially volume, specific gravity, colour, reaction), chemical examination for abnormal constituents (especially sugar and protein), microscopic examination (especially for blood and pus) and bacteriological examination. The commoner urinary abnormalities are discussed below.

Assessment of renal function
A precise assessment of renal function is a complex matter but sufficient information may be gained in many cases by measuring the ability of the kidney to produce a concentrated urine and by determining the level of urea in the blood (normal 15 to 40 mg per 100 ml or 2.5 to 7.0 mmol per l).

After fluid restriction the normal kidney will produce a concentrated urine (specific gravity not less than 1·025) while after a copious fluid intake the urine will be dilute (specific gravity around 1·004 to 1·002). In the presence of impaired renal function the specific gravity range becomes progressively less until finally the specific gravity becomes fixed at about 1·010.

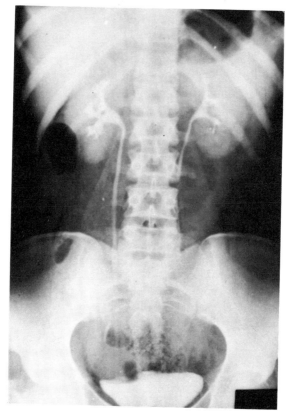

Fig. 10.3 A normal intravenous pyelogram (IVP) showing kidneys, ureters and bladder

Radiology and endoscopy

A straight X-ray of the abdomen may reveal the presence of opaque renal calculi or of enlargement of the kidneys. Additional information is gained by radiology, either after the intravenous injection of a radio-opaque dye which is excreted by the kidney (intravenous pyelography, see Fig. 10.3) or after injection of the dye directly into the ureters following uretetic catherization under direct vision through a cystoscope (retrograde pyelography). Cystoscopy also permits visual examination of the bladder mucosa and the taking of biopsy specimens.

COMMON ABNORMALITIES OF URINE

Polyuria

An increased volume of urine occurs physiologically after a high fluid intake, therapeutically after the administration of a diuretic, and pathologically in diabetes mellitus, diabetes insipidus, and chronic nephritis. When there is polyuria the specific gravity is low; the only exception to this is in diabetes mellitus, where, owing to the sugar present in the urine, the specific gravity is high.

Oliguria

A decreased volume of urine follows as a natural consequence of a low fluid intake. The commoner disease states associated with oliguria are acute nephritis, congestive cardiac failure, and excessive fluid loss from conditions producing diarrhoea and vomiting. Anuria, which is much less common than oliguria, means a complete cessation of urine formation.

Oliguria and anuria must always be differentiated from retention of urine caused by some obstruction to urinary outflow (a common example of this is prostatic gland enlargement).

Proteinuria

This is often referred to as albuminuria, but the term 'proteinuria' is more accurate since globulin is also present. Protein in the urine may be detected by the appearance of a while coagulate on heating acidified urine; the reaction is the same as that which occurs on boiling an egg. A simpler test involving a colour change on a specially treated strip of paper which is dipped into the urine is now in general use.

The causes of proteinuria may be considered in three groups.

1. Due to kidney disease of which the most important is nephritis.

2. Associated with a disease process elsewhere, e.g. congestive cardiac failure or any febrile illness.

3. Orthostatic proteinuria which is seen in adolescents and young adults. It is believed that a postural defect (undue lordosis of the lumbar spine) leads to kinking of the veins concerned with venous return from the kidney when the individual is upright and the consequent passive congestion causes proteinuria. Protein is present in the urine formed when the patient is ambulant but is absent from the urine formed during recumbency; there is no other urinary abnormality. There is no renal lesion and the prognosis is good. No treatment is required.

Haematuria

Copious blood in the urine produces a frankly blood-stained urine, lesser amounts lead to a smoky-brown appearance, while small quantities are detectably only by microscopy.

Haematuria may result from medical or surgical disorders of the renal tract (e.g. acute nephritis, tumour, renal calculus, trauma), from haemorrhagic disorders (e.g. acute leukaemia, purpura, haemophilia) or from subacute bacterial endocarditis.

Glycosuria
Sugar in the urine may be detected by a simple tablet test or even simpler dip strip test.

The most important cause of glycosuria is diabetes mellitus. It is important to differentiate diabetes mellitus from the harmless condition of renal glycosuria which is due to a low renal threshold for glucose (see also p. 277).

NEPHRITIS (BRIGHT'S DISEASE)

The subject of nephritis, or glomerulonephritis, is an extremely complex one but, from the dental student's viewpoint, it will be sufficient to give a very simplified account of the main clinical types of the disorder.

Acute proliferative glomerulonephritis
Other terms which are used are acute nephritis and acute haemorrhagic nephritis, and Type I nephritis. The condition is, in a sense, akin to rheumatic fever in that it is caused by an immunological reaction to recent infection with haemolytic streptococci. The glomeruli of both kidneys show acute cellular proliferation which may be very marked.

Clinical features
The condition is seen most commonly in young people. A history of sore throat about 10 to 14 days before is frequently present. The onset is abrupt usually with headache and vomiting; there may be pain in the loins. There is a slight degree of generalized oedema which is most evident below the eyes in the morning, leading to a puffy appearance of the face (Fig. 10.4). The blood pressure is slightly or moderately elevated. The urine is reduced in amount and contains protein and blood. The blood urea is raised as a result of impaired renal function.

Course
The great majority of patients with acute nephritis get completely better after an illness lasting a few weeks. A small number die in

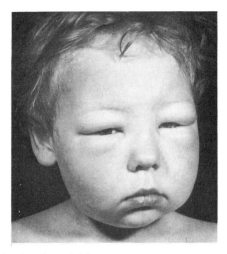

Fig. 10.4 Facial oedema in nephritis.

the acute stage, either from renal or cardiac failure, while others develop chronic nephritis with progressive renal damage.

Treatment
No curative measures are available, the cause of the disorder being unaffected by the use of antibiotics or immunosuppressives. The intake of fluid, potassium, salt and protein will require careful regulation as long as renal function is seriously impaired. Careful follow-up is indicated and any further upper respiratory infections should be treated energetically.

Membranous glomerulonephritis
This has also been known as subacute nephritis or Type II nephritis. The aetiology is obscure. The main pathological change is in the basement membrane of the glomerular capillaries which become much thickened.

Clinical features
The condition has an insidious onset and no history of previous sore throat is obtainable. The most striking clinical feature is oedema (Fig. 10.4). This may be extremely marked and, in addition to involving the limbs and the trunk, may produce ascites and pleural effusions. Pallor is usually prominent and may be out of keeping with the degree of anaemia which is usually present. The blood

pressure is usually normal in the early stages of the disorder but may become elevated later.

The urine contains very large quantities of protein and this leads to a fall in the plasma proteins which results in a diminution in the colloid osmotic pressure of the plasma; this is the main factor in the pathogenesis of the oedema (Fig. 6.5). The blood urea may be normal in the early stages but later it becomes elevated.

Course

The prognosis is rather less favourable than in acute nephritis. Although some patients recover spontaneously, others may die from intercurrent infection to which these individuals are more prone, while others develop progressive renal failure.

Treatment

It is customary to give a high protein diet in an attempt to replace the protein lost in the urine. The salt intake is restricted. The oedema can often be controlled by the use of a diuretic (a drug which acts on the renal tubules to increase the volume of urine).

The combination of gross proteinuria leading to low plasma proteins and hence to oedema is termed the *nephrotic syndrome* and membranous glomerulonephritis is an important cause in adults. In children the principal cause is a rather different lesion affecting only a part of the basement membrane and this variety of the nephrotic syndrome responds to steroid therapy.

Chronic nephritis

Chronic nephritis may follow a small proportion of cases of acute nephritis or it may develop in patients with membranous nephritis who do not die from intercurrent infection. In some instances there is no definite history of previous renal disease. A similar clinical picture results from chronic pyelonephritis.

The kidneys are smaller than normal, scarred, and granular. Microscopic examination reveals that many of the nephrons are replaced by fibrous tissue.

Clinical features

These are due to a combination of impaired renal function and hypertension. In the early stages of the disorder the kidney compensates for its inability to produce a concentrated urine by forming large quantities of more dilute urine and, in this way, the waste products of protein metabolism may be excreted. At this stage the main symptoms are polyuria and nocturia. The urine specific gravity is around 1·010 and there is little alteration from this figure following fluid restriction or increase. The urine contains protein, often in small amount, and a variable number of red cells and casts.

As the disease progresses, more and more nephrons go out of action and the kidney loses its ability to form a large volume of urine. When this occurs there is an inevitable retention in the body of the nitrogenous end products of protein metabolism associated with electrolyte imbalance and acidosis. Anaemia develops and may be severe. The features of this stage of chronic nephritis are essentially those of uraemia which is described in the following section.

The blood pressure elevation leads to arteriosclerotic changes in the blood vessels and to left ventricular hypertrophy; breathlessness and headache are the commonest symptoms. Cardiac failure may ensue. Changes in the optic fundi (narrowing of arteries, exudates, haemorrhages) are due to the hypertension.

Death may occur from uraemia, from cardiac failure or from a cerebrovascular catastrophe.

Treatment
The hypertension is controlled with drugs and the diet is modified particularly in respect of the protein content which requires to be progressively reduced as the renal failure progresses.

A new lease of life can now be afforded to many patients with 'end-stage' chronic nephritis by twice or thrice weekly treatment with an artificial kidney machine (regular dialysis therapy) or by renal transplantation. Reference has already been made (p. 189) to the possibility of hepatitis B virus infection in patients on regular dialysis. The dentist should also be aware that some patients on regular dialysis may be receiving anticoagulants and also that renal transplant patients will be receiving steroid therapy to minimise the possibility of rejection of the graft.

URINARY INFECTION AND PYELONEPHRITIS (NON-TUBERCULOUS)

Infection of the lower urinary passages (cystitis) is a very common condition. In some cases the infection also involves the upper renal tract, causing pyelonephritis, and this is a much more serious disorder since it may lead to renal failure and to hypertension.

Aetiology
The majority of cases are due to Gram-negative organisms, especially *E. coli*. The organisms may reach the kidney via the blood stream or from the lower urinary passages.

Important predisposing factors, which interfere with urinary flow, are pregnancy, prostatic gland enlargement, renal stone, hydronephrosis, congenital abnormalities and disease of the nervous system (e.g. disseminated sclerosis). A further factor is catheterization; unless this is done with meticulous care, infection is likely to follow. Many cases of urinary infection, however, occur without any apparent predisposing factor.

Clinical features

The patient with acute urinary infection usually has frequency of micturition, pain on micturition (dysuria), and sometimes haematuria. If the infection is severe, the temperature will be elevated. Suprapubic discomfort is present if the bladder is inflamed (cystitis) and loin pain is present if there is acute pyelonephritis.

Many patients with chronic urinary infection affecting the lower urinary passages or with chronic pyelonephritis have relatively little or even no urinary symptomatology. In these cases the condition may be detected on some routine examination of the urine, because the patient has an unexplained febrile illness or vague ill health, or, in the case of chronic pyelonephritis, because of the presence of renal failure or hypertension.

Diagnosis

The diagnosis is made in most cases by the demonstration of bacteria and pus in the urine. In acute cases there may be some confusion with abdominal emergencies such as appendicitis. In chronic pyelonephritis characteristic structural changes occur in the pelvis and these may be detected by radiology.

Treatment

Acute infections usually respond promptly to treatment with a sulphonamide or antibiotic to which the organism is sensitive, but recurrences are common. The infection tends to be more difficult to eradicate in cases of chronic infection and repeated courses of treatment may be required. In all cases it is important to consider and correct any underlying predisposing factor. If chronic pyelonephritis progresses to the stage of producing terminal renal failure regular dialysis or transplantation may be undertaken as in chronic nephritis.

URAEMIA

Uraemia, which literally means urine in the blood, is the term used to describe 'the metabolic disaster consequent upon renal failure'.

Aetiology
The causal factor may be primarily prerenal, renal, or postrenal; illustrative examples are given below.

Prerenal—severe hypotension leading to a fall in the filtration pressure in the glomerular capillaries.

Renal—chronic glomerulonephritis or chronic pyelonephritis.

Postrenal—chronic obstruction to urinary outflow by an enlarged prostate.

Clinical features
Chronic renal failure leads to a characteristic clinical picture; the symptoms and signs are due to complex biochemical derangements the chief being retention of nitrogenous end products (e.g. urea, creatinine), accumulation of potassium, and acidosis.

Restlessness, apathy, mental confusion and drowsiness are common *nervous* manifestations. Anorexia, nausea, and vomiting are common *alimentary* symptoms. The tongue is characteristically dry and covered with a dirty brown fur while the breath is foul and may smell of ammonia. Stomatitis may be present and the gums may bleed. There is a characteristic alteration in the *respiration*; the breathing is deeper and louder than normal (Kussmaul respiration) due to stimulation of the respiratory centre by the retained acid products. Hiccough is a common and distressing symptom. Examination of the *cardiovascular* system usually reveals hypertension if the uraemia is of renal origin; pericarditis may occur terminally.

Treatment
In cases of prerenal and postrenal uraemia there is good prospect of recovery if the patient can, by skilled correction of the biochemical derangements, be tided over the renal failure until such time as there is a return of renal function or until a procedure such as prostatectomy may be performed. In end stage renal uraemia the outlook has been transformed by the introduction of regular dialysis and transplantation.

OTHER RENAL DISORDERS

There are many other renal disorders and some of these are common and predominantly of surgical interest.

Hydronephrosis
The renal pelvis is dilated, often to a very considerable size. The condition follows chronic obstruction to the urinary outflow, e.g.

by calculus, or by external pressure on the ureter or by an aberrant renal artery. In conditions of chronic obstruction to the outflow of urine from the bladder back pressure may result in bilateral hydronephrosis. Infection is very likely to supervene and the dilated pelvis becomes filled with pus (pyonephrosis).

If there is sufficient functioning renal substance remaining then an attempt to remove the obstructive lesion is worthwhile; and the saccular dilated renal pelvis may be reconstructed by means of a plastic surgical operation. If there is very little renal substance remaining then the dilated sac, which is often filled with pus, should be removed by nephrectomy.

Renal calculus

Renal stones may be composed of phosphates, calcium oxalate, uric acid or urates, or rarely cystine. The phosphatic variety is seen particularly as a complication of urinary infection, whereas the cystine variety is due to an uncommon metabolic error. The aetiology of other varieties is uncertain. The term decubitus stone is used for the calcium stone which forms in the kidney in patients confined to bed for long periods particularly with skeletal disorders; there is decalcification of the skeleton and increased urinary excretion of calcium. Calcium stones are common in hyperparathyroidism (page 246).

Renal stones may cause a dull loin pain but, if the stone becomes lodged in the ureter, extremely severe pain associated with vomiting and collapse, results (renal colic). There may be haematuria. Such stones are usually passed into the bladder and if small enough are voided in the urine and the patient is managed with analgesia until this occurs. However, it is important to make certain since continued presence of the stone within the ureter is associated with subsidence of the pain and may be followed by the development of hydronephrosis. Stones which become impacted in the ureter must be removed (ureterolithotomy). Large stones within the renal pelvis can also be surgically removed. The pain caused by stones within the kidney or ureter must be distinguished from other causes of abdominal pain (e.g. gallstones).

Pyelonephritis is a very important complication of renal stones and surgical removal of the stones can be of great help in avoiding this problem.

Tumour

The commonest symptom of a tumour in the renal tract is haematuria which is often painless and in all such cases the renal tract must be thoroughly investigated. This includes the performance of intravenous pyelography and cystoscopy. Urinary tract tumours can present with other features such as hydronephrosis due to blockage of a ureter or by the presence of a secondary tumour.

The most important tumours of the renal tract are adenocarcinoma (hypernephroma) of the kidney which is particularly liable to cause secondary deposits in the bones and lungs, papillary adenocarcinoma of the renal pelvis, and papilloma or carcinoma of the bladder. These latter tumours are not nearly so likely to metastasize.

Hypernephroma is managed by surgical excision and even solitary secondary deposits may be excised with success in some cases. Tumours of the renal pelvis are usually also managed by a nephrectomy but papilloma of the bladder can be treated for long periods by endoscopic (transcystoscopic) fulguration. They are also sensitive to radiotherapy and large tumours which have failed to respond to these means can be treated by cystectomy. In this instance the flow of urine must be diverted to a loop of bowel.

In men carcinoma of the prostate commonly presents with symptoms similar to those caused by simple hypertrophy of the prostate. Important differentiating features are hardness of the gland and biochemical (high serum acid phosphatase) and radiological evidence of metastases. Obstruction to flow of urine by a prostatic carcinoma can be managed by transurethral resection of tumour at the neck of the bladder. The tumour is hormone dependent in many cases (see Ch. 5) and oestrogens (stilboestrol) can be used to manage the advanced disease and particularly to alleviate pain in bony metastases.

Prostatic hypertrophy
Enlargement of the prostate gland is very frequent in elderly men. There is progressive interference with urinary flow and, if not treated, renal damage results from back pressure and the development of bilateral hydronephrosis.

The treatment is surgical and the prostate may be removed either by open operation (transvesical or retropubic prostatectomy) or by the use of a diathermy cutting knife introduced with a special instrument through the urethra (transurethral resection).

Polycystic disease
Polycystic disease of the kidneys is one of the less uncommon congenital abnormalities which may affect the renal system. The kidneys are enlarged due to the presence of many cysts which, as they

increase in size cause progressive damage to the renal tissues. Renal failure and hypertension are common developments.

Renal artery stenosis

Very occasionally stenosis of the renal artery is associated with the development of hypertension. It is important to recognize this form of hypertension since it may be treated by surgical correction of the stenosed vessels.

Rupture of the kidney

The kidney is quite frequently damaged as a result of trauma. This may occur as a result of a direct blow (non-penetrating injury) or from a penetrating wound such as that caused by a knife or bullet.

Non-penetrating injury is managed in the first instance by conservative means and cessation of bleeding usually occurs. If not then operation is necessary. Penetrating wounds frequently require operation and the kidney is often not the only organ damaged.

11

Disorders of the haemopoietic system

PHYSIOLOGICAL CONSIDERATIONS

The average healthy adult has a blood volume of approximately five and a half litres. If a sample of blood, to which an anticoagulant such as heparin has been added, is centrifuged or is allowed to stand in a tube, the cellular elements will separate from the fluid plasma as depicted in Figure 11.1. The plasma contains the proteins albumin, globulin, and fibrinogen; fat, particularly as cholesterol; various electrolytes of which the most important are sodium, potassium, chloride, and bicarbonate; and minerals such as calcium and phosphate. The formed elements of the blood are the red cells, and the platelets. The main steps in the formation of

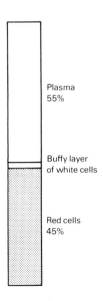

Plasma
55%

Buffy layer
of white cells

Red cells
45%

Fig. 11.1 The relationship between the formed elements of the blood and the plasma.

the red cells, white cells, and platelets are shown diagrammatically in Figure 11.2.

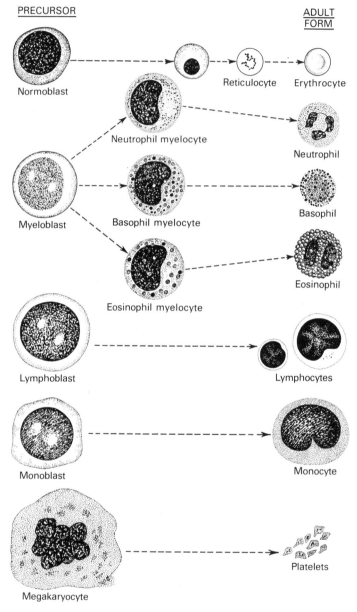

Fig. 11.2 The principal steps in the development of the red corpuscles, white corpuscles, and platelets.

Red cells

The red blood corpuscles, or erythrocytes, are non-nucleated biconcave discs with a transverse diameter of about 7 μ; they number approximately 4·5 to 5 million per cubic millimetre. They contain haemoglobin (composed of the iron-containing pigment haem and the protein globin) which has the ability to form a loose combination with oxygen and carbon dioxide. The red cells are thus enabled to transport oxygen as oxyhaemoglobin from the lungs to the tissues where oxygen is released and to remove carbon dioxide from the tissues to the lungs where it is excreted. The average normal haemoglobin content is 14·8 g per 100 ml sometimes expressed as 100 per cent.

Red cells are formed in the bone marrow from nucleated precursors called normoblasts. As the normoblast matures its cytoplasm becomes haemoglobinated and the nucleus becomes progressively smaller until it is extruded. For a period the very young red cell has a delicate structure of reticulum in the cytoplasm which may be demonstrated by a special staining technique; these young red cells, which are termed reticulocytes, are seen in the peripheral blood in cases of haemolytic anaemia and where an anaemia is actively responding to treatment, e.g. in pernicious anaemia following vitamin B_{12} therapy. The average life-span of a red cell is about 100 days and then the cells are broken down by the reticuloendothelial system, particularly in the spleen. The iron contained in the haemoglobin is conserved and used again for further haemoglobin formation; the non-iron containing residue goes to form the bile pigment bilirubin (see also p. 185).

The main substances known to be required for the formation of the red cells (erythropoiesis) are protein, iron, vitamin B_{12}, and folic acid. Vitamin C is also concerned with erythropoiesis but its precise role is less well understood.

White cells

The white blood corpuscles, or leucocytes, number some 4,000 to 10,000 per cubic millimetre. In contrast to the red cells they all possess a nucleus. The granular white cells, or polymorphonuclears, have granules in the cytoplasm and a lobed nucleus; depending on the staining reaction of the granules they are classified as neutrophil, eosinophil, or basophil polymorphs. Lymphocytes have a round nucleus and a clear blue cytoplasm. Monocytes have a kidney-shaped nucleus and a foamy blue cytoplasm. In health, a differential white cell count reveals that about 70 per cent of the white cells belong to the granular series, about 25 per cent are lymphocytes, while the remaining 5 per cent are monocytes.

The main function of the white cells is in dealing with infection and they usually increase in number (leucocytosis) in such circumstances. The polymorphonuclears are mainly increased in bacterial infections and the lymphocytes in viral infections. The white cells also deal with phagocytosis of necrotic or foreign material. The lymphocytes play an important part in antibody formation. The eosinophil polymorphonuclears are increased in certain allergic disorders such as hay fever, asthma, and urticaria, and in worm infestation.

The granular white cells are formed in the bone marrow and the lymphocytes in lymphoid tissue, particularly in the lymph nodes. The monocytes are also formed in the reticuloendothelial system but the exact details are uncertain. The primitive white cells are termed myeloblasts, lymphoblasts and monoblasts respectively; the myelocyte is an intermediate stage in the development of the adult polymorphonuclear from the myeloblast. Primitive white cells do not occur in the peripheral blood in health and their presence is always suggestive of leukaemia. The white corpuscles have a much shorter life than the red cells and the majority do not survive beyond a few days.

Platelets
The blood platelets, or thrombocytes, number about 250,000 to 500,000 per cubic millimetre. They are smaller than the red or white cells and have a varied shape. Platelets play an extremely important role in haemostasis (p. 230). They are formed in the bone marrow from the cytoplasm of megakaryocytes.

INVESTIGATION OF BLOOD DISORDERS

History
Many of the symptoms associated with anaemia are common to all varieties of the condition; they result from an inadequate supply of oxygen to the tissues consequent upon the low haemoglobin level and they disappear when the anaemia is corrected. In general, the more rapid the onset of the anaemia, the more severe the symptoms. The commonest symptoms are tiredness and breathlessness. Myocardial hypoxia may also produce palpitation and angina. Impaired gastric function leads to anorexia and, in some cases, to vomiting. Giddiness and mental confusion result from cerebral hypoxia.

After the history of the patient's immediate symptoms is elicited, enquiry is made regarding possible aetiological factors such as dietary deficiency (especially meat and vegetables), blood loss from the alimentary tract (haemorrhoids, peptic ulcer, and carcinoma of stomach or colon), menstrual disturbances, obstetric history, drugs which might cause bone marrow damage (e.g. chloramphenicol), or alimentary blood loss (e.g. aspirin). The family history is important in cases of haemolytic anaemia and haemorrhagic disorders. The ethnic background is important in haemolytic anaemia.

Clinical examination
Several clinical features of blood disorders are readily detected on general examination.

1. *Pallor* of the skin and mucous membranes is usually present in cases of anaemia but it is, at best, only a rough guide to the haemoglobin level; the colour of the conjuctivae is less misleading than the colour of the lips.

2. *Koilonychia*, a spoon-shaped depression of the finger nails, is diagnostic of iron deficiency anaemia (Fig. 11.3).

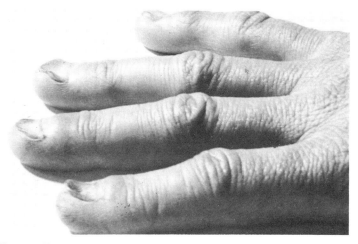

Fig. 11.3 Koilonychia.

3. *Glossitis* is present in about 50 per cent of cases of iron-deficiency anaemia and pernicious anaemia but it may occur also in certain vitamin B deficiency states (p. 265) in the absence of anaemia.

4. *Jaundice*, which is most readily detected in the sclera, is seen in cases of haemolytic anaemia; slight traces of jaundice producing

a lemon tint to the skin may be present in severe cases of pernicious anaemia.

5. *Petechial haemorrhages or bruising* of the skin is commonly present in acute leukaemia and in thrombocytopenic purpura.

6. *Lymph gland enlargement*, e.g. in the cervical region, should if local causes are excluded, suggest the possibility of leukaemia, Hodgkin's disease or infectious mononucleosis.

When the abdomen is examined, particular attention is paid to enlargement of the spleen or liver.

Laboratory investigations
Determination of haemoglobin level, red cell count, haematocrit (HCT or PCV) mean cell volume (MCV), mean cell haemoglobin (MCH), mean cell haemoglobin concentration (MCHC), white cell count, and scrutiny of a stained blood film form the basis for the initial laboratory investigation. Apart from the blood film all of these measurements are now readily available from a single blood sample using a modern electronic counter. Further investigations which may be required include platelet count, differential white cell count, bone marrow examination, red cell fragility, and tests of the coagulation mechanism.

The *erythrocyte sedimentation rate* (E.S.R.) or blood sedimentation rate may conveniently be described at this point although its application is greater in disorders other than those of the haemopoietic system. In the Westergren method a citrate anticoagulant solution is added to venous blood in a fixed proportion and the blood is drawn up into a long graduated tube which is allowed to stand vertically. The red cells sediment, leaving a top layer of clear plasma, at a relatively constant rate in normal individuals (not more than 15 mm in one hour). The principal factors which increase the E.S.R. are infections, other inflammatory processes such as rheumatic fever and rheumatoid arthritis, severe anaemia, malignant growths, other causes of tissue destruction such as fractures and surgical operations, and an increase in the globulin fraction of the plasma proteins. The E.S.R. is useful as a screening test for organic illness and in assessing the activity of a disease process and its response to treatment (e.g. tuberculosis and rheumatoid arthritis).

ANAEMIA

Anaemia, which is a common disorder, is present when there is a reduction in the level of haemoglobin: in most instances this is associated with a fall in the level of the red blood cells.

Classification and causes

The simplest classification is an aetiological one. In brief, anaemia may result from inadequate production of blood, from excess breakdown of blood, or from abnormal blood loss. The majority of cases of anaemia are due to iron deficiency, blood loss or vitamin B_{12} deficiency.

Disturbed production (dyshaemopoietic anaemia)

(a) Deficiency of iron, resulting in inadequate haemoglobin formation, causes hypochromic anaemia.

(b) Deficiency of vitamin B_{12} causes megaloblastic anaemia of which the main variety is pernicious anaemia. Megaloblastic anaemia may also be due to deficiency of folic acid, e.g. in pregnancy.

(c) Aplasia or hypoplasia of the bone marrow which may be primary, or secondary to certain drugs and industrial poisons or irradiation.

(d) Disturbed production of blood is an important sequel of severe infections, especially if they are chronic, and of certain metabolic derangements (e.g. uraemia).

Excess breakdown (haemolytic anaemia)

(a) Congenital acholuric jaundice which is due to increased fragility of the red cells.

(b) Haemolytic anaemia associated with certain infections (e.g. malaria), neoplasm, abnormal antibody formation, or drugs.

(c) Haemolytic anaemia due to the inherited disorders of haemoglobin synthesis, haemoglobinopathies.

Blood loss (posthaemorrhagic anaemia)

(a) Acute blood loss due to trauma, bleeding peptic ulcer or obstetric complications (Ch. 4).

(b) Chronic blood loss, which may be occult, from the alimentary tract or, in women, from the uterus.

Iron deficiency anaemia

Iron is an essential constituent of haemoglobin and when the iron content of the diet is insufficient to meet the demands of new blood formation, hypochromic anaemia results; this is still the commonest form of anaemia in Britain. It is most likely to occur where economic circumstances are poor because the iron-containing foods (meat, fish, vegetables) are the more expensive; in some cases, ignorance of a proper diet is the causal factor. Hypochromic anaemia is much commoner in women because their own iron requirements are greater due to the demands of menstruation, pregnancy, and lactation; in many cases hypochromic anaemia becomes evident during or after pregnancy. In some instances achlorhydria is a contributory factor; it leads to impaired absorption of iron.

When hypochromic anaemia occurs in men, or in postmenopausal females, serious consideration must be given to the possibility of an underlying source of chronic blood loss in the alimentary tract (haemorrhoids, peptic ulcer, carcinoma of stomach or colon); in some e.g. in elderly widowers, it results from dietary deficiency.

Clinical features

Any or all of the symptoms described on page 214 may be present. Pallor of the skin and mucous membranes is usually evident but the unreliability of pallor as a guide to anaemia has been stressed. Koilonychia (Fig. 11.3) should always be looked for as its presence is a sure indication of iron deficiency. Glossitis occurs in about 50 per cent of cases and, in a small number, is associated with dysphagia due to degenerative changes in the mucosa of the upper alimentary tract. The syndrome of hypochromic anaemia, glossitis and dysphagia, is termed the Plummer–Vinson or Kelly–Paterson syndrome or sideropenic dysphagia.

Investigations. The haemoglobin and the red cell level are both reduced, the MCV is low and the MCHC is low. Blood film examination confirms that the red cells are smaller than normal (microcytosis) and stain poorly (hypochromia) due to their low haemoglobin content.

Treatment

The majority of cases respond satisfactorily to the administration of an iron salt by mouth. A readily obtained, effective, and very cheap preparation is ferrous sulphate given in a dosage of one tablet (200 mg) three times daily. It should be taken after meals to minimize possible alimentary side effects and the patient should be warned that the faeces will become black due to the fact that not all of the iron is absorbed. If a fluid preparation of iron (e.g. iron and ammonium citrate) is used it may be taken through a straw to prevent blackening of the teeth. Iron is also available for intramuscular injection in patients who are intolerant of, or refractory to, oral iron therapy; it is also useful where a rapid response is desired. It is common practice to administer iron tablets during pregnancy and lactation because of the increased requirements.

In all instances consideration must be given to correction of any aetiologic factors, e.g. haemorrhoids, or ignorance regarding the composition of a normal diet. Where the main factor is financial hardship it will probably be necessary to supplement the diet with periodic administration of iron tablets.

In severe cases of the Plummer–Vinson syndrome the oesophagus may have to be dilated by bougies.

Megaloblastic anaemia

Certain anaemias are characterized by an alteration in the red cell precursors in the bone marrow termed megaloblastic erythropoiesis. Our understanding of this group of anaemias was helped greatly by the work of Castle and his associates who put forward the hypothesis that the normal maturation of red cell precursors in the bone marrow required the presence of an antianaemic factor (formed by the interaction of an extrinsic factor, derived from the food, and an intrinsic factor secreted by the cells of the gastric mucosa) which was absorbed from the gut, and stored in the liver until required by the bone marrow.

It is now known that vitamin B_{12} (cyanocobalamin) is the so called extrinsic factor, and that the role of the intrinsic or gastric factor is to promote the absorption of vitamin B_{12} from the alimentary tract. Vitamin B_{12} is present in protein foodstuffs and is formed by bacterial activity in the gut. The proper maturation of red cell precursors is also dependent upon the presence of folic acid, which is also a food constituent.

Pernicious anaemia

Pernicious anaemia is the most important variety of megaloblastic anaemia in this country. It is due to a defect in gastric function (intrinsic factor deficiency) whereby vitamin B_{12} cannot be absorbed from the alimentary tract. The gastric defect may be the result of an autoimmune mechanism (p. 243).

Clinical features

The disorder is seen particularly in middle age and in the later years of life. A family history is present in some instances. The onset is insidious and symptoms are often present for several months before medical advice is sought. Any of the symptoms described on page 214 may be present; the commonest are tiredness and breathlessness. In about half the cases there is soreness of the tongue due to glossitis. This may be limited to smoothness, due to papillary atrophy affecting perhaps only the sides of the tongue. In a smaller proportion of cases the tongue has a raw 'beefy' appearance. A sensation of pins and needles, or tingling, may be experienced in the hands and feet due to peripheral neuritis. In severe cases the pallor has a yellowish or lemon tinge.

Investigations. The red cell level is low, often markedly so; the haemoglobin level is not reduced to quite the same degree. The MCV is increased. Blood film examination confirms that the red cells are larger than normal (macrocytosis), and they tend to be oval or pear-shaped (poikilocytosis) and are well filled with haemoglobin.

Bone marrow examination revels that the red cell precursors are strikingly different from normal; the cells, which are termed megaloblasts, are larger, have a characteristic nuclear structure and other distinctive cytological features.

Examination of the gastric juice, obtained through a narrow rubber tube known as a Ryle's tube, invariably shows that there is no hydrochloric acid present even after the cells of the gastric mucosa have been stimulated by an injection of histamine. This histamine-fast achlorhydria, unlike the bone marrow findings, persists after the anaemia has been treated. Decreased absorption of vitamin B_{12} can be demonstrated by the Schilling test.

Complications

Slight degrees of peripheral neuritis are not uncommon in pernicious anaemia. A much more serious lesion of the nervous system, subacute combined degeneration of the spinal cord, may occur in cases of pernicious anaemia where treatment is inadequate or irregular, and is likely to produce permanent disability. There is muscle weakness due to involvement of the motor pathway or pyramidal tract, and sensory disturbance particularly of posture, due to involvement of the posterior columns.

Treatment

This disease was formerly invariably fatal and therefore deserved the name 'pernicious'. Now, however, if properly treated the patient can be restored to health and afforded a normal expectation of life. The first effective step in the treatment of pernicious anaemia was the demonstration in 1926 of the value of large quantities of raw or lightly cooked liver. At first these patients had to eat a half

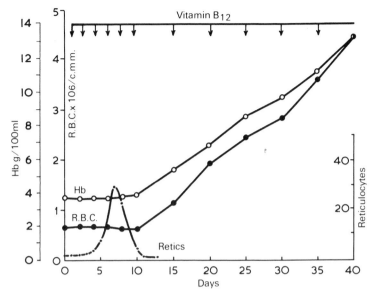

Fig. 11.4 Haematological response to vitamin B_{12} therapy in a case of pernicious anaemia. Note the initial reticulocytosis and the subsequent rise in haemoglobin and red cell levels.

to one pound of liver per day but soon oral liver extracts were available and these were followed by liver extracts suitable for intramuscular injection. The current treatment is to give frequent intramuscular injections of vitamin B_{12} (Fig. 11.4) until the blood levels have risen to normal and then to maintain normal blood levels with an injection every two to four weeks for the rest of the patient's life.

Other megaloblastic anaemias
The next commonest form of megaloblastic anaemia in this country occurs in the later stages of pregnancy. It is due to the combined effects of increased demands for folic acid and dietary deficiency. The therapeutic response to folic acid is excellent.

Other varieties of megaloblastic anaemia include those due to severe nutritional deficiency of protein, resection of the stomach, and impaired absorption as in steatorrhoea.

Hypoplastic and aplastic anaemia
In this variety of anaemia the bone marrow becomes progressively less cellular and fails to produce an adequate number of red cells.

The myeloid tissue and the megakaryocytes of the marrow are usually also involved so that low white cell and platelet levels are commonly associated.

Aetiology
Some cases are secondary to bone marrow damage resulting from certain drugs and industrial poisons (e.g. chloramphenicol, phenylbutazone, benzol derivatives), from exposure to X-rays and to radioactive substances. In other cases, termed idiopathic or primary, no cause for the bone marrow depression can be detected.

Clinical features
The clinical features result from a combination of anaemia, leucopenia, and thrombocytopenia. The main symptoms resulting from anaemia are tiredness and breathlessness, leucopenia causes an increased liability to infection, while thrombocytopenia leads to bruising, bleeding from the gums and purpura.

Treatment
Careful enquiry must be made regarding any possible aetiological factor and, if still operative, this should be removed. Repeated blood transfusions are necessary to sustain life and antibiotics may be required to control infection. With these measures life may be maintained for considerable periods even in the presence of irreversible bone marrow damage. In other cases a measure of bone marrow function returns. Corticosteroids occasionally are of benefit.

Congenital acholuric jaundice
Congenital acholuric jaundice is the most important form of haemolytic anaemia in this country. The basic abnormality is in the red cells which are spherocytic in shape and, in consequence, unduly fragile so that they are much more readily destroyed by the spleen. There is a compensatory hyperplasia of the bone marrow in its attempt to deal with the increased demands for new cells to replace those destroyed.

Clinical features
A family history of the disorder is readily obtained in most cases. The three main clinical features are anaemia, jaundice and enlargement of the spleen.

The anaemia is variable in degree; for long periods the level of haemolysis appears to be more or less balanced by new red cell formation, but from time to time, for reasons which are poorly understood, haemolytic crises occur during which the blood levels fall dramatically.

The degree of jaundice is closely related to the severity of the haemolytic process; between crises it is usually relatively slight. The condition is termed acholuric jaundice (i.e. without bile) because although the urine contains an excess of urobilinogen, which is derived from bilirubin, it does not contain bilirubin (Fig. 9.1).

Splenic enlargement is usually of moderate degree and readily detectable.

Treatment

During haemolytic crises blood transfusion is required. Once the crisis has settled, splenectomy should be performed. Although this does not alter the red cell abnormality it usually enables the individual to live a more or less normal life as the excessive haemolysis ceases.

POLYCYTHAEMIA

In polycythaemia there is an excess of red blood cells, haemoglobin, and a high blood volume. The condition may either be primary or secondary.

Primary polycythaemia or polycythaemia vera

The aetiology is unknown. The red cell count and the haemoglobin level become very high (e.g. R.B.C. 8–10 million/c.mm, (Hb 18–20 g per 100 ml) and in consequence the skin and mucous membranes are redder than normal and the conjunctivae are suffused. There is often cyanosis present as the increased viscosity of the blood leads to slowing of the circulation permitting increased reduction of oxyhaemoglobin. The sluggish circulation also predisposes to venous and arterial thrombosis. The spleen is commonly enlarged. The white cell count is often elevated and in some cases leukaemia develops.

Treatment consists of venesections followed by irradiation to damp down the excessive marrow activity. For this purpose conventional X-ray therapy has been largely replaced by the use of radioactive phosphorus (P^{32}).

Secondary polycythaemia

A compensatory or secondary polycythaemia occurs where there is chronic oxygen deficiency. It is seen in high altitude dwellers (e.g.

in the Andes), in cases of congenital heart disease associated with cyanosis, and in some cases of chronic lung disease. The condition must always be differentiated from primary polycythaemia.

LEUKAEMIA

Leukaemia is a disease characterized pathologically by a purposeless proliferation of white cell tissue and clinically by a progressive course leading to death in a few months to a few years. The condition is perhaps most readily understood if it is thought of as a form of tumour of the tissues which form the white cells.

Aetiology

It is now known that chromosomal abnormalities are present in leukaemia. The most consistent change is seen in chronic myeloid leukaemia in which the 21 chromosome, the Philadelphia chromosome, is defective. Ionizing radiation causes chromosomal damage and this is probably the mechanism of the occurrence of leukaemia in survivors of the atom bomb explosions in Japan and of the increased incidence of leukaemia in those children whose mothers had abdominal X-rays during the pregnancy. Radiological studies during pregnancy are now strictly limited.

Classification

Leukaemia may be classified morphologically into myeloid, lymphatic, and monocytic leukaemia or into acute and chronic forms depending on the rapidity of the disease; but, for practical purposes, it will be sufficient if we consider leukaemia under two headings.

1. Acute leukaemia—myeloid, lymphatic or monocytic.
2. Chronic leukaemia—myeloid, lymphatic.

Acute leukaemia

Acute leukaemia is seen at any age, but particularly in children, in whom it is the most common form of malignant tumour.

Clinical features

The condition has a rapid onset and within a few weeks pallor is evident and the child is listless and obviously extremely ill. Bruising of the skin and purpuric spots are common and there is a great tendency to bleeding within the buccal cavity and from the nose. Hypertrophy of the gums may occur and it is particularly a feature of monocytic leukaemia. Infection of the gums and of the throat is often present. Because of these changes in the buccal cavity the child may initially be taken for dental attention.

Examination usually reveals glandular enlargement but in many cases it is only slight or moderate. In the case of the cervical glands the enlargement may be partly due to the leukaemic process and partly to the associated infection in the mouth and throat. Enlargement of the spleen and liver may be found but again not of great degree.

Laboratory features. The white cell count may be moderately elevated but may be reduced. Examination of blood film shows that the great majority of the white cells are very primitive 'blast' cells and it is often impossible to state whether they are derived from myeloid, lymphoid or monocytic precursors. The haemoglobin and red cell levels are markedly reduced and in addition the platelet count is low. Normal marrow tissue is largely replaced with the primitive cells.

Treatment

Present day practice is to correct the anaemia with blood transfusions, control infection with antibiotics, and administer a combination of powerful cytotoxic drugs. Dramatic remissions may be induced and some patients may live for several years. The prognosis, however, remains grave and death occurs in the majority of patients within months or a few years.

Chronic leukaemia

Chronic myeloid leukaemia has its maximum incidence in the middle years of life while the lymphatic variety tends to occur rather later.

Clinical features

The onset is insidious and the patient usually presents with a complaint of tiredness, a dragging sensation in the upper left abdomen due to splenic enlargement, or of enlargement of lymph nodes. The splenic enlargement is often extremely great in chronic myeloid leukaemia and the spleen may come to fill the left side of the abdomen; it is less of a feature in chronic lymphatic leukaemia. Lymph node enlargement is usually prominent in the chronic lymphatic type of leukaemia and relatively slight in the myeloid variety.

Laboratory features. The white cell count is characteristically very high (e.g. 100–200,000 per c.mm). Examination of the stained blood film shows that the great majority of the white cells present belong either to the granular series (myeloid leukaemia) or are lymphocytes (lymphatic leukaemia). Most are mature. A slight or moderate degree of anaemia is usually present while the platelet count is normal or may be increased.

Prognosis

In most cases life may be maintained for some two to five years after the diagnosis of chronic myeloid leukaemia has been made and often rather longer in the lymphatic form. Towards the end of the illness the leukaemia may take on many of the characteristics of the acute variety, severe anaemia and haemorrhagic tendencies being prominent.

Treatment

Treatment may be with radiotherapy directed to the bone marrow, spleen, and lymph nodes or, alternatively, with an alkylating agent. In chronic myeloid leukaemia the drug is busulphan (Myleran) while in chronic lymphatic leukaemia chlorambucil (Leukeran) is employed.

AGRANULOCYTOSIS

In agranulocytosis there is a great reduction or complete absence of the granular cells of the blood.

Aetiology

The condition may be secondary to drug administration or X-ray irradiation in the same way as aplastic anaemia (p. 222). It also occurs as an accompaniment of idiopathic aplastic anaemia.

Clinical features

The essential clinical feature is a greatly increased liability to infection, particularly affecting the throat, the respiratory tract, and the skin. The total white cell count is low and differential white cell count shows that the granular series is virtually absent.

Treatment

Antibiotics are given to control infection (not chloramphenicol in view of the possible bone marrow damage which it may cause) and transfusions of fresh blood may sometimes be required. Any possibly harmful drug should, of course, be stopped.

LYMPHADENOPATHY

In this section a brief account will be given of the main steps taken in reaching a diagnosis. Cervical lymphadenopathy is of much greater importance of the dentist than lymph node enlargement in other areas and is discussed on page 255.

It is most important on finding enlarged lymph nodes in a patient, to consider whether (a) there is local disease within the nodes themselves, (b) the nodes are involved as a result of disease within their area of drainage (thus, for example, enlarged inguinal nodes may be associated with a lesion of the foot), (c) the enlargement of the nodes is part of a generalized disease (e.g. leukaemia).

Diagnosis of lymph node involvement is made by taking a detailed history and by examination including palpation of all the lymph node areas of the body, the spleen and in particular the areas drained by the affected group of lymph nodes.

Bacterial examination of any local infected lesions may be necessary and special diagnostic tests such as the Mantoux reaction in suspected tuberculous lymph nodes, the Wassermann reaction in syphilis and the Paul Bunnell reaction in glandular fever. The blood picture is often important as for example in acute leukaemia. In very many cases of lymph node involvement a precise diagnosis is not possible by these means and *biopsy* of the node with histology is necessary to establish a diagnosis. A small portion of any node removed should also be sent for bacteriological examination.

In some cases involvement of a lymph node with cancer is the first sign of disease elsewhere and a search must be made for the primary lesion utilizing other procedures such as a chest X-ray, barium meal examination and endoscopy.

LYMPHADENOMA (HODGKIN'S DISEASE)

Lymphadenoma is the commonest and most important form of the tumour-like conditions affecting primarily the lymph nodes and other parts of the reticuloendothelial system. The group term 'reticuloses' is used to describe these disorders; another example is lymphosarcoma.

Aetiology
Lymphadenoma has the proliferative characteristics of a malignant tumour and little more is known of its aetiology than of the aetiology of tumour in general.

Pathology

The normal lymph node structure becomes progressively replaced by a mixed proliferation of lymphocytes and large reticulum cells which may be multinucleated (giant cells or Reed–Sternberg cells); eosinophils and plasma cells may also be present. Caseation (softening) does not occur. Similar histological changes occur in the spleen and liver.

Clinical features

Hodgkin's disease is seen most commonly in young adults and it is more frequent in males. The onset is insidious and the individual usually presents with a history that for several weeks he has felt unduly tired and has then become aware of lymph node enlargement most often in the neck. Any of the superficial lymph nodes may be enlarged and, in addition, the glands in the mediastinum and abdomen are also commonly involved. The mediastinal enlargement may cause dyspnoea, cough, and cyanosis through pressure on the bronchi and great veins. The enlarged glands are firm and rubbery on palpation. They are usually discrete, are not painful, and there are no signs of inflammation associated; pus formation and sinus formation do not occur.

Enlargement of the spleen is a frequent occurrence and the liver may also be involved. Anaemia is usually slight at first but in the later stages of the disease may become very marked. The erythrocyte sedimentation rate is characteristically elevated. There is no characteristic alteration in the white cells although in a small proportion of cases there is an increase in the eosinophil level. Pyrexia is present in some cases and may have an intermittent nature, the temperature being elevated for a few days and then falling to normal for a period before becoming elevated again (Pel-Ebstein periodic pyrexia).

The prognosis in lymphadenoma is poor and even with treatment death usually occurs in a few years.

Diagnosis

The differential diagnosis of the various causes of lymph node enlargement is discussed in the preceding section. A definite diagnosis of Hodgkin's disease cannot be made until a gland is removed for histological examination.

Treatment

The method of treatment chosen depends on the extent of the disease. This is determined by chest X-ray and often by laparotomy involving splenectomy, liver biopsy and biopsy of the nodes along the abdominal aorta.

For localized disease treatment is by radiotherapy directed to the affected tissue but for more generalized disease chemotherapy is the treatment of choice.

MULTIPLE MYELOMA (MYELOMATOSIS)

Multiple myeloma is a tumour of bone marrow characterized by a local and diffuse overgrowth of plasma or myeloma cells. The main clinical features are bone pains, especially in the back, a tendency to pathological fractures, and anaemia. The sedimentation rate of the blood is very high and the urine may contain an abnormal substance termed Bence – Jones protein. Radiology of the skeleton shows numerous punched-out areas affecting particularly the skull, ribs, and spine.

The prognosis is poor. Palliative results may be obtained with radiotherapy and chemotherapy.

INFECTIOUS MONONUCLEOSIS (GLANDULAR FEVER)

Glandular fever is an acute infection due to a virus. The condition has its maximal incidence in young people.

Clinical features
The individual develops a febrile illness characterized by sore throat, enlargement of the lymph glands in the neck and elsewhere, splenic enlargement, and occasionally by a skin rash.

Investigations. The white cell count is elevated and examination of a blood film shows that the leucocytosis is mainly due to the presence of lymphocytes, many of which appear atypical. The blood findings associated with the clinical features may, in some cases, cause confusion with acute leukaemia. A serological test, known as the Paul Bunnell reaction, is frequently positive.

Treatment
None of the antibiotics currently available appears to influence the course of the disorder. The general measures applicable to any infectious disease should be employed.

THE HAEMORRHAGIC DISORDERS

Those diseases which are characterized by an undue tendency to haemorrhage are of great importance to the dentist. An account will first be given of the way in which bleeding is normally control-led (haemostasis) and will be followed by a description of the main clinical disorders.

Haemostasis

Haemostasis, or the control of bleeding, depends on the close in-teraction of a number of processes. The subject is an extremely complicated one and the following is only a brief and simplified account. If a vascular tissue is incised or otherwise traumatized the first reaction to the injury is adhesion of platelets to subendothelial collagen fibres which in turn leads to the release of platelet adeno-sine diphosphate (ADP) and serotonin. A platelet plug is formed which occludes the transected vessel and this is the main factor in the primary haemostatic process. The release of serotonin also causes contraction of small blood vessels and this secondary vascu-lar response augments the primary response. The third phase is the formation of fibrin partly as the result of liberation of platelet phos-pholipid and partly due to activation of the contact mechanism of the blood. The sequence of events leading to the production of fibrin is very complex and involves the interaction of many coagula-tion factors which have an agreed international nomenclature (Table 2). Fig. 11.5 gives a simplified version of the coagulation process following a dental procedure.

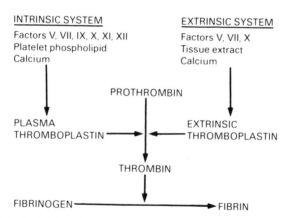

INTRINSIC SYSTEM
Factors V, VII, IX, X, XI, XII
Platelet phospholipid
Calcium

EXTRINSIC SYSTEM
Factors V, VII, X
Tissue extract
Calcium

PROTHROMBIN

PLASMA THROMBOPLASTIN ——→   ←—— EXTRINSIC THROMBOPLASTIN

THROMBIN

FIBRINOGEN ————————————→ FIBRIN

Fig. 11.5 A simplified version of the modern concept of the coagulation mechanism.

Fibrin removal

After the clot has served its purpose the fibrin is removed by a complex fibrinolytic system which maintains the patency of the

Table 2   International nomenclature of clotting factors

Factor I	Fibrinogen
Factor II	Prothrombin
Factor V	Ac-globulin, proaccelerin, labile factor
Factor VII	Proconvertine SPCA
Factor VIII	Antihaemophilic factor
Factor IX	Plasma thromboplastin component (PTC) or 'Christmas factor'
Factor X	Stuart-Prower factor
Factor XI	Plasma thromboplastin antecedent (PTA)
Factor XII	Hageman factor
Factor XIII	Fibrin stabilizing factor

vascular tree. In health there may be a dynamic equilibrium between the fibrinolytic enzyme system and the coagulation system.

Classification of haemorrhagic states

A simple classification of the haemorrhagic states with an indication of the nature of the defect is given below. The term purpura is a purely descriptive one for any condition characterized by haemorrhages into the skin and mucous membranes. The haemorrhages may be very small (punctate, pin-point, purpuric spots) or, in severe cases, may be confluent so that large bruises, or ecchymoses, are formed.

  I. Due to deficiencies of clotting factors
    A. Genetic defects
      1. Haemophilia—deficiency of antihaemophilic factor (AHF or Factor VIII).
      2. Christmas disease—deficiency of Christmas factor (Factor IX).
    B. Acquired defects
      1. Anticoagulant therapy.
      2. Liver disease—complex defect with deficiency of Factors II, VII, IX, X.
  II. Due to defects of platelets
      1. Thrombocytopenia—either primary or secondary.
      2. Impaired platelet function—scurvy, uraemia.
  III. Defects in vessel wall
      1. Anaphylactoid purpura—allergic capillary defect.
      2. Hereditary telangiectasia—focal capillary defect.
      3. Senile purpura—defect of supporting tissues.

HAEMOPHILIA

Haemophilia is the most important of the hereditary haemorrhagic disorders. It is due to a defect in the production of the high molecular weight protein (factor VIII) which is synthesised abnormally. The condition is not particularly common; in the West of Scotland it occurs about once in every 10,000 of the population.

Family history
The condition is transmitted as a sex-linked recessive Mendelian trait. The gene responsible is contained in the X chromosome of the reproductive cells. The inheritance of haemophilia can be understood by a study of Figure 11.6 which shows a typical family tree. The main points regarding the inheritance of the disorder which should be remembered are:

1. If a haemophilic male marries a normal female none of his sons will have the disorder but his daughters will be carriers of the disease.

2. If a normal male marries a carrier female there is a 50 per cent chance of the sons being affected with the disease and a 50 per cent chances of the daughters being carriers.

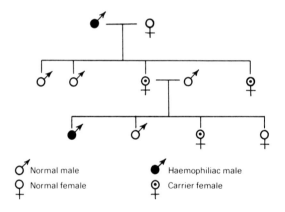

Fig. 11.6 A haemophiliae family tree.

In clinical practice about one-third of the individuals with haemophilia have no knowledge of a family history of the disorder. This is probably due to the passage down through several generations of female carriers without occurrence of the disease, or possibly due to gene mutation.

Haemophilia is extremely rare in the female; such cases as have occurred have been from the marriage of an affected man and a carrier female, many such marriages being consanguineous.

Clinical features

The bleeding tendency is not usually clinically apparent until the child is 1 to 2 years of age or even older. Once the disease does manifest itself the characteristic feature is bleeding after injury; the injury may be so trivial as to be scarcely noticed. If the defect is severe bleeding can occur spontaneously. Bleeding into the joints (haemarthrosis) is particularly common, the main joints involved being the knees, elbows, and ankles. The affected joint becomes swollen and very painful and the individual may be incapacitated for considerable periods. Permanent joint damage with limitation of movement (ankylosis) is likely to occur following repeated haemarthrosis and may be severe. Haematomata commonly occur in the subcutaneous tissues and in the muscles and, apart from causing bruising and pain, they may produce serious damage from pressure on vital structures such as nerves. Following cuts or any surgical procedure there is persistent bleeding which may be so prolonged as to endanger life. Thus after a dental extraction the individual may bleed from the tooth socket for days or even weeks and may, over this period, lose from a very small area many pints of blood. Tonsillectomy which leaves a large raw area, is a particularly hazardous procedure in haemophiliacs while more major surgical procedures may have a fatal outcome unless skilled replacement therapy is available.

While the above is the typical history of the average haemophiliac it should be appreciated that milder cases do occur in whom there is no past history of an undue haemorrhagic tendency and the condition is first suspected when the individual bleeds for an excessive time after a surgical procedure such as dental extraction. Indeed there is a spectrum of clinical severity in haemophilia with severe, moderate and mild grades which correspond with the assayed level of AHF.

Investigations

The diagnostic finding in haemophilia is a deficiency in antihaemophilic factor which in severe cases may be manifest as prolongation of the whole blood clotting time but in milder cases may be revealed only by more sensitive tests of the coagulation mechanism such as the kaolin cephalin clotting time.

Treatment

The haemophiliac should avoid injury as far as possible and he should be guided in his choice of occupation with this factor in mind. The dental implications in haemophilia are twofold and comprise the conservative dental care of the haemophiliac and the management of the haemophiliac in whom dental extraction is essential.

Many haemophiliacs previously reached early adult life with carious teeth and unhealthy gums because they had not received any conservative dental treatment of early caries. This deplorable fact was partly due to fear on the part of the patient to go for dental treatment and partly due to fear on the part of many dentists to undertake even the simplest forms of dental work in anyone stating that he is a bleeder. It cannot be stressed too much that the haemophiliac is possibly the patient most in need of conservative dental care and if the dental practitioner is not prepared to undertake this himself then he should certainly arrange for the patient to attend a dental hospital if this is at all possible. The majority of the new generation of haemophiliacs have excellent teeth.

The young haemophiliac should receive intensive instruction regarding the personal care of the teeth, e.g. regular brushing of teeth, avoidance of sweets, regular visits to the dentist. There is a good case for the use of fluoride to minimize the development of caries and if this has not been added to the local water supply the patient may add fluoride tablets to the drinking water or use fluoride-containing toothpaste.

Extraction of teeth in the haemophiliac should only be performed in conjunction with a doctor skilled in the management of this condition. The following is a summary of the procedure currently used in the Glasgow Royal Infirmary in cooperation with the Glasgow Dental Hospital.

On the day of extraction the patient is seen at 11.00 am and given either epsilon amino-caproic acid (Epsikapron) or tranexamic acid (Cyclokapron) and an oral antibiotic (tetracycline). An hour before extraction the patient is given a dose of anti-haemophilic factor concentrate. Extraction is carried out using appropriate local anaesthetic. No special precautions are needed as the patient is haemostatic. The patient may return home and will usually not require any further therapy except for continuation of the antibiotic and the fibrinolytic inhibitor, epsilon amino-caproic acid. Should further bleeding occur a further administration of Factor VIII is indicated. With such a routine it is now rare for blood transfusion to be required following dental extraction in haemophiliacs.

Christmas disease

Christmas disease is a haemorrhagic disorder which is clinically and genetically indistinguishable from haemophilia. The unusual name is derived from the surname of the first patient studied. The missing coagulation factor is termed the Christmas factor or Factor IX. The treatment is essentially as for haemophilia, except that concentrates of Factor IX are used and not of Factor VIII. AHG is ineffectual.

Thrombocytopenia

Thrombocytopenia, or reduction in the number of platelets, may be either primary or secondary. Haemorrhagic phenomena are likely to occur when the platelet count is 40,000 per cubic millimetre or less (the normal level is 250,000 to 500,000 per c.mm).

Idiopathic thrombocytopenic purpura

This disorder is seen particularly in young people. The cause is uncertain but there may be increased destruction of platelets within the spleen. Small haemorrhagic spots develop in the skin and mucous membranes and they may also occur in the internal organs, particularly the brain. The gums bleed unduly after brushing the teeth and nose bleeding is frequent. Dental extraction is a potential hazard because of haemorrhage although the problem is not of the same magnitude as that in haemophilia. Larger areas of bruising into the subcutaneous tissues are common after trivial injuries. Secondary anaemia commonly develops. Slight splenic enlargement may occur. The platelet count is very low, capillary fragility is increased, and the bleeding time is prolonged.

The acute stage is treated by transfusion of fresh blood and by the administration of corticosteroid drugs. Splenectomy, which must only be performed during a remission, often leads to considerable improvement.

Secondary thrombocytopenia

Reduction in the platelet count, with resultant purpura, occurs in several diseases of which the more important are acute leukaemia, primary aplastic anaemia, and bone marrow damage from drugs or irradiation.

Liver disease

An undue tendency to haemorrhage is an important accompaniment of many forms of liver disease. In obstructive jaundice the absence of bile from the intestine leads to impaired absorption of the fat soluble vitamin K and, in consequence, to a low prothrombin level, but the coagulation defect, as in parenchymal liver disease, is more complex and involves Factor VII, Factor IX (Christmas factor), and Factor X, in addition to prothrombin.

Before any form of surgery in patients with liver disease it is customary to give injections of vitamin K_1 (Konakion).

Anticoagulant therapy

The dentist should have some knowledge of anticoagulant therapy as a number of people are receiving this form of treatment, on a long-term basis, as a prophylactic measure in atrial fibrillation, in obliterative vascular disease, and in those with artificial heart valves or synthetic arterial grafts. The drug most commonly employed is warfarin which produces reduction of Factor II, VII, IX and X. An earlier anticoagulant called phenindione (Dindevan) is now seldom used. In clinical practice the patient who is receiving warfarin will require to attend hospital regularly for measurement of the effect of the drug on the clotting factors (Thrombotest) and the dosage of the drug is adjusted accordingly.

If dental extraction is required in an individual receiving anticoagulant therapy, it should be performed only after consultation with the doctor in charge of the case and may involve temporary correction of the clotting defect by injection of vitamin K_1.

Hereditary telangiectasia

This is an uncommon disorder in which there are areas of dilated blood vessels particularly on the mucous membranes of the lips, tongue, and nose. They may also be seen in the skin, especially of the face. A family history of the condition is usually obtained.

The commonest complaint is of frequent epistaxis and the chronic blood loss produces secondary anaemia. Undue haemorrhage after dental extraction may theoretically occur if there is telangiectasia in the operation field.

Senile purpura

In elderly people there is decreased elasticity in the skin and subcutaneous tissues resulting in diminished support for the small blood vessels; these are more liable to rupture following minor injuries and small purpuric areas result. These are seen particularly on the dorsum of the hands and forearms. The condition is not a serious one and there is no particular dental implication.

Anaphylactoid purpura (Henoch-Schönlein)

In this condition there is an undue permeability of the capillary endothelium as a consequence of some allergic reaction; the factor responsible is most frequently bacterial infection, especially streptococcal, and a history of a sore throat before the onset of the purpura is commonly obtained. In other instances an article of food is responsible while in some cases no cause can be detected.

The illness commonly starts with vomiting. Purpuric spots which are palpable as well as visible (in contrast to idiopathic thrombocytopenic purpura) occur on the skin, particularly of the legs, and may be very numerous. Joint effusions with pain may be present (purpura rheumatica or Schönlein's purpura) while in other instances bleeding from the alimentary tract is the main feature (Henoch's purpura). Renal involvement, shown by proteinuria and haematuria, may also be present. The lesion is a vascular one and the platelet count is normal. The degree of blood loss is seldom great.

Corticosteroids and antihistamine drugs have been tried but without proven benefit.

12

Endocrine disorders

THE THYROID GLAND

The thyroid gland is situated at the front and sides of the lower part of the neck. It consists of two lateral lobes, each about four centimetres long, joined across the midline by a narrow isthmus. The gland is partly covered by the muscles of the neck in front. Posteriorly and medially the main relationships are to the trachea, the recurrent laryngeal nerve, and the oesophagus. The parathyroid glands lie along the posterior surface of the lobes. The thyroid gland has a fibrous sheath which is fixed to the larynx and trachea so that the gland moves with these structures on swallowing. The blood supply is derived from the external carotid artery (superior thyroid artery) and the subclavian artery (inferior thyroid artery).

The gland is composed of many follicles which are usually lined by a single layer of cubical epithelium; the follicles contain colloid. The size of the follicles, the colloid content, and the epithelial lining vary considerably in the different thyroid disorders.

The thyroid gland manufactures, stores and secretes the two thyroid hormones, thyroxine (T_4) and triiodothyronine (T_3), of which iodine is an essential constituent. The synthesis of the hormones is regulated by the thyroid stimulating hormone (TSH) of the anterior lobe of the pituitary. The thyroid hormones stimulate the metabolic activities of the body generally, increase the heart rate, play a part in carbohydrate metabolism, and affect growth.

The first step on examination of the thyroid gland is a close inspection, in good light, of the lower neck, the patient's head being tilted slightly backwards; on swallowing the gland is seen to move upwards. Palpation is best carried out from behind, the patient's head being inclined slightly forward to relax the sterno-mastoid muscles; the swallowing test is repeated. If the vascularity of the gland is much increased there will be a systolic murmur, easily audible on auscultation, and it may be possible to feel a thrill.

Developmental anomalies

The isthmus and the medial parts of the lobes are formed from a central downgrowth from the floor of the primitive oropharynx; in adults the site of the downgrowth is represented by the foramen caecum. The downgrowth forms a hollow stalk called the thyroglossal duct, the lower end of which enlarges and forms thyroid tissue, while the upper end atrophies and disappears. On either side of the central downgrowth cells from the entoderm of the fourth arch proliferate to form the remainder of the lateral lobes.

The gland may not descend fully (lingual thyroid), may descend too far (retrosternal thyroid), may develop elsewhere, or the thyroglossal duct may persist in whole or part. None of these anomalies is common. The term ectopic thyroid refers to any portion of thyroid tissue which does not lie in the normal situation.

Lingual thyroid

This term is used where the thyroid does not descend as described above but develops in close proximity to the foramen caecum. The diagnosis is not usually made until after the gland enlarges at puberty. The gland may be completely buried in the root of the tongue or it may cause a rounded swelling on the posterior surface of that organ. If it is of considerable size it will produce dysphagia and dyspnoea and surgical excision will be indicated; if there is no thyroid tissue elsewhere the patient will subsequently require to take sodium thyroxine.

Retrosternal thyroid

If the developing gland descends too far an intrathoracic, or retrosternal, thyroid is formed. Should the thyroid become enlarged in this situation, pressure symptoms (dyspnoea and dysphagia) are very likely.

Other ectopic thyroids

Ectopic thyroid tissue may rarely be found in other sites, e.g. within the pharynx or laterally in the neck. In most cases thyroid tissue is also present in the normal thyroid situation.

Thyroglossal tract remnants

These are described under swellings of the neck (Ch. 13).

GOITRE

The term 'goitre' is used to describe enlargement of the thyroid gland. It may be a manifestation of several different disease processes which may be classified as follows:

1. Non-toxic, simple, or colloid goitre.

2. Toxic goitre, exophthalmic goitre, or thyrotoxicosis.
3. Thyroiditis.
4. Thyroid neoplasm.

Non-toxic goitre

Simple or non-toxic goitre is usually divided into endemic and sporadic categories according to whether many or few of the population are affected. The patient presents no other clinical evidence of disturbed thyroid function.

Deficiency of iodine is probably the principal factor in the production of endemic goitre. The deficiency is most commonly due to a low iodine content in water and locally produced foods. The cause of sporadic goitre is uncertain. In many instances it is possible that a combination of factors is responsible, for example disordered synthesis of thyroid hormones due to genetically determined defects, and iodine deficiency either primary or conditioned by certain goitrogenic substances in the diet.

Whatever the basic cause of simple goitre it is generally believed that the enlargement is due to a compensatory thyroid hyperplasia initiated by inadequate circulating thyroid hormones. The hyperplasia is most likely to develop when metabolic demands are increased, particularly during the period of reproductive life in the female. Hence non-toxic goitre is much commoner in females than in males.

The enlargement may be relatively slight or of such degree that the gland forms a large, disfiguring swelling causing pressure

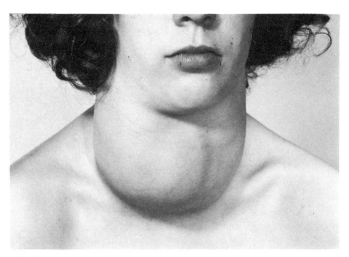

Fig. 12.1 Large simple goitre.

symptoms (Fig. 12.1). The surface of the gland may be smooth at first but it is likely to become increasingly nodular.

Prophylaxis by the addition of iodide to salt greatly diminishes the incidence of endemic goitre. In established cases of goitre the administration of sodium thyroxine may reduce the size of the gland but, if it is large and producing pressure symptoms, surgery is indicated.

Toxic goitre or thyrotoxicosis

Toxic goitre, thyrotoxicosis, or hyperthyroidism, is more common in women. Although it may occur at any age, it is seen more frequently in early adult life. The precise cause of the condition is uncertain but there is probably an underlying autoimmune dysfunction, which may be inherited. In predisposed subjects the illness may apparently follow a period of emotional disturbance.

Clinical features

Loss of weight occurs and, in contrast with most disorders which produce weight loss, it is associated with increased appetite. The patient is nervous, irritable, emotionally labile, and can be observed to be restless and jumpy. The eyes are often staring and prominent (Fig. 12.2) and a rim of white sclera may be visible around the iris. Sometimes the eyeballs protrude (exophthalmos). The thyroid gland is diffusely enlarged and, owing to its increased vascularity, a murmur is usually audible over the gland and a thrill may be present. The pulse is rapid even when the patient is asleep. Extrasystoles or atrial fibrillation may occur in older patients. The

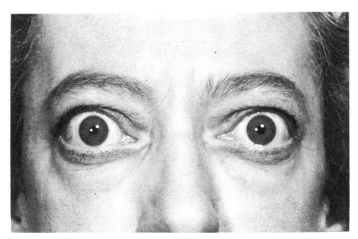

Fig. 12.2 Lid retraction in thyrotoxicosis.

skin is warm and moist and there is a fine tremor of the outstretched hand.

The clinical features are not always so clear cut. In some, particularly those of middle age or older, there may be little or nothing in the way of eye signs or thyroid gland enlargement and the diagnosis may not be immediately obvious. Atrial fibrillation and heart failure are commoner in this occult type of thyrotoxicosis. In most of these cases the thyroid is nodular (toxic nodular goitre or toxic adenoma).

Diagnosis

In classical cases diagnosis presents little difficulty but other causes of nervousness and irritability (e.g. anxiety state) or of weight loss (e.g. tuberculosis) must always be borne in mind. The diagnosis may be confirmed by measurement of the serum T_4 level, which is elevated, and also by measurement of the serum T_3 level since, in a proportion of hyperthyroid patients, there is increased secretion of T_3 but not of T_4.

Treatment

Three methods of treatment are available.

Drugs. Drugs such as carbimazole or methylthiouracil, have an antithyroid action and achieve satisfactory control of thyrotoxicosis in many cases by blocking the production of thyroxine. Treatment requires to be continued for a long period under careful supervision and good results are achieved in many cases. Drug treatment needs a cooperative patient and carries a slight risk of drug reaction, especially agranulocytosis and skin rashes.

Surgery. Partial thyroidectomy is an effective and relatively quick method of treatment which gives good results in skilled hands. Careful preoperative drug treatment is necessary to bring the thyrotoxicosis partly under control. Damage to the recurrent laryngeal nerve and inadvertent removal of the parathyroid glands are potential hazards. Surgical treatment is particularly useful where the gland is very large, where drug treatment has failed or where there are complications of drug treatment.

Radioactive iodine. Radioactive iodine is concentrated in the thyroid gland and the radiation liberated reduces thyroid activity. It is usually reserved for those of 40 years or over as, with other forms of radiation there is a remote possibility of cancer developing many years afterwards. The method is extremely useful for patients who are poor risks for surgery. Many patients subsequently become hypothyroid and they should therefore be kept under supervision.

Hashimoto's thyroiditis

Hashimoto's thyroiditis is characterized pathologically by lymphoid hyperplasia in the gland and clinically by goitre and sometimes by hypothyroidism. Administration of thyroxine, on a long term basis, will usually reduce the size of the gland and will correct any coincidental hypothyroidism. In a minority of patients surgery may be required for cosmetic reasons if the gland is large or if it is producing pressure symptoms.

In Hashimoto's thyroiditis there is evidence in the patient's serum of antibodies to some components of thyroid tissue (especially thyroglobulin) which act as antigens. Why some individuals develop such an antibody reaction against components of their own body is not known but the process, once started, leads to characteristic tissue damage in the thyroid gland. This type of process is referred to as an autoimmune disorder. In all patients with thyroid disorders enquiry is made as to the possibility of other autoimmune disorders in the patient or in relatives, e.g., pernicious anaemia and rheumatoid arthritis.

Thyroid neoplasm

Adenocarcinoma of the thyroid gland may commence in a pre-existing nodule of what apparently has been a simple goitre. It may arise from a solitary nodule of the thyroid gland (adenoma) or it may develop in a previously normal gland. There are three main types. The papillary type usually occurs in the young and the first manifestation may be the presence of an enlarged cervical lymph node. The lesion is often localized, perhaps in one lobe, but there may be other lesions throughout the gland. Lymph node spread is common but blood spread rare. Treatment is by a partial thyroidectomy on the affected side together with dissection of the adjacent lymph nodes and thyroxine is usually given postoperatively to decrease pituitary stimulation.

The follicular form is a tumour usually occurring in patients over 40 years old and the pattern of the tumour is characterized by thyroid follicles. The tumour is more aggressive than the papillary form and spreads by the blood stream to lungs and bones as well as by lymphatics. A more anaplastic form occurs in the elderly and is made of sheets of undifferentiated cells spreading locally so that the gland becomes hard and fixed to surrounding structures and causes local pressure effects. There are metastases to bones and lymph nodes. Treatment of the follicular form is by total thyroidectomy in order to remove the tumour and functioning thyroid tissue and then secondary lesions, if present, are irradiated. The more anaplastic tumours can sometimes be removed by radical surgery but are more often inoperable and deep X-ray therapy must be used.

Prognosis in the papillary form is extremely good but the outlook in the anaplastic form is poor. While the follicular type may have a good prognosis this is not so if distant spread has occurred.

Myxoedema

Myxoedema is the term commonly used to describe adult hypothyroidism arising from primary degenerative changes in the thyroid gland. Hypothyroidism may also result from over-energetic treatment of thyrotoxicosis or it may be due to Hashimoto's thyroiditis.

Clinical features

Thyroxine deficiency leads to a slowing down of all the body activities. The patient lacks energy, is mentally slowed, sleeps excessively, and feels the cold unduly. The weight increases due to deposit of mucin in the subcutaneous tissues; this may give the superficial appearance of oedema but there is no pitting on pressure.

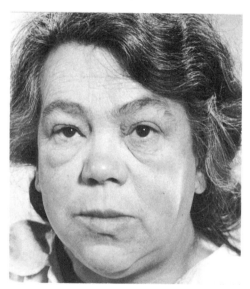

Fig. 12.3 Puffiness of face in myxoedema.

The features become heavy, the skin dry and rough, the hair coarse and sparse, bags may develop under the eyes (Fig. 12.3), while the eyebrows may become thinned in the outer third. The pulse rate is slowed, e.g. to 50 to 60 per minute.

Diagnosis
The diagnosis is confirmed by finding a low serum T_4 level.

Treatment
Substitution therapy is readily available in tablet form as sodium thyroxine. The initial dosage should be low and increases should be made gradually as cardiac function is often impaired.

Cretinism
Cretinism is the term used to describe hypothyroidism occurring in the early years of life. There is physical and mental retardation and the child is slow to reach the usual stages of childhood development such as sitting, crawling, walking, talking, etc. The face is heavy and dull, the expression is vacant, the mouth is usually open, the tongue large and protruding and the hair coarse and sparse. The abdomen is protuberant and umbilical hernia is common. Primary and secondary dentition is seriously delayed. An example of cretinism is shown in Figure 12.4.

It is important that the diagnosis is made early otherwise there

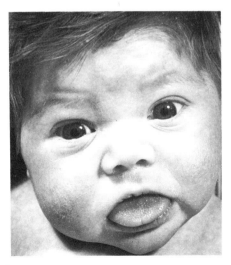

Fig. 12.4 Cretinism.

may be permanent mental and physical retardation. Treatment consists in administration of sodium thyroxine.

THE PARATHYROID GLANDS

The four parathyroid glands are situated along the posterior surface of the thyroid, usually outside the capsule, but occasionally just within the substance of the gland. The secretion of the glands, parathormone, controls the renal excretion of phosphorus so disordered function of the parathyroids is associated with profound alterations in phosphorus and calcium metabolism.

Hyperparathyroidism

This is a relatively rare disease but the dentist should be aware of it as it produces important skeletal changes which may involve the jaws.

Primary hyperparathyroidism is usually due to an adenoma of one or more glands, or occasionally hyperplasia of all four glands. Secondary hyperparathyroidism occurs as a complication of severe chronic renal failure.

The excess parathormone causes increased urinary excretion of phosphorus and, in consequence, the serum phosphorus level falls. Phosphate, as calcium phosphate, is mobilized from the skeleton in an attempt to restore the blood level of phosphorus and decalcification results. In a typical case the principal biochemical findings are a lowered serum phosphorus, an elevated serum calcium, and a high urinary calcium. The serum alkaline phosphatase level, which is an index of activity of bone breakdown and formation, is also raised.

Clinical and radiological features

The decalcification of the skeleton may show as a diffuse rarefaction or there may be multiple cysts present in addition (osteitis fibrosa cystica). The jaws are often decalcified but not the teeth. Compression of the vertebrae, pathological fractures, and deformities of the thorax and limbs may be present in severe cases. The bones may be aching and tender.

The excess calcium excretion by the kidney leads to the formation of renal calculi and progressive renal damage.

Treatment

If a tumour of the parathyroids is present it should be excised while if a diffuse hyperplasia is found three of the four glands are removed.

Hypoparathyroidism

Hypoparathyroidism, which is uncommon, may be congenital, idiopathic or may follow inadvertent removal of the glands during thyroidectomy. There is insufficient parathormone, the excretion of phosphorus decreases, the serum phosphorus rises and the serum calcium falls. The lowered serum calcium results in tetany which is characterized by increased neuromuscular excitability.

Tetany

Tetany may be due to hypoparathyroidism or more commonly to a lowered serum calcium from other causes such as rickets, osteomalacia and steatorrhoea. It may also occur in alkalosis probably as a result of lowering of the level of the ionized portion of the serum calcium. Alkalosis can be caused by abnormal losses of acid radicals as in severe vomiting, by a prolonged intake of readily absorbed alkalis such as sodium bicarbonate, or by overbreathing which causes increased carbon dioxide excretion. The latter may be seen in hysterical individuals.

In severe cases there is spontaneous muscle twitching, convulsions, and in children, a high-pitched cry due to spasm of the larynx (laryngismus stridulus). In less severe cases the neuromuscular excitability may be shown by twitching of the facial muscles after tapping over the facial nerve (Chvostek's sign) and by spasm of the hand after temporary occlusion of the blood supply of the upper arm (Trousseau's sign).

THE PITUITARY GLAND

The pituitary gland is situated in the sella turcica with the sphenoidal air sinuses below, the optic chiasma above, and the third, fourth and sixth carnial nerves, the cavernous sinus, and internal carotid artery on either side. The anterior lobe contains chromophobe, eosinophil and basophil cells while the posterior lobe consists mainly of nerve cells and fibres. Although the pituitary gland is a tiny structure it exercises a dominating influence on development and through a variety of body function hormones:

1. Growth is controlled by the growth hormone secreted by the anterior lobe.

2. The activity of the suprarenal glands is controlled by the adrenocorticotrophic hormone (ACTH) of the anterior lobe.

3. Thyroid function is controlled by the thyroid stimulating hormone (TSH) of the anterior lobe.

4. The function of the ovaries and breasts are controlled by the

follicle stimulating hormone (FSH), the luteinising hormone (LH) and prolactin; and of the testes by FSH and LH. All these hormones are from the anterior lobe.

5. The antidiuretic hormone (ADH) of the posterior lobe promotes water reabsorption from the renal tubule and hence controls the volume of urine.

Clinical disorders of the pituitary gland are relatively rare and only a brief account is given of them largely for general interest; only acromegaly is likely to be of direct interest to the dentist.

Gigantism

This is due to hypersecretion of the growth hormone of the pituitary gland occurring in childhood, i.e. before the epiphyses of the long bones have united. Heights of 7 or even 8 ft may be reached. These individuals are seldom strong and the majority die in early or middle age. Some gain their livelihood in circuses.

Dwarfism

Deficiency of the growth hormone in childhood produces pituitary dwarfism. The patient is usually well proportioned in contrast to the achrondoplastic individual in whom the head and trunk are normal in size but appear very large in contrast to the short limbs.

Dwarfism may also result from a general stunting of development caused by chronic severe illnesses occurring during childhood years (e.g. tuberculosis of the skeleton). It also occurs in cretinism.

Acromegaly

The term 'acromegaly' is derived from the Greek 'acros' meaning terminal and 'mega' meaning large, and thus is descriptive of the enlargement of the hands and feet which is a characteristic feature of the disorder. It is caused by hypersecretion of the growth hormone of the pituitary occurring in adult life, i.e. after the epiphyses have united. In most cases there is a tumour of the eosinophil cells.

The facial features (Fig. 12.5) become very coarse and heavy due to increase in the subcutaneous tissues, especially of the lips and nose. The mandible becomes enlarged to a much greater extent than the maxilla so that the lower jaw becomes very prominent. The frontal ridges and other bony prominences become enlarged. The hands and feet increase in size and the patient finds that larger gloves and shoes are required and rings no longer fit. Headache is a common complaint and later there is interference with vision because the pituitary tumour causes pressure on the optic chiasma.

No alteration takes place in the size of the teeth but they become

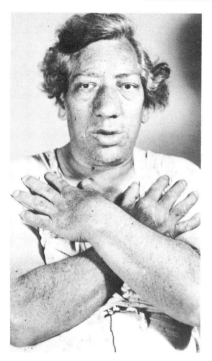

Fig. 12.5 Acromegaly. Note heavy features, large jaw, large hands.

well spaced because of the enlargement of the jaw. The lower teeth project beyond the upper often to a considerable extent. If the patient has dentures they will become progressively more ill-fitting as the lower jaw increases in size.

In the early stages of the disorder the diagnosis may often be made clear if comparison is made with a photograph of the patient taken some time before.

X-ray of the skull shows the enlarged lower jaw, prominent frontal ridges and enlarged air sinuses; in some cases enlargement and erosion of the pituitary fossa by the tumour is evident.

X-ray therapy directed to the pituitary gland is often successful in reducing the activity of the tumour. Surgical resection or cryosurgery (tissue destruction by extreme temperature reduction) are alternative forms of treatment.

Simmonds' disease

Severe haemorrhage associated with childbearing is the usual aetiological factor. For some ill-understood reason the shock leads to necrotic changes in the pituitary gland and thus to deficiency of several of the pituitary functions. Another term for the disorder is panhypopituitarism.

In the fully developed picture there is depressed thyroid function producing the features of hypothyroidism, depressed suprarenal function, and depressed sexual function producing sterility and amenorrhoea. Considerable improvement occurs following replacement hormonal treatment.

Cushing's disease

This is due to a basophil adenoma of the pituitary. The main clinical features are obesity, polycythaemia, hypertension, glycosuria and osteoporosis.

Fröhlich's syndrome

This syndrome is characterized by obesity, disturbances of the natural sleep rhythm and sexual retardation. It has been suggested that the fat boy in *Pickwick Papers* may have been an example of this condition.

Diabetes insipidus

Deficiency of the antidiuretic hormone, which controls the urinary volume, results in diabetes insipidus. The patient passes a very large volume of urine, possibly five or six times the normal amount, and, in consequence, suffers considerable inconvenience, loses sleep, and is constantly thirsty. The urine is of low specific gravity but does not contain any abnormal constituents. Diabetes insipidus can be controlled by supplying the antidiuretic hormone either by injection or as a snuff.

THE ADRENAL GLANDS

The adrenal, or suprarenal, glands are two in number, one lying on the upper pole of each kidney. The gland is composed of a medulla and cortex which have a different embryological origin and different physiological activities.

The medulla

The hormones of the adrenal medulla are adrenaline and noradrenaline. Both substances cause constriction of blood vessels and elevation of the blood pressure. Adrenaline also has a powerful effect on carbohydrate metabolism causing mobilization of liver glycogen and a rise in blood sugar. Adrenaline may be used in the treatment of asthma since it relieves bronchospasm.

Disorders of the adrenal medulla are rarely encountered. *Phaeochromocytoma* is an actively secreting tumour which causes the hypertension.

The cortex
A large number of steroid hormones secreted by the adrenal cortex have now been identified. The cortical hormones are secreted in response to stimulation by corticotrophin (ACTH) of the anterior pituitary. The steroid hormones play a vital role in many body functions and they have a range of therapeutic usefulness which far extends beyond the replacement therapy of adrenal insufficiency. The principal actions of the steroid hormones may be grouped as follows:

1. Carbohydrate metabolism. The so-called glucocorticoids (especially cortisol or hydrocortisone) produce increased glucose formation from protein and possibly fat and decreased glucose utilization through an anti-insulin effect.

2. Sodium metabolism. The so-called mineralocorticoids (especially aldosterone) produce retention of sodium and increased excretion of potassium through effects on the renal tubule. There is a tendency to fluid retention and hypertension.

3. Sex hormones. The adrenal cortex produces male hormones (androgens) and female hormones (oestrogens) which are largely responsible for the development of the secondary sex characteristics.

Acute hypocorticalism
Acute adrenal insufficiency is a very serious condition which may occur as a rare complication of severe infections with septicaemia, or as an adrenal crisis in Addison's disease. The principal features are acute circulatory collapse, dehydration, hypoglycaemia and vomiting. Intensive fluid, salt, glucose, and hormonal replacement therapy is required.

Chronic hypocorticalism
The principal form of chronic adrenal insufficiency is Addison's disease which is of dental interest because of the buccal changes. It may be caused by tuberculosis of the adrenals or idiopathic degenerative changes.

The main clinical features are marked loss of energy, hypotension (e.g. a blood pressure of 90/50 mm of Hg), anorexia and vomiting, and pigmentation of the skin and mucous membranes. The skin pigmentation is more marked on exposed areas and may appear as a slaty-blue colour or, in some instances, like sunburn. Slaty-blue or dark-grey pigmentation frequently occurs in the buccal mucosa particularly along the line of closure of the teeth. It is practically pathognomonic of Addison's disease provided physiological pigmentation of racial origin is excluded. The deficiency of mineralocorticoids leads to excessive renal losses of salt and thus to characteristic alterations in the biochemical pattern of the urine and blood.

It is important for dentists to appreciate that patients with Addison's disease tolerate anaesthesia, surgical procedures and infection very poorly. Injudicious surgery may precipitate an adrenal crisis which may prove fatal unless skilled replacement therapy is promptly instituted.

Mild cases may be controlled by the administration of salt supplements but it is often necessary to provide replacement of the deficient hormones, e.g. by giving cortisone or a related substance.

Hypercorticalism

Overactivity of the adrenal cortex, which may result from tumour or hyperplasia, is relatively uncommon. The clinical effects are largely determined by the steroid hormone which is preponderant. Excess secretion of the cortisol group (glucocorticoids) has features similar to those of Cushing's disease (p. 250). Excess secretion of aldosterone (mineralocorticoid) produces sodium retention, potassium loss, and hypertension (Conn's syndrome). Excess secretion of androgens produces masculinization in the female (virilism) and excess of oestrogens produces feminization in the male.

Diagnosis is by laboratory estimations of the steroid hormones and by radiological studies of the adrenals. If a tumour is found it is removed. If hyperplasia is found then bilateral adrenalectomy or subtotal removal of the adrenal mass is carried out.

13

Swellings of the head and neck

It is important that the dentist has a clear appreciation of the various disorders which may be responsible for producing swellings in relation to the head or neck and they are summarized in this chapter. Diseases of the salivary glands (Ch. 8), of the thyroid gland (Ch. 12), and certain disorders affecting the lymph nodes (Ch. 11) have already been dealt with.

Physical examination of swellings of the head and neck
The precise anatomical situation of the swelling is important. It is particularly important to note whether the swelling is attached to surrounding tissue and to determine the plane in which it lies. Skin swellings are most likely to be sebaceous cysts or boils whereas lesions infiltrating the skin are much more likely to be cancerous in origin.

Thyroid swellings (Ch. 12) occur below or on either side of the thyroid cartilage and move on swallowing. Thyroglossal cysts on the other hand lie in the midline but also move on swallowing or on protrusion of the tongue.

The common lateral swelling in the neck is due to lymph node enlargement but in the upper third of the neck anterior to the sternomastoid muscle branchial cyst must be considered.

Submandibular swellings characteristically appear just below the body of the mandible and swellings of the parotid gland behind the angle of the mandible and anterior to the mastoid process. If there is intermittent obstruction to a salivary duct then the relevant gland becomes tense and enlarged after a meal.

The *consistency* of the swelling is important as is its *shape*. These may give a clue to its origin and to the cystic nature or otherwise of the swelling. Fluctuation can often be very difficult to elicit in the neck but tenderness usually indicates inflammation. The only neck swelling that transilluminates brilliantly is a cystic hygroma.

Branchial fistula and branchial cyst
These two conditions are congenital in origin and arise from the

remnant of the second branchial cleft. The lowermost opening of the remnant of this cleft is at the anterior border of the sternomastoid muscle just behind and below the angle of the jaw. The track of the remnant then passes upwards between the internal and external carotid arteries and its inner opening is located in the region of the tonsil.

A branchial fistula stretching from the tonsillar fossa to the skin is most unusual. More commonly there is a sinus opening anteriorly and lined with squamous and occasionally columnar epithelium. The opening of the track may be very tiny and only as the child grows and the track becomes infected the orifice become evident, usually because of an intermittent discharge. Treatment is by excision of the entire track.

A branchial cyst is lined by squamous epithelium and the fluid contains cholesterol crystals. The cyst lies in the track of the second branchial cleft and presents in adult life protruding from the anterior border of the sternomastoid muscle. There may be a fibrous track passing upwards as in branchial fistula. Infection may occur particularly if attempts are made to aspirate the cyst. Treatment is again by complete excision.

Thyroglossal cyst

This is a cystic remnant in the length of the thyroglossal tract stretching from the junction of the anterior two thirds with the posterior one third of the tongue to the thyroid gland in the midline. The cyst lies anywhere in the midline above the thyroid cartilage and moves on swallowing or on protrusion of the tongue.

The track of the cyst runs anterior to and then curls up for a short distance behind the hyoid bone before descending to the thyroid gland. Excision of the cyst involves removal of the track; this often necessitating removal of the central portion of the hyoid bone.

Cystic hygroma. This is a multilocular cyst, often very large, and consists of a cavernous lymphangioma. The majority of cases present in early childhood or indeed may be evident at birth. Unlike many other swellings of the neck, a common site is in the posterior triangle or supraclavicular region. There are often deep extensions even reaching into the chest or axilla, and excision can be extremely difficult.

Skin lesions of the head and neck

Boils and carbuncles are extremely common, especially on the back of the neck, and the scalp is the most common site of the sebaceous cyst. This is a cystic swelling lying in the skin and lined by a squamous epithelium. The cyst arises from the sebaceous glands related to the hairs and may occur anywhere on hair-growing areas of the body. The cyst is filled with sebum and there is always a small orifice (punctum) visible on the surface. Sebaceous cysts commonly become infected and discharge intermittently. Treatment is by surgical excision.

Skin tumours have been dealt with elsewhere (Ch. 5) but it should be remembered that nearly all varieties of the common skin tumours occur very frequently about the face.

Cervical lymphadenopathy

Swellings of the cervical lymph nodes are of great importance to the dentist. Some of these have already been referred to in discussing disorders of the haemopoietic system (Ch. 11). The following are common causes of lymph node enlargement in the neck.

Lymphadenitis

The cervical lymph nodes and in particular the submental, submandibular and jugulodigastric glands are commonly infected from inflammatory lesions of the scalp and face, the tongue, oral cavity, nasal cavity, tonsils and pharynx. The infected nodes are swollen, painful and tender to touch, and as the inflammation progresses, they become adherent. Abscess formation may occur with the formation of fluctuant swellings and reddening of the skin, and these abscesses may discharge spontaneously.

Diagnosis is dependent on tracing the source of infection and this involves full examination of the head and neck, including a detailed examination of the teeth. Treatment consists of attention to the source of infection and appropriate antibiotic therapy. Abscess cavities in the neck may require incision and drainage. Long continued chronic infected foci, as for instance a chronic periapical abscess, may result in chronically enlarged slightly tender cervical nodes which may resolve on appropriate treatment of the primary source of infection.

Tuberculous and syphilitic lymphadenitis have already been discussed.

Glandular fever

This is an important cause of lymph node enlargement, the main diagnostic points being the blood picture and the Paul Bunnell reaction.

German measles or rubella

This may similarly be associated with enlargement of the glands in the upper part of the posterior chain of cervical lymph nodes.

Reticuloses and leukaemia

Cervical lymph node adenopathy is commonly seen in acute leukaemia, being due partly to the leukaemia per se and partly to the infection which occurs in the mouth and throat in these cases. The main diagnostic points are the presence of anaemia, bruising and the characteristic blood and marrow findings. Cervical lymph node enlargement is common in chronic lymphatic leukaemia, examination of the blood yielding a diagnosis readily. Lymph node enlargement is much less common in other leukaemias.

Lymphadenoma, lymphosarcoma and the other reticuloses may also lead to enlargement of the glands of the neck and differentiation is on the basis of histological features.

Secondary carcinoma

The cervical lymph nodes are commonly enlarged as a result of a secondary spread from cancer anywhere in the upper alimentary or upper respiratory tracts. It is important to recognize that enlargement of the supraclavicular group of nodes, particularly on the left, can occur in cancer of the stomach or pancreas. Diagnosis involves appropriate investigation of the alimentary or respiratory tract but excision biopsy with histology is usually necessary.

Carotid body tumour

This is a tumour arising from the carotid body at the bifurcation of the common carotid artery. It is a slowly growing tumour and may occlude the carotid vessels.

The tumour does not move on swallowing and characteristically pulsates and is mobile in a horizontal but not in a vertical plane. Treatment is by surgical removal.

14

Disorders of nutrition and metabolism

It is important, for several reasons, that the dentist should have a clear understanding of what constitutes a well-balanced diet.

1. Proper nutrition throughout childhood is an essential factor in the development of sound primary and secondary teeth.

2. Dietary factors are of definite importance in regard to the causation and prevention of dental caries.

3. Several deficiency disorders have important manifestations in the buccal cavity.

4. Resistance to infection, including dental infection, is lowered in states of faulty nutrition and the powers of recovery from illness are impaired.

A sound diet may be defined as that which will enable the body to develop to its full potentiality, yield sufficient energy for work and play, maintain the body weight at a proper level, and aid in keeping the individual in good health. The constituents of a well-balanced diet are protein, fat, carbohydrate, minerals, vitamins, water and electrolytes.

CALORIE CONTENT

It is generally recommended that a young healthy adult male, of average weight, engaged in an occupation entailing moderate physical effort, should have a calorie intake of about 3,000 calories per day. The comparable figure for a young housewife is about 500 calories less. It should be appreciated that these are average figures and that there are considerable individual variations in energy expenditure among persons engaged in apparently similar occupations.

An increased calorie intake is required for those doing heavy manual work, during infection, during pregnancy and lactation, in hyperthyroidism, and in cold climates. Thus some heavy manual workers require about 5,000 calories per day. The calorie requirements decrease with advancing years.

One may calculate the calorie content of the diet in a simple way by remembering the following approximate figures.

1 gram carbohydrate	yields 4 calories
1 gram protein	yields 4 calories
1 gram fat	yields 9 calories

PROTEIN

Protein, which is composed of various amino acids, is an essential constituent of all living cells. A certain intake is therefore necessary for growth, for the replacement of tissues, and also for the formation of some enzymes and hormones. Those amino acids which are termed 'essential' cannot be readily synthesized by the body from other sources whereas the 'non-essential' amino acids can be. The essential amino acids are eight in number—lysine, tryptophan, phenylalanine, leucine, isoleucine, threonine, methionine and valine. Protein foodstuffs which supply all the essential amino acids are classified as first-class protein; those lacking some of the essential amino acids are referred to as second-class proteins.

For the average adult the protein intake probably should not be less than 60 to 70 g per day. A higher intake is required in pregnancy and lactation. In children the figure is relatively higher because of the demands of growth. The main animal sources of protein are meat, fish, milk and milk products, and eggs; peas, beans, lentils, oatmeal, and soya beans are good vegetable sources.

Kwashiorkor is a disease caused by gross protein deficiency in children. It is widespread in Africa. The main features are wasting, severe liver dysfunction, oedema, and a failure to thrive.

FAT

Fat is important in the diet because it is a rich source of calories, it contains some fatty acids which are essential for health, and it contains the important fat-soluble vitamins A, D and K. The wide use of fat for cooking renders many foods more palatable. The amount of fat in the diet varies considerably according to individual taste, to racial customs, to the time of year, and to the climate. In Britain a daily intake of around 100 g per day is common. The intake is usually higher in cold countries.

Fat may be of animal origin such as meat and milk products, or vegetable origin such as margarine and many cooking fats. The possible role of a high animal fat intake in the pathogenesis of coronary artery disease has already been referred to (p. 104).

CARBOHYDRATE

Carbohydrate is the main source of energy in the diet and the daily intake should depend largely on the required calorie expenditure. Obesity will inevitably result if an excess is taken.

Given a protein and fat intake of 70 to 100 and 100 to 120 g per day respectively, this leaves approximately 1,600 calories to be supplied by carbohydrate—i.e. an intake of about 400 g.

Carbohydrate foods are less expensive than either protein or fat and their proportion in the diet usually increases as the family income falls. Main sources of carbohydrates are sugar, bread, other flour products such as buns, scones, biscuits, cakes, potatoes, jams and other preserves.

MINERALS

Iron

Iron is an essential constituent of haemoglobin. The daily requirements are about 12 to 15 mg. A considerably greater amount of iron is present in an average diet, but the body absorbs from the gut only what it needs. The principal dietary sources of iron are meat, fish, egg yolk and green vegetables.

Deficiency of iron leads to hypochromic anaemia which is fully discussed in the chapter on blood diseases.

Calcium

Calcium is required for the formation of bone and teeth. It also regulates neuromuscular excitability and, if the level of calcium in the blood falls, tetany may be produced (p. 247). In addition, calcium is one of the factors necessary for the coagulation of the blood.

The chief sources of calcium are milk, milk products such as butter and cheese, cereals, green vegetables, and eggs. The average adult requires about 0·75 g of calcium per day and up to twice this amount in pregnancy and lactation.

About 25 per cent of the calcium in the food is absorbed from the small intestine. Absorption is largely controlled by vitamin D and the parathyroid glands. Deficient absorption occurs if there is inadequate intake of vitamin D or if the hydroxyalation of vitamin D in the kidney to its active metabolite is deficient as a consequence of chronic renal disease. Calcium absorption may also be impaired if there is defective absorption of fat (steatorrhoea) due to the fact that the inabsorbed fats combine with the dietary calcium to form insoluble soaps. It can be shown in experimental animals that phytic acid decreases calcium absorption although the significance of this in human dietetics is debated. Calcium carbonate is added to bread made from flour with a high phytic acid content, as a precautionary measure.

The blood level of calcium is normally 2·2 to 2·6 mmol per litre (9 to 11 mg per 100 ml). The calcium level bears an inverse relationship with the serum phosphorus level so that the product Ca:P tends to remain a constant.

Iodine

Iodine is an essential constituent of thyroxine, the hormone of the thyroid gland. The daily requirement is about 0·25 mg. Normal sources of iodine are drinking water, fish and vegetables. Deficiency of dietary iodine is an important cause of simple goitre.

Phosphorus

Phosphorus, like calcium, is an essential constituent of bone and teeth. The diet should contain 1 to 2 g per day and the requirement is increased in pregnancy and lactation. Phosphorus is found in similar foodstuffs as calcium and a diet adequate in the one mineral will be adequate in the other.

The normal serum inorganic phosphate level is 0·8 to 1·4 mmol per litre (3 to 4·5 mg per 100 ml). Organic phosphate is to be found mainly within the cells where it is the principal anion. The organic intracellular phosphates are connected with energy exchange and with the metabolism of fats and carbohydrate. The cells also contain phosphorus in the nucleoproteins, phosphoproteins and phospholipids.

Fluorine

Fluorine is a substance which has a considerable dental interest. It is present in the bones and teeth, especially the dentine, in higher concentration than in other tissues of the body. The arguments for and against fluoridation of water supplies will be well known to the dental student and need not be repeated in this text.

WATER AND ELECTROLYTES

Water

It will be seen from a study of Figure 14.1 that water comprises more than half of the total body weight. The amount in the average adult is approximately 40 litres, of which 25 litres is within the cells and 15 litres is extracellular.

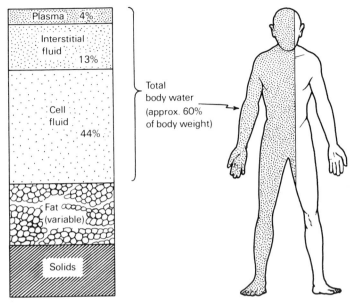

Fig. 14.1 The composition of the body.

The water intake is derived from the fluid drunk and from the water content of food. To this must be added the metabolic water derived from the oxidation of foodstuffs. The total water available from those sources is, on average, about 2½ litres per day. This intake is balanced by insensible loss of water from the skin and lungs, by the urine, and by the faecal water.

In health, the body does its own regulating, largely through the medium of thirst and variation in urinary volume, but in diseases these mechanisms may be deranged. It is of critical importance to maintain a proper fluid balance in all who are ill.

Salt
Sodium and chloride are widely distributed through the body and, in health, their concentrations are kept within narrow limits. Sodium is the principal cation of the extracellular fluid and is one of the main agents responsible for controlling the acid-base balance of the body. Chloride is the main anion of the extracellular fluid.

The normal salt intake is about 5 to 15 g per day but there is considerable individual variation. The main route for salt excretion is the urine. Excess sweating may be an appreciable factor in very hot atmospheres and salt depletion is now known to be the cause of 'heat-exhaustion'. Very large amounts of salt may be lost by diarrhoea and vomiting as in cholera and dysentery. The hormones of the adrenal cortex play an important part in regulating salt metabolism, and abnormal salt loss in the urine is a characteristic feature of Addison's disease.

Potassium

Potassium is the principal cation of the intracellular fluid. Hypokalaemia causes a form of muscle paralysis while hyperkalaemia leads to impaired cardiac function which may prove suddenly fatal.

THE VITAMINS

Historical

Probably the first clear-cut demonstration of the relationship between deficiency of foodstuffs and the development of a specific disease was the work of James Lind, the British naval surgeon. His *A Treatise of the Scurvy* published in 1753 showed clearly the value of fresh fruit in preventing scurvy among the crews of sailing-ships and his work was responsible for the introduction of fruit juice in seamen's rations. The subsequent compulsory issue of lime juice in the British Merchant Service led to the use, by Americans, of the term 'limeys' for British seamen; it is still sometimes employed, often in a derogatory sense, for the English.

In the early years of this century Hopkins and Funk published separate papers dealing with certain accessory food factors which were necessary for life. Funk coined the name 'vitamine' in the belief that the substances were amines; the 'e' was later dropped when it became apparent that this was not so. A tremendous amount of knowledge has now accumulated about the vitamins and they have been tried, often quite irrationally, as therapeutic agents, in practically every disease. Their use is indicated only where there is definite deficiency or at least a reasonable suspicion of deficiency.

Definition

Vitamins may be defined as organic substances which are essential for normal growth and the maintenance of health, are effective in very small amounts, do not yield energy directly, but are essential for the transformation of energy.

Classification of the vitamins

1. Water-soluble vitamins

Vitamin B complex, the more important components being thiamine, riboflavine, nicotinic acid, vitamin B_{12} and folic acid.

Vitamin C or ascorbic acid.

2. *Fat-soluble vitamins*
   Vitamin A.
   Vitamin D.
   Vitamin K.

Normal requirements
The average daily requirements of vitamins are given in Table 3. These are increased in pregnancy, lactation, and childhood. The figures are internationally accepted and, owing to American influence, they are generous by the standards of many countries.

Causes of deficiency
Vitamin deficiency may result from one or more of the following causes.

   1. Inadequate intake. This may be due to economic factors, faulty cooking (especially vitamin C), food faddism and alcoholism.

   2. Diminished absorption from the gut. This may be caused by steatorrhoea, in which case the deficiency is multiple, or the absence of bile from the gut, in which case the deficiency is limited to the fat-soluble vitamins.

   3. Increased requirements. There is an increased requirement for vitamins in infection, pregnancy, lactation and hyperthyroidism.

   4. Impaired synthesis. Antibiotic or sulphonamide therapy may lead to the destruction of the bacteria in the gut which normally synthesize vitamins of the B complex.

The vitamin B group
The vitamin B complex is now known to comprise at least 12 individual components but only thiamine, riboflavine and nicotinic acid will be considered here. Vitamin B_{12} and folic acid are described in the chapter on blood diseases.

   All the components of this group of vitamins are concerned with fundamental enzyme systems which control the later stages of energy production and cellular metabolism. Good plant sources of vitamin B are yeast, peas, beans and grain, while satisfactory animal sources are egg yolk, liver and milk. A simple and relatively inexpensive way to ensure a high intake of all the vitamin B group is to give three or four yeast tablets three times daily.

Thiamine (aneurine or vitamin B_1)
Deficiency of thiamine produces a disorder termed 'beriberi', which is endemic in the Far East in people who live almost exclu-

Table 3 Recommended daily dietary allowance of vitamins

	Vitamin A I.U.	Thiamine mg	Riboflavine mg	Nicotinic acid mg	Ascorbic acid mg	Vitamin D I.U.
Moderately active man	5,000	1·5	1·8	15	25	*
Moderately active woman	5,000	1·2	1·5	12	25	*
Woman in pregnancy or lactation	6–8,000	1·5	2·5–3·0	15	100–150	400
Child up to 12 years†	2–5,000	0·4–1·2	0·6–1·8	4–12	30–75	400
Child over 12 years	5,000	1·3–1·7	1·8–2·5	12–17	80–100	400

* It is doubtful if the average adult requires to supplement from dietary sources the vitamin D derived from the skin.
† The requirements in childhood increase progressively with age.

sively on highly polished rice. Beriberi has two main forms. The principal feature of wet beriberi is cardiac failure with oedema and dyspnoea. Dry beriberi is characterized by a severe polyneuritis with muscle wasting, paralysis, and limb pains; in severe cases mental confusion is present.

Riboflavine (vitamin B_2)

Riboflavine is especially concerned with the metabolism of the cells of the buccal cavity, cornea and skin. Deficiency causes glossitis, the tongue often being magenta in colour, angular stomatitis, increased vascularity of the cornea producing photophobia and keratitis, and a scaly, greasy change in the skin around the nose, lips and ears.

Nicotinic acid (niacin)

Deficiency of nitotinic acid produces a disorder termed 'pellagra'; the word is derived from the Italian for rough skin 'pelle agra'. Pellagra is endemic in areas where maize, which may contain a toxic factor, is the staple item of diet. The main features are dermatitis, maximal in areas exposed to light, diarrhoea, and mental confusion progressing to complete dementia.

Occurrence of vitamin B deficiency

It is commoner to see cases showing deficiency of several of the components of the B complex rather than isolated deficiencies. Furthermore, there is often a deficiency of other substances, e.g. protein, iron and minerals.

Vitamin B deficiency may occur as follows.

1. Endemic in certain areas of the world due to dietary inadequacy.

2. In special circumstances of deprivation such as Japanese POW camps in the 1940–45 war, famine and drought.

3. Secondary to absorption defects such as steatorrhoea.

4. In chronic alcoholics in whom it is largely responsible for the mental symptoms of delirium tremens.

5. As a complication of antibiotic therapy.

Vitamin C

Sources

Vitamin C, or ascorbic acid, is present in good concentration in fresh fruits and in green vegetables. Although relatively small quantities are present in potatoes, we obtain a substantial proportion of our vitamin C requirements from this source because of the amount eaten. Vitamin C is destroyed by overcooking and by alkalis. The basic requirements are 25 to 30 mg per day.

Functions

Vitamin C is essential for the formation of intercellular substances in connective tissues, capillary walls, bone and dentine. It plays a part in the development of red blood cells although its precise role is uncertain. Vitamin C is also concerned with the reactions of the body to infection and stress; in this connection it may be noted that it is present in high concentration in the adrenal glands.

Scurvy

Scurvy is caused by a deficiency of vitamin C. It used to be a very serious cause of disease among the crews of sailing vessels, and in the British Navy scurvy was probably responsible for more deaths than enemy action. In large towns such as Glasgow it is now seen particularly in elderly people, especially men, who are living in poor circumstances on a very limited diet often largely consisting of bread and tea. It may be seen occasionally in peptic ulcer patients adhering to a very rigid bland diet without proper supervision.

The main clinical features of scurvy are as follows:

1. Marked loss of energy.

2. Changes in the gums of those who still possess their own teeth. The gums become spongy, swollen, and bleed very readily, e.g. on brushing the teeth or after mastication. The changes are usually first evident in the interdental papillae. Infection of the gums is frequently superimposed leading to halitosis.

3. Bruises after trivial injuries. The bruises may be extensive and very painful. They are most often seen on the legs.

4. Small haemorrhages around the hair follicles especially on the thighs. Roughening of the skin at the base of the hair follicles also occurs (hyperkeratosis).

5. Delayed wound healing and a tendency for recently healed wounds to burst open.

6. A moderate degree of anaemia often largely due to an associated dietary deficiency of iron.

7. Subperiosteal haemorrhages, which may cause considerable pain, are a feature of severe scurvy in infants.

Scurvy responds to intensive treatment with oral vitamin C, e.g. 200 mg three times daily of the synthetic preparation. The essential step in prophylaxis is a liberal intake of properly cooked vegetables and of fresh fruit or fruit juices.

Vitamin A

Sources
Vitamin A is fat-soluble and is present in high concentration in fish liver oils, dairy products and eggs. Carotene, which is converted to vitamin A in the body, is present in certain vegetables, especially carrots and tomatoes.

Functions
Vitamin A plays an important part in the regulation of the growth of epithelial tissue, and it is essential for the formation of visual purple.

Deficiency
If there is deficiency of vitamin A the main effect is shown on the epithelial tissues. The skin becomes hardened, scaly and roughened ('toad skin'), the cornea becomes dry (xerophthalmia) and in severe cases ulcerated, and there is impaired vision in the dark causing night blindness.

Uses
There is a popular belief that the administration of regular supplements of vitamin A and D gives protection against the common cold and other respiratory infections but the scientific basis for this view is very insecure.

Vitamin D

Sources
Vitamin D is fat-soluble and, like vitamin A, is found in high concentration in fish liver oils, in dairy products and in egg yolk. It is also formed in the skin from a precursor 7-dehydrocholesterol under the influence of ultraviolet light. It may be prepared synthetically from ergosterol by irradiation.

Functions
Vitamin D is essential for the proper absorption of calcium and phosphorus from the gut and for their subsequent utilization in bone formation. Deficiency leads to rickets in the child and osteomalacia (p. 286) in the adult.

Rickets

Aetiology
Deficiency of vitamin D in the growing child is usually due to a

faulty diet. Lack of sunlight often plays an important contributory role. Calcium absorption is impaired and, in many cases, an associated dietary inadequacy increases the deficiency of this mineral so that there is insufficient calcium for the body's needs. Calcium salts are not deposited in normal amounts in growing cartilage and newly formed bone which remains soft. These changes are particularly evident at sites of very active bone formation such as the ends of long bones and at costochondral junctions. The soft osteoid tissue is liable to be deformed according to external stresses. The lack of calcium also leads to loss of tone in the skeletal muscles and hyperexcitability of the nerves.

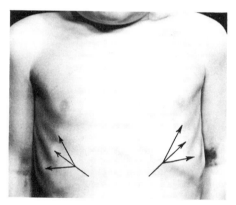

Fig. 14.2 Rachitic rosary.

Clinical features

The main clinical features (Figs. 14.2 and 14.3) which may be found in florid cases can be grouped as follows:

1. The limb bones. The earliest change is thickening of the wrists and ankles due to enlargement of the epiphyses caused by the pull of muscles and tendons. As the child begins to crawl and walk, the softened long bones become curved and deformed.

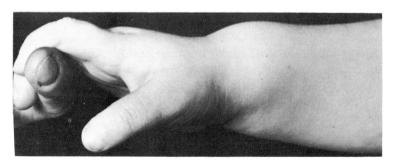

Fig. 14.3 Thickening of wrist in rickets.

2. *The pelvis.* The bones of the pelvis become deformed when weight bearing occurs and in females this causes, in later years, serious mechanical obstruction to childbearing.

3. *The skull.* Softening of the skull bones of the infant is one of the earliest skeletal changes in rickets. The change is usually most evident in the occipital and parietal regions where it may be relatively easy to depress the softened bone with finger pressure. Delayed closure of the fontanelles is another important sign. Later there is abnormal thickening of the skull in the region of the frontal and parietal eminences so that the head may have a relatively square shape.

4. *The thorax.* Enlargement of the costochrondral junctions produces a line of swellings along the chest wall termed 'rachitic beading' or the 'rachitic rosary'. The sternum often projects unduly giving the chest a 'pigeon shape', and in severe cases the chest may be almost triangular on cross-section.

5. *The teeth.* Delayed dentition is invariable and the teeth when they appear are poorly calcified.

6. *Other points.* The nutrition may appear quite good owing to a high carbohydrate intake, but rachitic children are usually underheight for their age. The muscle hypotonia leads to a pot belly and weakness of the limbs.

Biochemical changes
The most consistent biochemical change in active rickets is elevation of the serum alkaline phosphatase level. There may be a fall in one or both of the calcium and phosphorus levels.

Radiological changes
The changes are most evident at the lower ends of the radius and ulna. The epiphyseal line becomes irregular or frayed, concave, and splayed out owing to the widening of the bone ends (Fig. 14.4). The bones are less dense than normal. The deformity of the long bones is confirmed. A thin white line develops in the epiphyseal area when healing occurs following treatment.

Prevention and treatment
Severe rickets is now uncommon in Britain due to the general adequacy of nutrition and the ready availability of additional milk and vitamin D in pregnancy and childhood. Less severe rickets still occurs, however, and perhaps especially in immigrant children in whom the dietary intake of vitamin D is inadequate to compensate for the reduced amount derived from the skin in our duller climate.

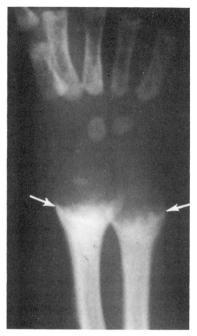

Fig. 14.4 Rickets—irregular, concave, epiphyseal line with widened bone ends.

For the treatment of active rickets vitamin D is usually pre-scribed (as calciferol) to give a daily dose of about 2,000 i.u. per day. A satisfactory calcium intake is also required.

Vitamin K

Sources
Vitamin K is fat-soluble. It is found in green plants, especially spin-ach, and it is formed in the large bowel by the normal bacterial flora.

Functions.
Vitamin K is essential for the formation in the liver of prothrombin which is one of the factors necessary for coagulation of the blood.

Deficiency
Deficiency of vitamin K often develops in obstructive jaundice be-cause absence of bile from the gut causes impaired absorption of fat, including the fat-soluble vitamin K. Deficiency of prothrombin results and there is undue tendency to bleed.

Uses

Vitamin K should be given by injection before any form of surgery in patients with jaundice. A suitable preparation is Synkavit.

Vitamin K_1, which is an analogue of vitamin K, is an efficient antidote to the oral anticoagulant drugs such as phenindione and warfarin.

EMACIATION

The principal conditions which may produce marked loss of weight are listed below. A careful history and physical examination will frequently yield a presumptive diagnosis but, in many cases, other investigations will be required.

1. Inadequate food. Starvation is now rare in Britain but it is still a major problem in many areas of the world.

2. Diabetes mellitus.

3. Thyrotoxicosis.

4. Chronic infection, specially tuberculosis.

5. Malignant neoplasm of any site.

6. Obstructive lesions of the alimentary canal (e.g. pyloric stenosis) or impaired absorption (e.g. steatorrhoea).

7. Anorexia nervosa. This is a psychiatric disorder which most often affect girls or young women. There is profound loss of appetite and weight loss.

SIMPLE OBESITY

The term 'simple obesity' is used to describe an excess of fat unassociated with any apparent endocrine disorder. The condition, which is a common one, is more frequent in women and the incidence rises with age.

Aetiology

The basis of simple obesity is always a prolonged intake of calories in excess of the calories expended in energy, a state of affairs graphically described as a plethora of calories. Carbohydrate is the main source of the unnecessary calories.

Many individuals tend to put on weight as they get older because they do not decrease their food intake commensurate with the reduction in physical exercise which normally occurs in middle age and later. In other persons the appetite, for reasons which are not fully understood, is grossly excessive and, even although the individual may remain quite active, he (or more frequently she) becomes obese. Some consider that gluttony is often determined by psychological factors and that the pleasure derived from excessive eating is a substitute for some deep-seated unsatisfied desire.

Fat people commonly shelter behind the belief that they have some ill-defined glandular upset over which they have no control, but, as far as is known at the present time, there is no evidence that this is so in the vast majority of cases.

Prognosis

The obese may suffer little disability for many years apart possibly from breathlessness on exertion and some limitation of physical activity. In middle age and in the later years of life, however, they are much more prone to develop coronary artery disease, gallbladder disease, diabetes mellitus, cerebrovascular catastrophes, osteoarthritis and varicose veins. Furthermore, the obese are greater risks for surgical operations and anaesthetics. It is not surprising, therefore, that the expectation of life is distinctly shorter for the obese. Life insurance societies are well aware of this fact and adjust their premiums accordingly.

Treatment

Treatment is extremely simple in principle but often difficult in practice. The calorie intake is reduced principally by cutting down on carbohydrates. A diet yielding about 1,000 calories per day with a carbohydrate content not greater than 100 g is satisfactory in most cases until the body weight is near normal; it can then be carefully increased to a level which keeps the weight steady. Even lower calorie intakes may be used but, if so, careful supervision is necessary.

Difficulty arises because many fat people strongly deny that they eat excessively while others have a genuine problem in adhering to the diet. Firm handling of the patient is necessary together with frequent visits and remonstrations. The use of the amphetamine group of drugs to depress appetite is undesirable; they have serious side effects and may lead to addiction.

DIABETES MELLITUS

The term 'diabetes mellitus' is derived from two of the cardinal features of the disorder, namely the passage of a large volume of urine which contains sugar. Patients with diabetes mellitus may be divided into two categories:

1. Those in whom the diabetes develops in early life (say up to

40 years), who lose weight, and who require insulin therapy.

2. Those in whom the diabetes develops in later life, who are obese, and who do not require insulin therapy.

Insulin deficient diabetes mellitus

Aetiology

The islets of Langerhans in the pancreas lose the ability to produce adequate amounts of insulin. The disorder may develop at any age. A family history is present in about 25 per cent of cases.

As a consequence of insulin deficiency carbohydrate metabolism is seriously affected; the tissues cannot utilize glucose and the liver cannot store glucose as glycogen. The level of glucose in the blood increases (hyperglycaemia) and some of the excess is excreted in the urine. Protein and fat are utilized as sources of energy and wasting therefore occurs. Fat metabolism is also impaired and there is accumulation of ketone bodies which are excreted in the urine and breath.

Clinical features

Polyuria occurs due to the osmotic effect of the sugar present in the urine, and the increased fluid loss causes thirst. Pruritus, or itch, results from irritation of the urinary passages by the sugar. There is loss of weight and loss of energy. The breath may have the characteristic fruity odour of acetone.

The urine is of high volume, pale, and contains sugar which gives it a high specific gravity. Ketonuria is a feature of severe, uncontrolled cases.

Diagnosis

The urinary findings plus a high blood sugar are usually sufficient to make a diagnosis, but a glucose tolerance test is necessary in doubtful cases. The fasting blood sugar is determined, the patient is given at least 50 g of glucose in water to drink, and the blood sugar is estimated at half-hourly intervals for 2½ hours. In the diabetic subject the fasting level is high, the curve rises out with the normal range, and does not return to normal (Fig. 14.5). The normal fasting blood sugar is 4·0 to 5·5 mmol per litre (80 to 120 mg per 100 ml) and the non-fasting range is 5·5 to 10 mmol per litre (120 to 180 mg per 100 ml).

Complications

Diabetes mellitus, especially if it is poorly controlled, may be

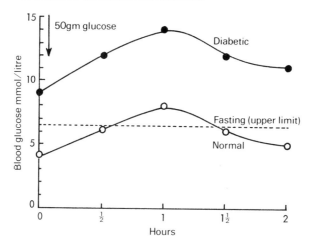

Fig. 14.5 Glucose tolerance curves in a diabetic subject and a normal person.

associated with complications affecting practically every system. There is a greatly increased liability to sepsis. This may show itself as boils and styes, while, from the dental point of view, infection and hypertrophy of the gingival tissues is important. There is an increased incidence of pulmonary tuberculosis. Arteriosclerotic changes occur earlier and more severely in the diabetic, causing an increased tendency to coronary artery disease and peripheral arterial disease with gangrene. Peripheral neuritis is not uncommon while the eyes may be affected by cataract (loss of translucency of the lens) and by changes in the retina. Kidney function may be seriously impaired by a special variety of glomerular lesion. Autonomic neuropathy is common and may cause nocturnal diarrhoea, postural hypotension and, in men, impotence.

Prognosis
Despite the formidable list of complications that may afflict the severe and the poorly controlled diabetic, the student should remember that properly regulated insulin therapy now permits the majority of diabetics to live long and useful lives.

Treatment
The basic principle of diabetic treatment is to give a diet yielding sufficient calories for the patient's needs and sufficient insulin to enable carbohydrate and fat metabolism to proceed normally.

The number of calories required varies with the age, sex, weight, occupation and personal habits of the patient. The aim should be to keep the body weight at, or preferably just below, the ideal body weight as it has been found that 'a thin diabetic is healthier than a fat diabetic'. Consideration is given to a proper balance between carbohydrate, fat and protein, particular attention being paid to the carbohydrate content. In most cases, once stabilization has been achieved, it is sufficient for the patient to rely on simple measurements, e.g. an average slice of bread is equivalent to 15 g of carbohydrate.

Insulin is given by subcutaneous injection in gradually increasing dosage until glycosuria is controlled. The diabetic must be instructed in the measurement of the dose, and self-injection; the majority learn to do this very well. Soluble insulin, the natural product, may be used for long-term treatment but as it has a short duration of action two or three injections per day are required to ensure diabetic control. A number of longer acting modified insulins are available which have the advantage that they need be administered only once or twice daily. Insulin is available in different strengths and the patient must be fully aware of this, otherwise serious errors in dosage will occur.

The patient is taught to test the urine for sugar regularly and to keep a careful weight record so that modifications in insulin dosage and diet may be made as required.

Hypoglycaemia

A blood sugar below the lower limit of normal (4·0 mmol per litre or 80 mg per 100 ml) may occur in a diabetic in the following circumstances:

1. An overdose of insulin either through an error in measurement, or an error in the strength of insulin.

2. Correct insulin dosage but insufficient food, e.g. due to being late for a meal.

3. Unexpected exercise or emotional upset leading to increased metabolism of glucose.

The early stages of hypoglycaemia are characterized by mental confusion, slurred speech, headache, incoordination of movement, profuse sweating, and a full strong pulse. In some instances there may be confusion with drunkenness, a point of considerable legal importance. Unless corrected at this stage, unconsciousness will follow in all but mild cases. The urine is free from sugar and the blood sugar is low.

If seen and recognized in its early stages, hypoglycaemia responds quickly to the oral administration of carbohydrate, e.g. a glucose drink, sweetened tea, lump sugar, etc. If the patient is unconscious, glucose must be given by intravenous injection. An alternative treatment is to convert the liver glycogen to glucose by the subcutaneous injection of 0·5 ml of a 1 in 1,000 solution of adrenaline hydrochloride.

Diabetic ketosis or diabetic coma

This is a gross metabolic derangement which develops in diabetes mellitus when insulin dosage is inadequate. It used to be seen as the inevitable terminal event in preinsulin days. When it occurs now it is usually associated with infection, which increases insulin requirements; in the presence of infection the diabetic should increase insulin dosage, but he may do the reverse because he is eating less due to poor appetite and vomiting.

The features of diabetic ketosis develop over many hours, or even a few days, and not suddenly as in hypoglycaemic coma. Nausea and sickness are prominent and drowsiness merging into coma occurs. The skin and tongue are very dry due to dehydration, the breathing deep due to acidosis, the blood pressure low, and the pulse weak; the breath has the fruity odour of acetone. The urine is loaded with sugar and acetone, and the blood sugar is high.

Diabetic ketosis calls for urgent treatment which is a skilled procedure requiring intravenous soluble insulin and intensive fluid and salt replacement.

Obese variety of diabetes mellitus (Maturity onset diabetes)

Aetiology

This usually occurs in men or women of middle age and over who have eaten excessively for many years and become progressively more obese. At first the excess carbohydrate is converted into fat and stored as such, but later this mechanism for disposing unnecessary carbohydrate becomes overwhelmed and the blood sugar rises leading to glycosuria. There does not appear to be a primary deficiency of insulin; the pancreas is doing its best but it simply cannot deal with the prolonged excessive intake of carbohydrate.

Clinical features

Polyuria, thirst and glycosuria are present but, in contrast to the other variety of diabetes, the patient is overweight. The complications mentioned above may occur, but they are usually less prominent.

Treatment

The essential step in treatment is to reduce the carbohydrate content of the diet and so ensure weight reduction, as described under simple obesity. In some patients an oral hypoglycaemic drug such as tolbutamide or chlorpropamide may be required.

Other causes of glycosuria

Renal glycosuria
In this disorder the kidneys have a low threshold for sugar, and glycosuria occurs even although the blood sugar level is perfectly normal. No symptoms are associated and the condition usually remains undetected until the individual has some routine medical examination, e.g. for the Armed Services or for insurance purposes. The diagnosis is confirmed by a glucose tolerance test (Fig. 14.5).

Alimentary glycosuria
After short-circuit operations on the alimentary tract, such as gastroenterostomy, carbohydrate may be more quickly absorbed than normal leading to a transiently high blood sugar after meals. If the urine should be tested at this time it will be found to contain a trace of sugar. The condition is not important.

GOUT

Gout is a disorder of purine metabolism in which there is an accumulation of urates in the blood and the periodic deposition of urate salts in the tissues, especially of the joints. It is commoner in men and there is often a family history.

The individual experiences periodic attacks of acute pain in the joints, especially the great toe, and after a time this produces permanent damage. Deposits of urates also occur in the subcutaneous tissues, particularly of the ears, causing small firm swellings, termed gouty tophi, which contain a chalky material. The blood uric acid is high.

An acute attack may be relieved by a variety of drugs including colchicine. Further attacks can be prevented or minimized by the regular administration of drugs, such as allopurinol, which increase the urinary excretion of uric acid.

15

The allergic disorders

The term 'allergy' describes an abnormal form of tissue reaction to a variety of agents (allergens) which in similar amounts are harmless to the majority of individuals. A family history is commonly present in those affected. The range of allergens is extremely wide and includes articles of the diet, microorganisms, drugs, topical applications, various chemicals and pollens of grasses. The precise nature of the tissue reaction is not known with certainty, but many authorities believe that histamine, or a histamine-like substance, is liberated by contact between the allergens and specific antibodies which have developed as a result of previous exposure. Histamine causes vasodilatation of the capillaries of the skin, mucous membranes and constriction of the smooth muscle of the bronchi.

HAY FEVER

Hay fever is caused by allegy to the windborne pollen of grasses, and of some weeds and trees. It is seen especially in young people and it tends to lessen in severity with age. The maximum incidence of the attacks is in the early summer months.

The principal symptoms are a profuse, watery nasal discharge, paroxysms of sneezing, conjunctival irritation and lachrymation, headache and depression.

Those who are severely affected should try to avoid contact with the causative pollen. The use of the antihistamine drugs (*vide infra*) gives a high degree of symptomatic relief. Steroids may be given in severe refractory cases. Specific desensitization by a series of injections of gradually increasing doses of an extract of the pollen is often valuable. The injections should be started several weeks before the pollen season and may have to be repeated yearly.

Allergic rhinitis may be due to causes other than hay fever. It is then termed vasomotor rhinitis. The allergens include bacteria and viruses, house dust, and locally applied drugs. The clinical features are essentially the same as in hay fever except that the disorder does not have a seasonal incidence.

ASTHMA

Aetiology

In this condition there are recurrent attacks of acute breathlessness due to intense spasm of the smooth muscle in the walls of the bronchi, swelling of the bronchial mucosa, and an exudate of mucus. These three changes lead to marked interference with the flow of air during inspiration and expiration; expiration is affected to a greater degree since it is a less powerful action.

In many patients it can be shown that they are abnormally sensitive, or allergic, to various substances commonly inhaled, such as vegetable or animal particles in the atmosphere, or ingested in the food. Emotional or psychological factors may also play an important aetiological role. In many instances the precipitating factor is an upper respiratory tract infection.

There is frequently a family history of asthma or other allergic condition such as hay fever or urticaria.

Clinical features

The typical asthmatic attack is sudden in onset. The patient becomes intensely breathless and inspection shows that the main difficulty is in expiration. There is a short forceful inspiration, aided by the accessory muscles of respiration, followed by a longer, easily heard, wheezing expiration. Expiration is not successful, however, in deflating the chest which becomes distended and fixed in the position of full inspiration. The face is pallid, sweating and anxious while the lips, ears, nose and extremities show cyanosis. The attack may last from half an hour or so up to several hours. Very prolonged attacks are termed status asthmaticus.

Sometimes the bronchospasm is not so severe and the individual is able to get about although he is limited somewhat in his activities because of breathlessness. The wheezing expiration may be readily audible.

Course and prognosis

Childhood asthma sometimes becomes less severe in adult life and, indeed, may even disappear. In other cases recurrent attacks of asthma occur throughout life and in those patients emphysema is likely to develop leading to severe incapacity.

Treatment

The treatment of asthma may be divided into the control of the acute attack and the general management of the patient.

Should a dentist be faced with the problem of dealing with a patient suffering from an *acute attack* of asthma he should first stop whatever dental procedure is going on, check that the airway is patent, loosen tight clothing around the neck, permit the patient to sit upright, and ensure that the atmosphere in the room is airy and cool. Many asthmatics carry a remedy of proven value to them and, if this is found to be so, it should be used.

The common remedies for self-administration are:

1. A pressurized aerosol, containing isoprenaline or salbutamol (Ventolin), or an insufflator containing sodium cromoglycate (Intal). These are made in small containers which can be readily carried in the pocket or handbag.

2. Ephedrine or salbutamol tablets for oral use, or isoprenaline tablets for sublingual use.

3. Subcutaneous injection of ½ to 1 ml of a 1 in 1,000 solution of adrenaline hydrochloride.

In severe or prolonged attacks other measures may have to be employed such as oxygen inhalations, the intravenous injection of aminophylline, or a course of steroid drugs. An antibiotic is given if there is any suspicion that infection has precipitated the attack. Sedation is often helpful.

In the *general management* of asthma it is always helpful to instruct the patient in breathing exercises which should be performed regularly. A commonsense appraisal of the individual and his environment will usually reveal any major emotional factor which may be operative. A careful history may reveal a substance to which the patient is allergic. He should try to avoid this substance, if possible, or an attempt may be made to desensitize him by the use of repeated injections of gradually increasing amounts of the substance, although the results of this procedure are often rather disappointing. Sedation is helpful at times of emotional stress, as for example prior to dental procedures.

DRUG ALLERGY

Allergic reactions may occur to a very large number of drugs and, in some cases, may be very serious and even fatal. The incidence is likely to be higher in those with a history of other allergic disorders such as asthma, and possibly in those receiving the drug for long periods of time. The reactions may develop after the first administration of the drug or, sometimes, only after the drug has been given on one or several prior occasions.

Important examples of common drugs which may produce allergic reactions are penicillin, barbiturates, aspirin, and local anaesthetics. Although the percentage of individuals reacting in this way is small, these drugs are used so frequently that the problem is a real one. Prior to their administration it is wise to ask if the patient has had any untoward drug reactions in the past.

Clinical features
Drug allergy may take any of the following forms singly or in combination:

1. Systemic upset with sickness, fever, joint pains, lymphadenopathy.

2. Sudden fatal collapse as a result of cardiac arrest.

3. Skin eruptions ranging from transient reddening of the skin (erythema) or urticaria to severe exfoliative dermatitis.

4. Haematological abnormalities including agranulocytosis, aplastic anaemia, haemolytic anaemia, and thrombocytopenia.

5. Oedema of the glottis which may lead to asphyxia.

Treatment
If there is any suspicion that drug allergy is developing, the drug should be stopped immediately and an intihistamine preparation given in full dosage. The subcutaneous injection of ½ to 1 ml of 1 in 1,000 solution of adrenaline hydrochloride is a valuable emergency measure in severe case. Steroids are of definite value in severe cases. The management of cardiac arrest is described on page 111. Prevention of further attacks by avoidance of the causal drug is important for the individual in the future.

URTICARIA

Aetiology
Urticaria is an allergic reaction of the skin to a variety of factors which include foods such as shellfish, nuts and fruits, drugs; bacterial infection; and infestation with intestinal parasites. Of dental interest is the view of some authorities that bacterial infection of the teeth and throat is an important cause of chronic urticaria.

Clinical features
Multiple, elevated weals, which are intensely itchy, develop quickly on the skin. They last from an hour or two to a day or two. In

severe cases a systemic upset shown by sickness, fever, and joint pain is associated.

Treatment
The measures described under drug allergy apply. Calamine applied to the skin gives symptomatic relief. In chronic or recurrent cases consideration should be given to the possible role of bacterial infection in the mouth and throat.

Angioedema (angioneurotic oedema)
Angioedema is characterised by recurrent episodes of intense localised subepithelial oedema. The condition may affect many sites but is most serious when the soft tissues of the buccal cavity are affected as obstruction of the airway, with fatal outcome, may result. Physical trauma, which may be relatively minor or even trivial, is the commonest precipitating factor and dental extractions, in those afflicted with the disorder, can cause life-threatening attacks. Other precipitating factors include extremes of temperature, infection and emotional stress (hence the earlier term angioneurotic oedema). This puzzling disorder is now known to be due to an inherited defect in the functioning of the complement system and those affected have low serum levels of C_4, C_2 and C_1 esterase inhibitor. The frequency of attacks may be lessened by the oral administration of an antifibrinolytic agent, such as tranexamic acid, or an anabolic steroid such as danazol. Acute attacks do not respond to adrenaline, antihistamines or corticosteroids, in contrast to allergic reactions to drugs etc. (vide supra), but intravenous administration of fresh-frozen plasma, which supplies the deficient complement factor is beneficial.

CONTACT DERMATITIS

Aetiology
Contact dermatitis is an allergic reaction of the skin to contact with a very large variety of substances. The most important of these include soaps and detergents, antiseptics, local anaesthetics, sulphonamides or antibiotics applied topically, shampoos, cosmetics, hair dyes, dyes applied to fabrics, metals such as nickel and chromium, many chemicals used in manufacturing processes and some plastics. The disorder is of great importance in industry, while some doctors, dentists and nurses have the misfortune to react in this manner to substances they would customarily handle in their professional duties.

Clinical features

The initial reaction is swelling and redness of the skin followed by the development of small vesicles which rupture to produce a raw, oozing area. The lesion is itchy and secondary infection from scratching is common. The site of the lesion depends largely on the nature of the causal agent; the back of the hands and the face are common areas.

Treatment

Mild cases may settle once the cause is removed but serious cases require skilled treatment by a dermatologist. A barrier cream is often a helpful prophylactic measure.

STEVENS–JOHNSON SYNDROME

The Stevens–Johnson syndrome is usually considered to be a variant of a generalized allergic skin disorder known as erythema multiforme.

The principal features are the abrupt development, with fever, of ulcerative lesions of the buccal cavity and of the genital area, followed a day or two later by a generalized bullous eruption. The condition is treated by corticosteroids.

ERYTHEMA NODOSUM

Erythema nodosum is characterized by the development of red, tender swellings in the subcutaneous tissues, especially over the front of the lower legs. It is an allergic reaction to several processes including haemolytic streptococcal infection of the throat, tuberculosis, sarcoidosis and some drugs.

DRUGS IN ALLERGIC DISORDERS

It will be useful to summarize the drugs which are used to control the allergic disorders. They fall into three categories: adrenaline and allied substances, the antihistamines, and the corticosteroids.

Adrenaline

Adrenaline by subcutaneous injection of a 1 in 1,000 solution is a very effective drug for acute emergencies such as oedema of the glottis. It acts very quickly. It is useful in severe attacks of asthma but is less frequently used following the introduction of isoprenaline and the corticosteroids. Isoprenaline is quickly absorbed from the sublingual mucosa and is a very valuable preparation in bronchial asthma. It may cause unpleasant palpitations. It is also widely available in aerosol form.

Antihistamines

The antihistamine drugs largely prevent the reactive hyperaemia of the skin and mucous membranes caused by histamine, but they have relatively little effect on the smooth muscle constriction which histamine may produce. The majority of cases of hay fever, vasomotor rhinitis, drug allergy, urticaria and mild forms of angioneurotic oedema respond favourably to the use of the antihistamines, both prophylactically and therapeutically, but as might be expected from their range of action, they give disappointing results in asthma.

Numerous preparations are available for oral use and some of the drugs are also available in a form suitable for parenteral administration in cases of emergency. The principal side effect is drowsiness and the patient should be warned that it may occur. Other side effects include dryness of the mouth and blurring of vision. There is considerable individual variation in the response to these drugs and the frequency of side effects.

Commonly used preparations are mepyramine maleate (Anthisan) in a dosage of 100 to 200 mg daily, promethazine (Phenergan) 25 to 100 mg daily, and cyclizine (Marzine) 25 to 50 mg daily.

Corticosteroids

These are very valuable in the treatment of acute allergic emergencies such as oedema of the glottis, sudden collapse due to drug allergy or insect stings, and status asthmaticus. Treatment usually commences with the intravenous injection of hydrocortisone (100 to 300 mg) followed by oral prednisone.

16

Musculoskeletal and connective tissue disorders, including fractures

OSTEOMALACIA AND OSTEOPOROSIS

The first stage in bone formation is the laying down by the osteoblasts of an extracellular matrix, termed the osteoid, which is composed of nitrogenous substances. This is followed by the deposition in the osteoid of calcium salts—i.e. calcification.

Osteoporosis

Osteoporosis is characterized by a decrease in the bone matrix. There is no detectable abnormality of calcium or phosphorus metabolism and the blood levels of these substances, and of the alkaline phosphatase, are normal. Osteoporosis may occur in the following circumstances:

1. After disuse as in prolonged immobilization.

2. In old age probably as the result of androgen deficiency.

3. In some women after the menopause due to oestrogen deficiency.

4. In malnutrition due to deficiency of the nitrogenous components of the matrix.

5. In thyrotoxicosis due to increased metabolic demands.

6. Where there is an excess of certain steroid hormones of the adrenal cortex as in Cushing's syndrome or prolonged steroid therapy.

7. In fragilitas ossium, or osteogenesis imperfecta, which is a rare congenital disorder characterized by osteoporosis, multiple pathological fractures, hypermotility of the joints, deafness due to otosclerosis, and blue sclerae; dentine formation is usually defective and the teeth are malformed and prone to caries.

The principal bones involved in osteoporosis are the vertebrae, the pelvis and the long bones. Radiological studies show increased translucency, thinning of the cortex and, in many cases, compression collapse of the vertebral bodies. Low back pain and kyphosis are common features. Characteristically the skull does not show radiological changes and the lamina dura around the teeth are not affected.

The main therapeutic aspects are correction of causal factors, the provision of a well-balanced diet and, in some cases, the carefully supervised use of hormones (androgens and oestrogens) which encourage matrix formation. No curative treatment is available for osteogenesis imperfecta.

Osteomalacia

Osteomalacia is due to defective deposition of calcium and phosphorus in the developing bone matrix of the adult. Rickets is the comparable condition in the child. The abnormality of calcium and phosphorus may be due to

1. Dietary inadequacy of calcium and vitamin D, which is still responsible for many cases of osteomalacia in under-developed countries.

2. Defective absorption of calcium and vitamin D as in steatorrhoea.

3. Renal disorders which lead to chronic renal failure.

In most varieties of osteomalacia the serum calcium is low and the alkaline phosphatase high. The skeleton is much softer than normal and deformity of the weight-bearing bones commonly ensues. Bone pain and tenderness are usually present. The bones show increased translucency and, unlike in osteoporosis, this may be apparent in the skull where the lamina dura around the teeth may be absent.

Treatment varies to some extent with the cause but, in general, correction of any deficiency of calcium and provision of a vitamin D preparation which will promote calcium absorption are indicated.

PAGET'S DISEASE (OSTEITIS DEFORMANS)

Paget's disease is a chronic bone disorder, of unknown aetiology, which is not uncommon in elderly people. The long bones (Fig 16.1) the pelvis, the skull and the spine are chiefly affected.

The initial process appears to be a patchy decalcification leading to areas of softening and this is followed by a rather disorderly recalcification. As a result of these two processes the affected bones are considerably thickened and deformed. In severe cases pathological fractures may occur.

The skull becomes enlarged and the face may become deformed by involvement of the maxillae and mandible. Rarely a 'leonine'

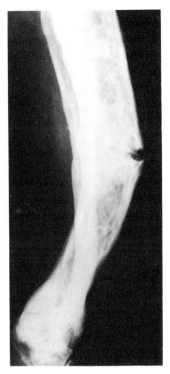

Fig. 16.1 Advanced Paget's disease of the tibia showing a pathological fracture

appearance results. Changes in the bone around the roots of the teeth may cause their partial destruction. Bowing and deformity of the legs are commonly present. Involvement of the spine leads to kyphosis and a stooping posture. The only biochemical abnormality is an increased serum alkaline phosphatase. Radiological studies show areas of decalcification, areas of increased density, thickening of the cortex, and deformity. Osteosarcoma is a late complication.

No generally effective treatment is available but calcitonin may produce some improvement in certain cases. Regular analgesics may be required to relieve the discomfort which many of these patients experience. If the jaws are markedly involved the teeth may have to be extracted, dentures refashioned, and excess bone removed.

ACHONDROPLASIA

Achondroplasia (Fig. 16.2) is an hereditary disorder of the skeleton due to defective cartilage growth and endochondral bone forma-

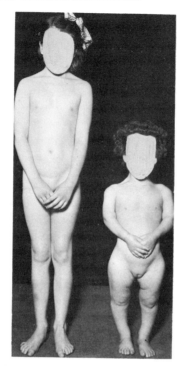

Fig. 16.2 Achondroplastic child with normal child of same age.

tion. The individual is dwarfed due to marked shortening of the limb bones. The gait is waddling. The limbs are often very powerful and muscular and the fingers short and thick. The trunk is relatively normal in size while the head is often rather enlarged.

The lips are thickened and the bridge of the nose sunken.

OSTEOARTHRITIS

In osteoarthritis, or degenerative arthritis, the cartilage which normally provides a smooth articular surface becomes thinned, irregular, and eventually worn away. The exposed bone becomes hardened and eburnated and bony outgrowths tend to form at the articular margins producing 'lipping'. The weight-bearing joints, especially the hips, knees, and small joints of the spine, are mainly involved.

Aetiology
Minor osteoarthritic changes may be noted radiologically in a con-

siderable proportion of elderly individuals and, to some extent, may be taken as a more or less inevitable accompaniment of ageing. More severe degrees of osteoarthritis are often largely caused by the abnormal strain which obesity throws on the weight-bearing joints. In other instances faulty weight bearing such as may occur after a badly aligned fracture or direct damage to the joint by a fracture extending into the joint and leaving residual distortion, are responsible.

Clinical features
The dominant symptoms are stiffness and pain in the affected joints, and these are usually worse when movement occurs after a period of rest. In severe cases pain may be almost continuous. There are no signs of inflammation around the joint and no constitutional upset as shown by fever, anaemia, or elevation of the sedimentation rate. Small bony outgrowths, called Heberden's nodes, develop on the dorsal aspect of the terminal joints of the fingers in many cases (Fig. 16.3).

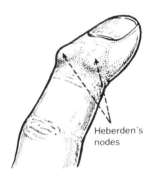

Heberden's nodes

Fig. 16.3 Heberden's nodes.

Treatment
The main principles of treatment are correction of any aetiological factor such as obesity, the provision of a suitable analgesic drug such as aspirin, paracetamol or codeine, and the use of physiotherapy to improve joint function. In severe cases surgery may offer relief, particularly for osteoarthritis of the hip or knee joint. The joints are either realigned and in the case of hip the insertion of a prosthesis to form a new hip joint (replacement arthroplasty) is possible. Such developments are now feasible in the knee joint also. Occasionally, surgical fusion of the joint (arthrodesis) is necessary.

RHEUMATOID ARTHRITIS

Rheumatoid arthritis is a chronic disorder characterized by inflammatory changes in the synovial membrane, the capsule, and the surrounding soft tissues of the joints, leading to progressive destruction of the joint structures, deformity, and loss of function. The condition occurs at all ages and women are affected about three times more frequently than men.

Aetiology

The aetiology of rheumatoid arthritis remains obscure. Reaction of the joint tissues to foci of chronic infection, infection of the joints with an as yet unidentified agent, an autoimmune disorder and hornonal imbalance resulting from abnormal adaptation to stress are the principal hypotheses which have been advanced. The evidence for all is inconclusive. Obesity is not a factor in the production of rheumatoid arthritis.

Clinical features

The main joints involved are the small joints of the hands, wrists and feet, with the elbows and knees being next in order of inci-

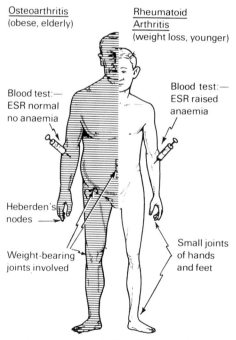

Osteoarthritis
(obese, elderly)

Rheumatoid
Arthritis
(weight loss, younger)

Blood test:—
ESR normal
no anaemia

Blood test:—
ESR raised
anaemia

Heberden's
nodes →

Weight-bearing
joints involved

Small joints
of hands
and feet

Fig. 16.4 Difference between osteoarthritis and rheumatoid arthritis.

dence. In contrast to osteoarthritis there is local evidence of an inflammatory process revealed by tenderness and swelling of the affected joints. There is also evidence of a constitutional upset shown by pyrexia, elevation of the sedimentation rate, anaemia and loss of weight (Fig. 16.4).

Movement of the joints is limited at first largely by pain and swelling, later by fibrous ankylosis, and still later by bony ankylosis. Progress of the condition is characterized by periods of activity, as shown by exacerbation of joint pain and constitutional disturbance, and periods of relative inactivity.

The appearance of the hands is often sufficiently characteristic to permit a diagnosis to be made at a glance (Fig. 16.5). The interphalangeal joints of the fingers are enlarged and there is wasting of the intermediate soft tissues of the fingers leading to a spindle-shaped deformity. The finger joints are usually held slightly flexed, the patient is unable to close the fist properly and the grip is weakened. Ulnar deviation of the hand at the wrist is commonly present.

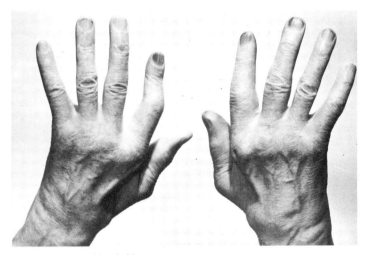

Fig. 16.5 Rheumatoid arthritis.

Marked involvement of the knee joints may, in the absence of vigorous treatment, lead to the joints becoming fixed in a position of semi-flexion and the patient becomes bedridden; similar deformity may occur in the elbow joints. In some cases firm, painless nodules develop in the subcutaneous tissues, especially around the elbows (Fig. 16.6). Temporomandibular joint involvement is discussed on page 308 and Sjögren's syndrome on page 161.

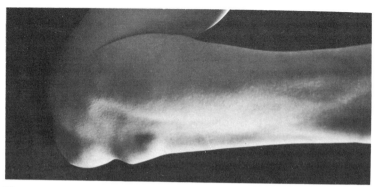

Fig. 16.6 Rheumatoid nodule in region of elbow.

A variant of rheumatoid arthritis is psoriatic arthropathy. The patients have a relatively common chronic skin disorder termed psoriasis together with a polyarthritis which resembles rheumatoid arthritis.

Prognosis
Rheumatoid arthritis is a chronic disease which leads to serious disablement in about 50 per cent of cases. The disorder is particularly disabling should it affect those whose livelihood depends on the skilled use of the hands, e.g. dentists.

Treatment
No specific treatment exists for rheumatoid arthritis. Most authorities agree that the following measures are applicable to all cases and that their long-term use will help to control the disease and lessen disablement:

1. The use of analgesics to control the pain and stiffness of the joints.

2. The employment of *physiotherapy* to prevent deformity of the joints and to maintain as full a range of movement as possible. Heat and exercises are the main measures. Splinting may also be required.

3. The use of *rest* when the disease process is active, care being taken to avoid stiffness and loss of joint function from immobility.

4. Attention to the *general health* including the provision of a nutritious diet and the correction of anaemia.

Several *drugs* have been tried in the hope that they might have a specific effect on the disease process but none are curative. Examples are gold, which is given in a course of intramuscular injections, phenylbutazone which is a moderately powerful analgesic, indomethacin which has anti-inflammatory properties in addition to being an analgesic, and corticosteroids. Corticosteroids should be used only if the disease is actively progressing despite the use of the other measures referred to. If any of these drugs are employed, the patient should be under careful medical supervision as there are important toxic effects.

Surgical removal of the inflamed synovial membrane in the early stages of the disorder (synovectomy) is producing encouraging results in some cases while surgical correction of established joint deformities can be of considerable value in long-standing severe cases. Joint replacement, even of the finger joints, is also now a feasible exercise.

Focal sepsis used to be considered as a possible aetiological factor in rheumatoid arthritis and the dentist was not uncommonly asked to perform multiple extractions in the hope of curing the joint disorder. It is now generally agreed that this concept is not a valid one, and that teeth should never be sacrified in this fashion. Any dental abnormality in a patient with rheumatoid arthritis should be carefully treated on its own merits.

Anklylosing spondylitis

Anklylosing spondylitis is a disorder of unknown aetiology which has its maximum incidence in young men. Some authorities consider that it is a variant of rheumatoid arthritis.

The small joints of the spine, especially in the lumbosacral region, and the sacroiliac joints become affected by pathological changes similar to those of rheumatoid arthritis. In addition, there is a tendency for calcification to develop in the intervertebral ligaments leading to characteristic radiological appearances of the spine (bamboo spine).

The main symptoms are pain and progressive stiffness of the back. The normal thoracic curvature of spine becomes exaggerated and the patient develops an increasingly bent forward posture. Eventually the spine may become entirely rigid.

Radiotherapy produces benefit in many instances but, in view of the possible relationship of such treatment to the subsequent development of leukaemia, it should not be employed unless the disorder is severe and has failed to respond to physiotherapy and analgesics.

Other forms of arthritis

Several other forms of arthritis are merely local expressions of some systemic disorder or infection which is described elsewhere.

1. Arthritis due to infection, e.g. tuberculosis, gonorrhoea.
2. Arthritis associated with rheumatic fever.
3. Arthritis due to a metabolic disorder such as gout.
4. Arthritis due to recurrent bleeding into joints as in haemophilia.
5. Arthritis due to neurological conditions which cause loss of sensation in the joint structures—e.g. the Charcot joints of tabes dorsalis.

FIBROSITIS

Fibrositis, or muscular rheumatism, is a very common disorder. Exposure to draughts, a sudden chilling or wetting, chronic muscular strain, and upper respiratory infections are all well-known predisposing factors, but the nature of the soft tissue changes is obscure. Focal sepsis is no longer held to be of any aetiological significance.

The principal clinical features are aching pain, stiffness, and tenderness in the muscles and related soft tissues. Any of the fibromuscular tissues may be affected but the commoner sites are the lumbar area (lumbago), the shoulder and the neck.

The main aspects of treatment are the provision of rest, warmth and analgesics. Injection of local anaesthetic into the affected area may give valuable symptomatic relief.

COLLAGEN DISORDERS

The connective tissue of the body, which provides a framework of considerable stability, is composed of fibres largely formed of protein, set in a polysaccharide ground substance. Collagen is one of the main protein constituents of connective tissue representing about 30 per cent of the total body protein.

The collagen disorders are characterized by extensive fibrinoid degeneration of collagen. The clinical manifestations are very varied and usually involve many organs, as might be expected from the widespread distribution of connective tissue in the body, but certain features tend to be common to all, namely a more or less profound constitutional upset, elevation of the plasma globulin level, and marked acceleration of the erythrocyte sedimentation rate. The corticosteroid drugs are of value in treatment but are not curative.

Examples of collagen disorders are systemic lupus erythematosus, in which there is often a red rash on the cheeks, polyarteritis nodosa, in which there are widespread lesions of the small arteries, and scleroderma, in which the skin becomes thickened and indurated.

FRACTURES

A fracture (Fig. 16.7) is a break in a bone. It may be *simple*, in which case the skin overlying the bone is not breached, or *compound* where there is disruption of overlying skin. This carries the risk of infection and compound fractures are therefore much more serious.

A fracture may be incomplete, the bone breaking along one border but remaining intact on the opposite side. Such fractures are prone to occur in young children and are known as *greenstick fractures*. More usually, however, the bone is completely broken; if

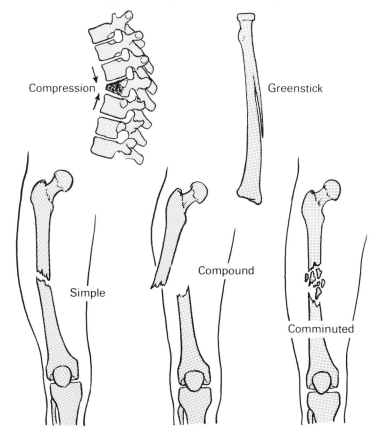

Fig. 16.7 Different kinds of fractures

many fragments are produced the fracture is known as *comminuted*. Occasionally, compression causes the bone to shatter and impact (this is a particularly common form of fracture in the vertebral column and in the calcaneum of the heel).

Healing of bone

Following a fracture in the bone bleeding occurs and a *haematoma* forms. The blood lost into this haematoma can be very considerable. For example, in a fracture of the femur, as much as 2–3 litres may be involved. As in healing of wounds (see Ch. 3) the haematoma is organized from the periphery and from the broken bone ends by ingrowth of new blood vessels and connective tissue cells which follow closely the macrophages which absorb the haematoma. The *granulation tissue* in this instance, however, contains many osteoblasts. Once the granulation has formed the osteoblasts begin to lay down immature (woven) bone and this mass uniting the bone ends is known as *callus*. The callus matures, the woven bone being gradually replaced by mature bone which forms so as to support the reconstituted structure. Gradually the callus is remodelled by osteoplastic and further osteoblastic activity. The time for healing to occur varies in different bones.

Factors affecting the healing of bone are similar to those affecting wound healing. However, there are special circumstances in osseous tissue. Firstly, good reduction of the fracture with alignment of the bone so that there is not a large gap between the free ends is important. Secondly, movement tends to disrupt the forming callus so that a degree of immobility is of importance, and thirdly, infection is of particular importance in this instance since it is extremely likely to be followed by osteomyelitis and a protracted delay in healing. In addition, some bones have a peculiar blood supply such that the fracture produces avascular necrosis of a segment of the bone. This makes healing impossible. Well known examples are fracture of the neck of the femur which may be followed by necrosis of the head of the femur and fracture of the scaphoid bone of the wrist which can be similarly complicated.

Clinical features

A history is always useful, since it may not only help in the diagnosis of fracture but be of value in the assessment of associated injuries. Furthermore, a good description of the force and direction of the blow that produced the fracture is of value. Thus a fall on the chin can produce a bilateral fracture of the neck of the mandible.

The patient complains of pain and swelling and on clinical examination the affected bone may show obvious deformity. This is not always present but local tenderness overlying the fracture is an invariable sign. There may be swelling and bruising of the surrounding structures and in compound fractures laceration of the skin through which a fragment of bone may protrude. Movement of the bone causes pain and may be accompanied by a grating sound (crepitus). Fracture of major bones (e.g. femur, pelvis) may produce sufficient haemorrhage to cause hypovolaemic shock.

It is extremely important to assess damage to adjacent structures caused by the fracture. Examples of nerve damage associated with bone fractures are damage to the radial nerve in fracture of the humerus, damage to the inferior dental nerve in fracture of the mandible and damage to the lateral popliteal nerve in fractures of the neck of the fibula. Failure of the surgeon to detect such palsies before treatment are serious since the residual paralysis may well be attributed by the patient (and by his legal advisers) to the result of therapy. Major blood vessels may be damaged by fractures and assessment of the circulation of the limb distal to a fracture is essential. The fractured bones may also penetrate body cavities and damage underlying viscera such as the brain, lungs, liver, spleen or bladder.

Treatment
The object of treatment is to produce a good functional end result. The management of a fracture can be considered under three headings.

1. *Emergency treatment.* The object is to lessen pain, prevent blood loss, treat shock and prevent infection in compound fractures. This is achieved by the administration of analgesia and by a temporary splinting of the fracture (this not only relieves pain but slows blood loss). Blood is taken for grouping and cross-matching and blood transfusion used as required. Any wounds are covered with sterile dressing for later debridement (see Ch. 3) in the operating theatre. Tetanus toxoid and penicillin is given for tetanus and gas gangrene prophylaxis as outlined previously. An assessment is then made of peripheral nerve and vascular function and of visceral damage. In particular the need to maintain an airway is important and the passage of an endotracheal tube may be necessary in the severely injured. Assessment of associated injuries to the brain, contents of the chest, or of the abdomen is made. If such injury is suspected the appropriate specialists are immediately consulted and management of severe thoracic, abdominal or cerebral

injury takes precedence over definitive management of the fracture.

In facial fractures, particularly the airway may be threatened and tracheal intubation and even tracheostomy may be necessary early in the course of management.

2. *Reduction*. When a bone is fractured the fragments may be severely displaced, not only by the fracturing force, but also by the pull of muscles attached to the bone fragments. For example, in some fractures of the mandible traction by the pterygoid muscles can produce quite marked displacement.

X-rays are taken to show the displacement and degree of comminution. It is important to take X-rays in two planes otherwise the extent of the fracture may not be revealed. It is important to realize that fractures on X-ray may show up, not only as a break in the bone but as a line of increased density if two fragments overlap.

Reduction of deformity usually requires general anaesthesia, both to relieve pain and to relax muscle spasm. The fragments are reduced as much as possible but it is important to realize that good alignment is more important than perfect X-ray apposition. This ensures subsequent good function, particularly of related joints. Nevertheless, it is desirable to have the bones as closely approximated as possible without intervening muscle or other tissues. In the case of compound fractures debridement is performed at this time and any small detached fragments of bone are removed but such removal should be conservative since bony defects are difficult to close. In most instances of compound fracture the overlying wound is repaired as outlined previously but if gross infection is present then the wound may be left open and dressed for subsequent management. Reduction having been achieved some means must be used to maintain the bones in correct position.

3. *Immobilization*. This may be affected by external splinting, by traction or by internal fixation. *External splinting* is usually applied in the form of a plaster of Paris cast which should extend far enough beyond the lines of fracture to maintain the immobilization. However, as much function as possible should be allowed to surrounding joints so as not to unduly weaken the muscles in the area or to allow stiffness to develop in these joints. It is extremely important that plaster casts are accurately applied and checked frequently after the application since compression of the soft tissues with vascular impairment and subsequent gangrene can result. Splinting fractures of the jaw is performed by the application of cap splints or splints formed from dentures (Gunning splints) to the fractured segments of bone. The fractured mandible or maxilla

may also be fixed by penetrating struts and splinted by these to a skull appliance. This is a form of external splinting.

Traction is used to effect relative immobilization in fractures where muscle spasm is a major factor in the production of the initial deformity. The outstanding example is in fracture of the femur where the powerful thigh muscles tend to produce overriding of the fragments. Traction to the legs and the application of an external splint (Thomas's splint to the thigh) is usually sufficient. *Internal fixation* can be effected by wiring the fragments of bone together or by plating them with metal plates screwed to the opposing fragments or by insertion of a metal bar into the medullary cavity.

4. *Rehabilitation* following fracture is of great importance. A good functional result, not necessarily perfect alignment of bones, is the aim. To this end, appropriate exercises are commenced, sometimes during the period of fracture immobilization and are then continued in the phase following healing of the fracture. Thus, for example, in fracture of the femur, it is possible to achieve appropriate splintage and at the same time to allow exercise of the knee. This allows exercise of the great muscles of the thigh, which can be continued in the follow-up period. Function of the leg and its joints are preserved and recovery hastened. Rehabilitative exercises of this sort are particularly important in the hand where prolonged immobilization can lead to permanent damage and muscle contracture.

Facial fractures

Facial fractures are of very considerable importance to the dentist and are covered in detail during the course of maxillofacial and oral surgery. As with other fractures, they may be compound and extend either to communication with the external environment or communicate with the mouth or nasal sinuses. They are often accompanied by head injury. The fractures may involve the zygomatic arch, the maxilla, the mandible or all of the facial structures. The immediate urgent aspects of the management of facial fractures are occasionally the arrest of bleeding, the maintenance of a good airway, particularly in bilateral fractures of the mandible which allow the tongue to fall backwards and compromise respiration, and assessment of associated injuries and in particular of cerebral injury.

Examination of the patient should include a careful history and an assessment of displacement of bone. This can be especially difficult once gross facial swelling has taken place. Assessment of the occlusion may give important clues and abnormal mobility of segments of bone or of the alveolar arch may be detected. There may be areas of paraesthesia or anaesthesia due to entrapment of nerves by the fractured bone (e.g. an area of anaesthesia covering the upper lip and ala of the nose is not infrequent in fractured maxilla involving the infra-orbital nerve). There may be a disparity on examination of the eyes and the patient may complain of diplopia as a result of displacement of one or other of the orbital contents.

Special X-rays are taken to demonstrate the fractures and treatment is instituted as early as possible but may be delayed for a few days especially where other injuries take priority. However, if the condition of the patient is good and especially if the fracture is compound, treatment should be instituted early.

The aims of treatment are to restore good function, good occlusion and good appearance. In addition, if there are visual defects, these must be corrected. If there are associated tears of the dura mater resulting in rhinorrhoea or otorrhoea, then dural repair by a neurosurgeon is often necessary.

Fractures of the zygomatic arch are elevated by insertion of an appropriate instrument introduced through an incision in the hairline and passed down deep to the temporalis fascia.

Fractures of the mandible and maxilla are reduced and are fixed either with wires, splints fixed to the teeth with external bars, by internal fixation by means of screwing bars to the fragments of bone or by wiring methods. There is, of course, a necessity to treat associated soft tissue injuries and if there is skin loss extensive plastic surgical repairs may be necessary.

As with all fractures, a period of rehabilitation is necessary and any teeth damaged or lost at the time of injury must be adequately repaired or replaced by means of suitable prostheses.

17

Disorders of the nervous system including head injury and management of the unconscious

ANATOMICAL AND PHYSIOLOGICAL CONSIDERATIONS

General structure
The principal parts of the central nervous system are the cerebrum, the cerebellum, the brain stem, and the spinal cord (Fig. 17.1). The peripheral nervous system consists of the cranial and peripheral nerves.

The cerebrum is divided into two hemispheres each comprising a frontal, parietal, temporal and occipital lobe. The surface is mainly grey matter and within the substance of the hemispheres lie the

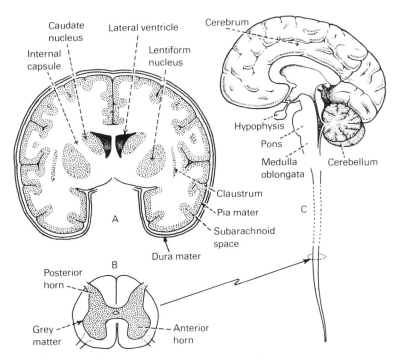

Fig. 17.1 A simplified diagram of the principal parts of the central nervous system.

basal ganglia, the third and lateral ventricles, the thalamus, and the internal capsule which contains many ascending and descending tracts (white matter), of which the most important is the pyramidal or motor pathway.

The cerebellum lies dorsal to the pons forming the roof of the fourth ventricle. The surface is composed of grey matter and the centre is mainly white matter containing three nuclei of grey substance. Tracts link the cerebellum with the spinal cord and other parts of the nervous system.

The brain stem is composed of the mid-brain which lies uppermost, the pons which lies ventral to the fourth ventricle and the cerebellum, and the medulla which is continuous with the spinal cord below. The brain stem contains ascending sensory and descending motor tracts, and the cranial nerve nuclei from which the cranial nerves arise and emerge as shown in Figure 17.2. In the medulla the pyramidal fibres cross from the anterior aspect of the brain stem to the lateral part of the other side and descend in the cord.

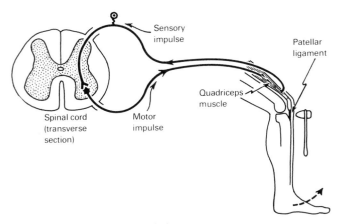

Fig. 17.2 The reflex arc of the knee jerk.

The spinal cord occupies the bony vertebral canal between the foramen magnum and the first lumbar vertebra. Thirty pairs of nerves arise from the cord, each being made up of an anterior motor root and a posterior sensory root. The grey matter forms a central column, which is H shaped on cross-section (Fig. 17.2), throughout the length of the cord. The white matter is composed of ascending sensory tracts, ascending cerebellar tracts, and the descending pyramidal and extrapyramidal tracts.

Reflex activity

A reflex occurs without conscious mental effort as an almost simultaneous response to a stimulus. There are many varieties of reflexes but in clinical neurology most use is made of the tendon reflexes, the plantar responses, and the reaction of the pupils to light.

The tendon reflexes, which include the knee, ankle, biceps and triceps jerks, are also termed deep or stretch reflexes. The reflex arc for the knee jerk, which is taken as an illustrative example, is shown in Figure 17.2. A tap on the patellar tendon below the kneecap causes a brisk forward movement of the lower leg due to contraction of the quadriceps muscle. Tendon reflexes are increased in pyramidal, or upper motor neurone lesions, and decreased or absent in lower motor neurone lesions.

The plantar response is a superficial reflex initiated by stroking the sole of the foot. In health there is plantar flexion of the great toe whereas in pyramidal tract lesions the toe dorsiflexes—the extensor or Babinski response.

The pupillary light reaction is a further superficial reflex. The pupil contracts in response to light. The light reflex is lost in many cases of neurosyphilis (Argyll Robertson pupil).

The motor system

The pyramidal pathway is composed of upper motor neurones and lower motor neurones.

1. Upper motor neurones commence in the motor area of the cortex, converge to pass through the internal capsule, traverse the brain stem giving connections to the cranial nerve nuclei of the opposite side, decussate in the medulla, and descend in the opposite side of the spinal cord, ending in synapses with the anterior horn cells.

2. Lower motor neurones are formed by the cranial nerve nuclei and the anterior horn cells of the cord, and the cranial and peripheral nerves respectively.

The difference between an upper and a lower motor neurone lesion is shown in Table 5.

Table 5 Comparison of the features of upper and lower motor neurone lesions

	Upper	Lower
Muscle power	decreased	decreased
Muscle tone	increased (spastic)	decreased (flaccid)
Tendon jerks	increased	absent
Plantar response	extensor	flexor
Muscle wasting	not present	present
Muscle fasciculation	never	sometimes

The extrapyramidal system is formed by the basal ganglia and certain nuclei in the brain stem from which tracts descend to end in relation to the anterior horn cells. Lesions of this system cause muscle rigidity and tremors but no paralysis.

Lesions of the cerebellar system cause incoordination of movement.

Sensory system

Sensory fibres pass in the sensory peripheral nerves to the cord via the posterior nerve roots, or via the sensory cranial nerves, and ascend to intermediate relay centres in the brain stem (deep sensation and position sense) and the thalamus (pain and temperature), from where fibres pass to the sensory areas of the cortex.

The cerebrospinal fluid

This is a clear, colourless fluid of similar composition to the plasma except that it contains very little protein. It is formed by the vascular choroid plexuses of the ventricles and the volume is about 120 ml. It circulates in the subarachnoid space providing a protective 'water-jacket' for the brain and spinal cord.

Cerebrospinal fluid may be obtained for diagnostic purposes by lumbar puncture in which a fine needle is passed, under local anaesthesia, between the spinous processes of the lower lumbar vertebrae (i.e. below the termination of the spinal cord) into the subarachnoid space.

PAINS ABOUT THE FACE AND HEAD

It is essential that the dentist should have a clear appreciation of the various disorders which may be associated with pain in the face and head. The symptom is a common one and, as with all forms of pain, it frequently leads the patient to seek advice. A simple classification of the causes is given in Table 6.

In patients with trigeminal neuralgia, and in many others with non-organic facial pain, a diagnosis may be made with reasonable accuracy on the basis of the history provided one takes the time necessary to obtain a full description of the pain, its site, mode of onset, duration, precipitating factors, etc.; but a careful clinical examination must never be omitted whether or not an organic basis is suspected and, in many instances, radiological studies and other special investigations will also be required.

Table 6 Classification of pains about the face and head

No organic pathology	Secondary to	Associated with

Trigeminal neuralgia
Migraine
Other 'functional'
   headaches and pains
	Disorders of—teeth
	   —sinuses
	   —ears
	   —eyes
		Hypertension
		Toxic and
		   febrile states
		Myocardial
		   ischaemia

Postherpetic neuralgia	—T.M. joint Other bone annd joint disorders Temporal arteritis Intracranial disorders Disorders of mouth and tongue	

Trigeminal neuralgia or tic douloureux

This is a disorder that affects elderly people. The pain is usually experienced in the second and/or third division of the fifth cranial nerve and very rarely in the first. It is always confined to one side of the face. The pain occurs in paroxysms which last for a few seconds and it may be extremely severe. It never radiates outside the distribution of the fifth nerve. A paroxysm may be triggered off by such simple factors as sitting in a cold draught, talking, swallowing, taking of hot or cold foods, washing the face, insertion of dentures, or by touching the side of the face. In trigeminal neuralgia there are no neurological signs and there is no numbness of the face.

Mild cases may be treated with analgesics or by a phenothiazine derivative called carbamazepine (Tegretol) but if the paroxysms are frequent and severe, more positive steps are required. The affected division or alternatively the Gasserian ganglion may be injected with alcohol or phenol, or destroyed by means of thermo-electro-coagulation and if this is not sufficient to produce long-lasting relief, surgical division of the pre-ganglionic part of the nerve is indicated. Loss of corneal sensation may follow such procedures and secondary corneal ulceration results. This must be prevented.

Migraine and migrainous neuralgia

This disorder is believed to be due to recurrent spasm followed by dilatation of the intracranial arteries; the pain results from stretching of nerve endings in the arterial wall. A family history is frequently present. Sufferers from migraine are often perfectionist individuals who are more prone to attacks in stressful situations. In its classical form migraine shows the following characteristics.

1. A family history.
2. An onset in childhood or adolescence and a tendency for the attacks to lessen in severity after middle age.
3. Premonitory visual symptoms such as blurring of vision, photophobia, or flashes of light in front of the eyes.
4. Headache, usually unilateral or mainly so, which may last for many hours, and is often severe.
5. Vomiting, especially towards the end of an attack.

Some patients do not have this classical pattern but experience neuralgic pain, usually less severe, on the side or front of the face, sometimes in the upper jaw and gums, and rarely in the lower jaw. The pain is sometimes episodic and sometimes more or less constant with periodic exacerbations. This is termed migrainous neuralgia.

Most migrainous patients find some measure of relief by resting in a darkened room and by taking an analgesic such as aspirin or codeine and an antiemetic. Severe attacks are often helped, or may be aborted, by the administration of ergotamine which constricts the dilated arteries.

Other 'functional' headaches and pains

Many patients with non-organic pain or discomfort in the face or head do not readily fit into the disorders described above. They are usually people who find difficulty in coming to terms with life and its problems and, in consequence, cannot relax, worry unnecessarily, sleep poorly, and are jumpy and irritable. A long history of the discomfort is usually present with periodic exacerbations at times of domestic or business upsets. The nature of the discomfort varies considerably; it may be described as a sense of pressure in the head, a feeling as if the head is going to burst, dull or sharp discomfort in the face, or stabbing pains in the vertex.

The pathogenesis of the discomfort may well be similar to that in migraine, but these patients often command less sympathy than those who suffer from classical migraine. The main therapeutic steps are reassurance that no organic disease is present, an explanation of the aetiology of the symptom, advice to try and relax more, and sedation; but it must be admitted that the symptoms continue, or recur, in many instances.

Postherpetic neuralgia

Elderly patients are more often affected with this disorder. The pain may be relatively mild or very severe. It is experienced in the area in which the vesicles occurred and the presence of scars from the vesicles may give a clue to the origin of the disorder.

Dental causes

The various dental abnormalities which may cause facial pain will not be enumerated, but the following general remarks are not out of place:

1. Even a detailed clinical examination will not always reveal dental caries, especially at contact points and small cavities below the gingival margin may be difficult to find. X-ray examination and particularly bite-wing films are necessary.

2. Pain of dental origin may be referred from the upper to the lower jaw and vice versa, but is never referred to the other side of the face. It may be referred to the temporal region on that side.

3. If a full clinical and radiological examination does not reveal any dental abnormality in a patient with facial pain, dental extractions should never be performed in the vague hope that this will produce a cure of the facial discomfort. It should always be remembered that just as dental pain may be referred elsewhere in the head and neck, so disorders elsewhere (such as maxillary sinusitis) may present as toothache.

Sinus disorders

Acute or chronic infection of the sinuses is a common complication of upper respiratory tract infection. Frontal sinusitis tends to cause pain in the first division of the trigeminal nerve and there is commonly tenderness on palpation over the affected sinus. Maxillary sinusitis is important to the dentist since it may produce pain in the teeth and indeed the upper teeth may be tender to percussion, the condition thus simulating periapical abscess. Sometimes the tenderness is confined to only one tooth. However, there is also pain on pressure in the infra-orbital region and above the apices of the upper pre-molar teeth intraorally. The presence of pus within the sinus is easily demonstrated on X-ray since the affected sinus is opaque. Suppuration in the sphenoidal or ethmoidal sinuses may be impossible to diagnose without careful radiological study; severe headache may be caused and some authorities have described anterior facial pain due to involvement of the sphenopalatine ganglion.

Treatment is by appropriate inhalations and postural drainage and the administration of antibiotics, but surgical drainage may be necessary, most frequently in the maxillary sinus (Caldwell-Luc operation), since the normal opening of the sinus is high on its posterior and medial wall so that natural drainage is difficult.

Neoplasm of the sinuses is a serious cause of facial pain but is less common than simple infections. Nevertheless, it is important to keep this possibility in mind. Facial swelling on the affected side, diplopia, unilateral nasal discharge, loosening of the teeth and perhaps the appearance of an ulcer in the mouth are all late signs. The diagnosis is confirmed by appropriate biopsy and treatment is by surgical excision with appropriate reconstruction (this may need the provision of complicated dental prostheses) or by radiotherapy or by a combination of the two.

Neoplasm of the sinuses is a serious cause of facial pain, but it is fortunately much less common than simple infection.

Aural disorders
Boils, acute otitis media, and mastoiditis cause local pain in the ear which may be intense. There is seldom any likelihood that these conditions will be confused with other causes of facial pain.

The geniculate ganglion of the facial nerve may be involved by herpes zoster or by chronic middle ear suppuration. Confusion may arise in these instances as the pain may be felt in the front of the ear and on the ipsilateral side of the tongue and hard palate, in addition to in the ear itself. Geniculate herpes is usually associated with facial paralysis through secondary involvement of the motor fibres of the nerve (Ramsay Hunt syndrome).

Ocular causes
Errors of refraction are so well recognized as a cause of headache that testing of the visual acuity is often one of the earliest special investigations requested in patients with this complaint. Glaucoma, which is an eye disorder characterized by increased intraocular pressure, is a less common, but very important, cause of facial pain; the condition may be acute or chronic.

Temporomandibular joint disorders
Arthritis of the temporomandibular joint may occur in a relatively small number of cases of rheumatoid arthritis or as an uncommon metastatic complication of several infectious diseases of which gonorrhoea is an example. However, pain arising from the temporomandibular joint is much more commonly caused by local factors which throw a strain on the joint structures and disturb the normal articular relationships. This is termed the temporomandibular joint

syndrome (or Costen's syndrome). It is usually associated with malocclusion of the teeth which may be of a relatively minor nature and follow loss of teeth with consequent drifting of others, unsatisfactory restorative procedures, improperly fitting appliances and abnormal stresses after injury to the jaws. Overclosure of the jaws is also an important associated factor and may result from dentures which allow such overclosure. The pain is experienced in the side of the face and particularly on movement of the joint to the external auditory meatus, the auriculotemporal nerve and the middle ear structures. Associated symptoms including discomfort in the ear, impairment of hearing, tinnitus (p. 314) and temporal pain are not uncommon. Examination will often reveal some tenderness over the affected joint and overclosure of the mandible or deviation to one side on final closure may be evident.

It is very difficult to be precise about the frequency of the temporomandibular joint syndrome since the discovery of a dental abnormality can often be found in patients who do not have pain in the face or who have pain for some other reason. Many may suffer from a form of non-organic pain such as described earlier in this section. However, careful dental appraisal is important and the eradication of minor occlusive abnormalities is not difficult. Careful consideration must be given before embarking on major oral rehabilitation programmes. In very severe cases osteotomy of the ramus of the mandible produces relief.

Tumours as a cause of facial pain
Tumours of the nasal sinuses have already been referred to. However, there are a variety of dental tumours and tumours of the jaws which, although they usually present with swelling of the bone or pathological fracture may occasionally present with facial pain. It is important to mention the rare tumours of the nasopharynx which are difficult to diagnose and may present with pain in the face, sometimes associated with ear symptoms consequent upon blockage of the Eustachian tube. Secondary tumours also may present with facial pain and if associated with the jaws may cause loosening of the teeth.

Other bone and joint disorders
Involvement of the bones of the face and skull by Paget's disease, myelomatosis or primary and secondary tumour (see p. 76) is likely to be associated with headache and facial pain.

Osteoarthritis of the small joints of the cervical spine is a common disorder in elderly people. It may cause occipital headache and troublesome stiffness and pain in the back of the neck radiating into the shoulders and arms.

Temporal arteritis

This uncommon condition is probably a local manifestation of a collagen disorder (p. 294). Other arteries of the head and neck may also be affected. The patient experiences severe temporal pain and headache. The diseased vessel may be palpable as a tender cord. Temporal arteritis is a serious disorder as it may cause blindness if untreated. Steroid therapy is almost always helpful and should be instituted without delay.

Intracranial disorders

The more important intracranial disorders which may be associated with headache are meningitis, cerebrovascular disorders, and cerebral tumour and abscess.

Hypertensive headache

Headache is often believed to be associated with hypertension but in many instances the headache does not develop until the patient has been made aware of the presence of high blood pressure.

Toxic headaches

Headache may be experienced in a large variety of febrile and toxic states ranging from simple respiratory infections and 'hang-overs' to severe disorders of the liver and kidneys.

Myocardial ischaemia

Reference has already been made (p. 113) to pain in the angle of the jaw resulting from myocardial ischaemia.

THE CRANIAL NERVES

The principal functions of the cranial nerves and their mode of emergence from the brain stem are shown diagrammatically in Figure 17.3.

First nerve

The olfactory nerve is of little clinical importance in disorders of the nervous system. Lesions of it give rise to loss of smell (*anosmia*) but this is also a feature of many local conditions of the nose due to mucosal changes.

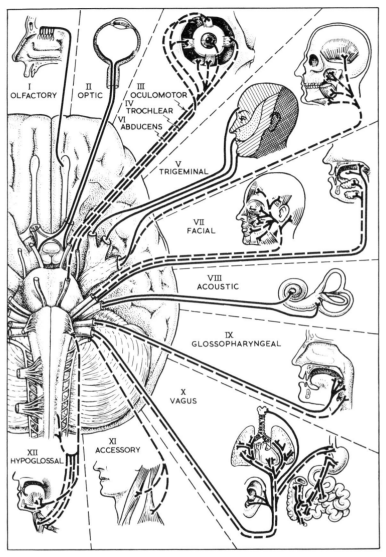

Fig. 17.3 The cranial nerves. An interrupted (— — —) indicates a motor pathway and a continuous line (———) a sensory pathway.
(After Frank H. Netter, M. D., The Ciba Collection of Medical Illustrations.)

Second nerve

The main steps on the visual pathway are the visual area of the cortex in the occipital lobe, the optic radiation which passes through the internal capsule, the optic tracts, the optic chiasma which is closely related to the pituitary gland, and the optic nerves.

The medial fibres cross in the optic chiasma and, as a result, the lateral half of the retina derives its fibres from the ipsilateral visual area whereas the fibres on the medial side come from the opposite occipital lobe.

The effect of a pituitary tumour, e.g. as in acromegaly, will be taken as an illustrative example of a lesion of the visual pathway. The central part of the chiasma is pressed upon, resulting in loss of vision in the lateral half of each visual field (bitemporal hemianopia). The term *papilloedema* describes the swollen ophthalmoscopic appearance of the optic disc which develops if the intracranial pressure is increased, e.g. in cerebral tumour or severe hypertension. A healthy disc has a distinct margin and a centrally depressed portion, or cup.

Third, fourth and sixth nerves

The oculomotor nerves are collectively responsible for the nerve supply to the extrinsic ocular muscles. The nuclei lie in the brain stem and the nerves pass through the cavernous sinus on their way to the eye muscles. The fourth nerve supplies the superior oblique muscle, the sixth nerve the lateral rectus muscle, while the third nerve supplies the four remaining extrinsic muscles, i.e. the inferior rectus, superior rectus, internal rectus and inferior oblique. The third nerve also supplies the voluntary part of the levator palpebrae superioris and the parasympathetic fibres to the muscles of accommodation, stimulation causing constriction of the pupil.

An isolated lesion of the fourth or sixth nerve on one side causes paralysis of one extrinsic muscle and this results in a squint, or *strabismus*. A third nerve palsy also causes a squint and, in addition, drooping of the eyelid (*ptosis*), and a dilated pupil which does not react to light or accommodation. Neurosyphilis produces a small, slightly irregular pupil which does not react to light.

Fifth nerve

The motor component is responsible for the muscles of mastication and the sensory component supplies sensation to the side of the face and head, including the cornea, and to the teeth and gums.

The principal disorders of the trigeminal nerve are trigeminal neuralgia (p. 305) and herpes zoster (p. 6 and Fig. 1.1).

Seventh nerve

The facial nerves supplies the muscle of facial expression and also the taste fibres to the anterior two-thirds of the tongue. The nucleus is in the pons close beside that of the sixth nerve. The nerve passes across the posterior fossa of the skull in proximity to the eighth nerve, traverses the bony facial canal in the petrous portion of the temporal bone where it is related to the middle ear and the mastoid air cells, emerges from the skull through the stylomastoid foramen, and passes through the parotid gland before dividing up into branches for distribution to the various facial muscles and to the mucosa of the tongue.

Paralysis of the facial nerve may be either supranuclear (upper motor neurone lesion) as in cerebral haemorrhage, or infra-nuclear (lower motor neurone lesion). The two varieties may be distinguished because in the lower motor variety the facial muscles around the eye are usually involved in the paralysis while they are spared in the upper motor variety as a result of their bilateral innervation.

Bell's palsy

This is the commonest variety of facial palsy. The lesion is lower motor in type. This cause of Bell's palsy is not known with certainty, but it is generally believed that there is a localized inflammation of the nerve (neuritis) and that the resultant pressure on the swollen nerve at the stylomastoid foramen leads to paralysis. In a fully developed case the appearance is characteristic (Fig. 17.4). All the

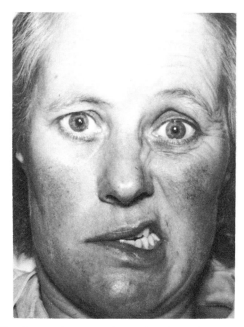

Fig. 17.4 Bell's palsy—patient attempting to show the teeth.

muscles of expression on one side of the face are paralysed. The patient cannot wrinkle the forehead, cannot close the eye properly, cannot purse the lips into the position for whistling, and when he attempts to show the teeth exposes less of them on the affected side. There is no sensory loss over the face, but if the fibres of the chorda tympani are involved, taste is lost over the anterior two-thirds of the tongue.

The majority of patients with Bell's palsy recover without any special treatment in a relatively short time. Corticosteroids are sometimes given with the aim of reducing the swelling of the nerve at the stylomastoid foramen. In severe cases it is desirable to fashion a simple splint which is hooked into the angle of the mouth and behind the ear to prevent stretching of the paralysed muscles. The paralysis is permanent in a few unfortunate individuals and they are left with disfiguring asymmetry of the face. Plastic surgery is often very valuable in such cases.

Surgical causes of facial palsy

Facial palsy is an uncommon complication of surgical procedures and most commonly occurs after operations on the parotid gland. Sometimes the mandibular branch of the facial nerve is damaged in excisions of the submandibular salivary gland. The facial nerve has also been reported damaged in operations involving the middle ear or the mastoid process after an ill-directed injection of local anaesthesia and sometimes after prolonged forced instrumental opening of the mouth.

Eighth nerve

The eighth nerve has an auditory component and a vestibular component. The principal symptoms which may follow lesions of the eighth nerve are vertigo, tinnitus (noises in the ears) and deafness. These may occur singly or in combination.

Vertigo

The patient has an illusion of movement or of visible objects moving about him. If he is on his feet he staggers and may fall. Vomiting is often associated. Vertigo is caused by disordered function of the labyrinthine mechanism which is responsible for normal equilibrium. It is a much less common symptom than giddiness or light-headedness. *Ménière's syndrome* is a special form of paroxysmal vertigo, of obscure aetiology, associated with tinnitus and deafness. Labyrinthitis, of infective origin, is another important variety which may occur in small outbreaks.

Deafness

Impairement of hearing may be due to lesions of the eighth nerve but more commonly it results from chronic suppuration in the middle ear.

Ninth, tenth, eleventh and twelfth nerves

Isolated lesions of these nerves are rare. *Glossopharyngeal neuralgia*, which is much less common than trigeminal neuralgia, is characterized by paroxysms of pain in the throat and ear. In *bulbar palsy* there is a lower motor neurone paralysis, due to degenerative changes in the nuclei of the muscles supplied by the lower cranial nerves. The tongue becomes small, atrophic, shows muscle fasciculation, cannot be protruded, and, in consequence, there is great difficulty in eating, speaking and swallowing. *Pseudobulbar palsy*, so-called because there is no wasting or fasciculation, is caused by a bilateral lesion, usually vascular, of the pyramidal fibres which supply the lower cranial nerve nuclei. *Unilateral hypoglossal paralysis* causes paralysis and atrophy of the muscles on the same side of the tongue. The tongue deviates to the paralysed side on protrusion (Fig. 17.5). Carcinoma of the tongue does not cause hypoglossal paralysis but fixes the tongue which protrudes to the side of the lesion.

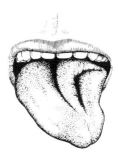

Fig. 17.5 The appearance of the tongue in a left hypoglossal paralysis.

VASCULAR DISEASES

Disease of the cerebral blood vessels is one of the commonest causes of disease of the nervous system.

Cerebral arteriosclerosis

Ischaemic changes in the brain, usually of patchy distribution, are common in old age as a consequence of narrowing of the cerebral arteries. Milder forms of cerebral ischaemia are the cause of the impairment of memory and deterioration of mental acuity which are prone to occur in many people with advancing years. More marked ischaemia may cause paralysis of a limb or limbs, disturbance of speech (dysphasia) and gross derangement of intellect.

Cerebral thrombosis and haemorrhage

The blood vessels situated deep in the cerebral hemispheres in the region of the internal capsule are commonly affected by thrombosis or haemorrhage. Atheroma and hypertension are common predisposing factors. Older people are most often affected.

Cerebrovascular catastrophes, or strokes, are typically sudden in onset. There may be loss of consciousness, the breathing is usually stertorous, and there may be incontinence of urine and faeces. The signs in the nervous system depend on the site of the lesion; in the majority of cases there is weakness of the limbs on the opposite side of the body due to damage to the motor pathway in the contralateral hemisphere (Fig. 17.6). If the lesion is extensive, death is likely to ensue. If a fatal outcome does not take place, the patient

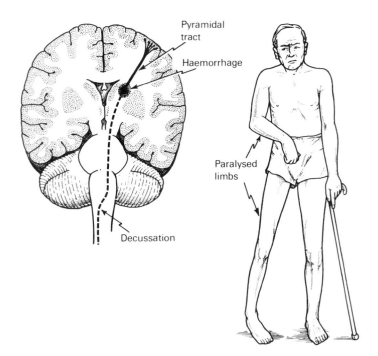

Fig. 17.6 The effect of a vascular lesion of the internal capsule. Note the decussation of the pyramidal fibres in the medulla.

gradually recovers consciousness and, thereafter, may regain some power in the paralysed limbs although residual weakness is common. In addition, there may be dysphasia, personality change, or other form of cerebral dysfunction.

Careful nursing is essential to prevent bed sores and pneumonia, and antibiotics may be of value in this respect. Physiotherapy and rehabilitative measures are required in those patients who survive.

Cerebral embolism
The two main causes of cerebral embolism are mitral stenosis with atrial fibrillation, and subacute bacterial endocarditis. The patient is usually younger than those affected by cerebral thrombosis or haemorrhage and shows evidence of a cardiac lesion. The clinical picture is otherwise similar to that in thrombosis or haemorrhage.

Cerebral aneurysm and subarachnoid haemorrhage
The blood vessels at the base of the brain form an anastomotic circle termed the circle of Willis. In some individuals there is a localized dilatation, or aneurysm, of one of these vessels. It may press on the adjacent cranial nerves, causing signs referable to the second, third, fourth, fifth, or sixth nerves usually associated with pain. If the aneurysm bursts, there is haemorrhage into the subarachnoid space. Severe headache is experienced and consciousness is often lost. Examination reveals evidence of meningeal irritation, as shown by stiffness of the neck, and lumbar puncture yields a bloodstained fluid. The prognosis is grave.

Surgical treatment by ligation of the affected vessel is possible in some cases.

Vertebrobasilar insufficiency
This is the term given to cerebral ischaemia resulting from obliterative changes in the vertebral or basilar arteries. The most characteristic clinical feature is of transient episodes of loss of consciousness and paresis probably resulting from small emboli derived from atherosclerotic patches in these extracerebral arteries.

INFECTIONS OF THE NERVOUS SYSTEM

During the present century there has been a steady reduction in the incidence of infectious diseases of the nervous system. Poliomyelitis, neurosyphilis and meningeal tuberculosis (Ch. 1) are now uncommon in developed countries.

Herpes zoster is described in connection with chickenpox (p. 6) since both diseases are caused by the same virus. There are a number of other infectious diseases of the nervous system but they will not be dealt with.

Poliomyelitis

Anterior poliomyelitis, or infantile paralysis, is due to a virus with an affinity for the anterior horn cells of the spinal cord and the cranial nerve nuclei. It has its maximum incidence in children and young adults and the incubation period is about 12 days. The virus normally gains access to the body via the upper alimentary tract, including the oropharynx.

Clinical features

Not everyone who becomes infected with the virus develops a serious illness with widespread paralysis; many develop immunity without experiencing any symptoms while others have a short pyrexial illness without paralysis.

In the unfortunate minority who became paralysed the usual sequence of events is influenza-like symptoms followed by paralysis, usually asymmetrical and especially of the limbs (Fig. 17.7). The paralysed muscles are tender and the tendon jerks are absent.

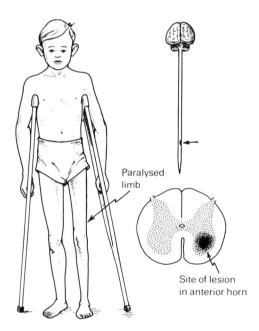

Paralysed limb

Site of lesion in anterior horn

Fig. 17.7 The lower motor neurone paralysis of poliomyelitis.

If the trunk is affected there is disturbance of respiration due to intercostal and diaphragmatic paralysis. Involvement of the cranial nerve nuclei causes difficulty in swallowing and further interference with respiration.

Prognosis

Mild paralytic cases may recover more or less completely, but if the paralysis is severe and extensive some permanent weakness is probable. The majority of children or young adults whom one sees with a drop foot, or other evidence of limb paralysis, have suffered from poliomyelitis. In fatal cases death is usually due to respiratory paralysis.

Treatment

The most important measure is prevention and the incidence of poliomyelitis has been greatly reduced by the widespread immunization of children.

During epidemics the chances of paralytic poliomyelitis are reduced by avoiding muscular fatigue, treating and observing carefully any upper respiratory tract infection, and by postponing operations on the throat, such as tonsillectomy, since these are believed to facilitate the entry of the virus.

Meningitis

Acute inflammation of the covering membranes of the brain and spinal cord may be due to many pathogenic organisms. One of the important varieties, which will be taken as an illustrative example, is *cerebrospinal fever* or meningococcal meningitis.

The maximum incidence is in children and young adults. Overcrowding is a predisposing factor. The incubation period is short. The onset is abrupt and the main features of the illness are headache, fever, and stiffness of the neck due to meningeal irritation. Lumbar puncture yields a purulent fluid containing the meningococci.

The prognosis has been much improved since the introduction of the sulphonamides and penicillin.

EPILEPSY

Epilepsy is due to paroxysmal bursts of uncontrolled cerebral activity and the nature of the attack depends on the area of brain involved and the intensity of the process.

In the majority of cases the cause of the disorder is quite unknown. In some instances epilepsy follows local damage to the brain from tumour, trauma or infection, and a cause such as this should always be considered when the disorder commences in middle age or over.

Clinical forms of epilepsy

In major epilepsy, or *grand mal*, the individual has recurrent convulsions. Sometimes there is a brief warning, or aura, but more frequently the seizure occurs without warning. Consciousness is suddenly lost and the patient may fall heavily to the ground and injure himself in so doing. For a few moments the limbs and trunk muscles are rigid and tense (the tonic phase) but this is quickly followed by violent uncontrolled movements of the limbs. Frothing at the mouth is common and the tongue may be bitten. Incontinence of urine often occurs. Each attack may last from a few moments up to many hours; the term status epilepticus is used when seizures persist for hours. Following the attack the patient is often drowsy and confused and may sleep deeply or be semiconscious for several hours.

Petit mal is characterized by a transient mental blank, but there is no convulsion. This form of epilepsy is more frequent in children. The attacks occur without warning and last for a few seconds to a minute or so. The child is quite unresponsive during the attack and may be scolded by teachers or parents unless the diagnosis is known.

Other forms of epilepsy include major non-convulsive seizures in which consciousness is lost but there is no motor activity, and temporal lobe epilepsy in which the patient does not lose consciousness but experiences peculiar sensory disturbances and may exhibit violent or other antisocial behaviour of which he has no recollection.

Treatment

The most important step during a convulsive seizure is to prevent the patient injuring himself. He should be dragged away from anything dangerous such as a fire, machinery or a cooking stove, a padded gag should be placed between the teeth if possible, dentures should be removed, and the collar or any other tight clothing should be loosened. After the attack, the patient should be kept under supervision until he has returned to normal. Depending on the circumstances and duration of the attack, this may necessitate hospital admission.

Management of the patient between seizures is very important.

Special schooling is often necessary for epileptic children and, later, a suitable occupation should be chosen so that if seizures occur while at work the chance of injury to the patient and others is minimal. The principal drugs employed to reduce frequency and severity of seizures are phenobarbitone, phenytoin (Epanutin, Dilantin) primidone (Mysoline) and sodium valproate (Epilim). These may be employed singly or in combination. The dentist should remember that hyperplasia of the gums (p. 150) may follow prolonged use of phenytoin. In petit mal the principal drugs used are phenobarbitone, troxidone (Tridione) and ethosuximide (Zarontin).

If dental treatment is required in a known epileptic the likelihood of seizures occurring will be lessened if attention is paid to the following points.

1. Ensure that prescribed anticonvulsant drugs are being taken regularly.

2. Sedate beforehand.

3. Use a local rather than a general anaesthetic since transient cerebral anoxia may occur with the latter and precipitate an attack.

MULTIPLE SCLEROSIS (DISSEMINATED SCLEROSIS)

Apart from the vascular disorders, multiple sclerosis is now probably the commonest serious disease affecting the central nervous system. The cause is unknown.

Pathologically the disorder is characterized by areas of demyelination scattered throughout the spinal cord, the cerebral hemisphere, and the cerebellum. Depending on the site of these lesions we may have a varied clinical picture but the commonest sequence of events is as outlined in the following paragraph.

Multiple sclerosis usually starts in early adult life. The first expression of the disease is most often a transient weakness of a limb, sensory disturbance affecting a limb, or disturbed vision such as diplopia. Characteristically these first symptoms are of short duration but later the individual develops more areas of demyelination throughout the nervous system, and although there may be some temporary improvement after each episode there gradually builds up a background of permanent disability. The fluctuating course of the disorder is of great diagnostic significance. In the fully developed case there is usually evidence of pyramidal tract involvement shown by weakness of the legs with increased tendon jerks and extensor plantar responses, loss of bladder control, slurring of the speech, and a tremor which is only apparent when the patient uses the hands. Euphoria, which is a sense of well-being or elation, is fortunately present in many cases.

No curative treatment is known for multiple sclerosis. Physiotherapy may help; sympathy and encouragement are essential. The duration and severity of acute episodes may be reduced by a course of ACTH. The disorder may be aggravated by anaesthetics or operations, even of a relatively minor degree, and this fact should influence the nature and extent of dental procedures in these patients.

PARALYSIS AGITANS

Paralysis agitans, or Parkinsonism, may follow a virus infection of the brain (encephalitis) in younger individuals, or may occur idiopathically in middle or later life. In both varieties the corpus striatum and related areas of the mid-brain and cerebellum are depleted of dopamine. This leads to unbalanced cholinergic activity.

The clinical picture is characteristic and includes some or all of the following features:

1. Slowness and poverty of all movements but especially of facial movements so that the expression is mask-like.
2. Stiffness or rigidity of limbs
3. Coarse tremors of limbs, especially the arms
4. A flexed posture of the trunk.
5. A shuffling gait.
6. Dysarthria.
7. Excess salivation (ptyalism).

The administration of levodopa (usually in combination with cardidopa as Sinemet) benefits many patients with Parkinsonism; it is converted into dopamine in the brain.

CEREBRAL TUMOURS AND ABSCESS

Primary tumours

The majority of cerebral tumours are malignant and they have the peculiarity that they never metastasize to other tissues.

The clinical features may be described conveniently in two groups:

1. Those due to increased intracranial pressure—headache, vomiting usually without nausea, visual upset due to papilloedema, and possibly bradycardia.
2. Those due to focal damage—muscle weakness, sensory de-

fects, personality changes, etc., depending on the position of the growth.

Further information regarding the site of the tumour may be obtained from highly specialized radiological studies, including ventriculography and cerebral arteriography or, more recently, by non-invasive scanning techniques.

Treatment may be by radiotherapy or surgery. The prognosis is poor in the majority of cases.

Secondary tumours
The brain is a common site for secondary tumour, and bronchogenic carcinoma especially deserves mention in this connection.

Cerebral abscess
An important cause of cerebral abscess is chronic infection of the middle ear but abscess may also follow infection of the face, particularly of the lateral angle of the nose, or may be metastatic in nature. The clinical features may be similar to those of cerebral tumour though the cause of the illness is usually more acute. Precise diagnosis allows the surgeon to perform drainage which may be curative.

PERIPHERAL NERVE DISORDERS

Mononeuritis
A neuritis involving a single nerve is usually due to some local pathological change in the tissues surrounding the nerve such as inflammation, tumour and pressure. Examples are brachial neuritis due to pressure by a cervical rib, compression of the median nerve in the fascial tunnel at the wrist, and sciatica, which will be described further.

Sciatica
This literally means pain in the distribution of the sciatic nerve. It is now appreciated that the majority of cases are due to pressure on the sciatic nerve by intervertebral disc protrusion (Fig. 17.8). This may follow some sudden muscular exertion such as lifting a heavy object. The patient experiences severe pain in the buttock and down the back of the leg. The pain is increased by attempting to raise the straight leg.

The majority of cases respond to rest on a firm mattress, analgesics, and spinal extension exercises. A plaster cast to hold the spine extended may be required in some instances. In refractory cases

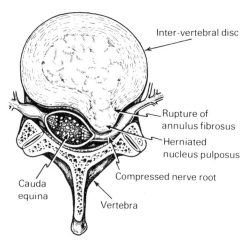

Fig. 17.8 Mechanism of production of sciatica by a prolapsed intervertebral disc.

surgical removal of the offending disc may be necessary before relief is obtained.

A few cases of sciatica are secondary to pressure from tumour deposits in the spine and this variety must always be carefully borne in mind.

Polyneuritis

This is a feature of many generalized toxic or metabolic disorders, and because of the diffuse nature of the cause many peripheral nerves are affected, usually symmetrically. It may occur in chronic lead poisoning, in poorly controlled diabetes mellitus, in chronic alcoholism, in deficiency states such as beriberi, while some cases are apparently due to a virus infection with a specific affinity for peripheral nerves.

The principal features are weakness of all limbs, wasting of muscles, loss of reflexes, sensory loss of all types over the distal parts of the limbs and tenderness of the calves.

Damage to peripheral nerves

Direct damage to peripheral nerves may occur as a result of involvement by tumour or their proximity to infected focci, but more usually due to trauma. There is paralysis in the affected group of muscles with wasting and in sensory nerves, associated sensory loss. Excision of the damaged ends with accurate suture can be followed by a remarkable degree of recovery. Dental examples of damage to peripheral nerves are the damage which may occur to the inferior dental nerve during extraction of teeth or to the lingual nerve during the removal of impacted lower molar teeth. The infra-orbital nerve may be damaged in fractures of the facial skeleton as may the inferior dental nerve.

OTHER DISORDERS OF THE NERVOUS SYSTEM

Horner's syndrome
This results from paralysis of the ocular sympathetic fibres which arise from the lower part of the cervical cord, e.g. by pressure from a tumour in the vicinity. The syndrome consists of slight ptosis, a small pupil, and retraction of the eyeball (enophthalmos).

Syringomyelia
In this disorder cystic areas develop within the spinal cord, usually at the cervical level. They cause pressure damage to both motor and sensory pathways within the cord. The sensory loss is often 'dissociated' in that pain and temperature sensation is lost while deep sensation is not affected.

Subacute combined degeneration of the cord
This is a serious disorder of the nervous system caused by deficiency of vitamin B_{12} and characterized by degenerative changes in the pyramidal tract and the posterior sensory columns. Peripheral neuritis is usually associated. It is liable to develop in inadequately treated cases of pernicious anaemia (p. 219), but in some patients the neurological lesions antedate the anaemia. Intensive vitamin B_{12} therapy is required.

Cervical spondylosis
In this disorder pressure damage to the cervical part of the spinal cord and the posterior nerve roots results from degenerative changes in the cervical intervertebral discs. The disorder may present because of pain in the back of the neck, shoulders and arms, or because of weakness and sensory disturbances in the legs.

Motor neuron disease (amyotrophic lateral sclerosis)
This is an uncommon disorder, of unknown aetiology, characterized by progressive degenerative changes in the anterior horn cells, the cranial nerve nuclei, and the pyramidal pathway. It causes severe disability. Bulbar palsy (p. 315) results from involvement of the lower cranial nerve nuclei.

Huntington's chorea

This rare form of chorea may be distinguished from chorea of rheumatic origin by a family history of the disorder and progressive dementia. The involuntary movements are often extremely marked.

Facial spasms

Involuntary spasms of the facial muscles may be due to either form of chorea, to habit spasms which are commoner in children and are usually bilateral, and to clonic facial spasm. The latter disorder is usually unilateral and is commoner in older people. It is believed to be due to an irritative lesion of the facial nerve; alcoholic injection of the nerve often gives prolonged relief.

MUSCLE DISORDERS

Myasthenia gravis

This is a disease in which the muscles show an abnormal fatiguability on exercise. It usually affects groups of muscles especially those innervated by the cranial nerves and common symptoms are double vision (diplopia), ptosis, and difficulty in chewing, swallowing or speaking. The symptoms are usually more prominent at the end of the day. The disease shows a tendency to remission and relapse.

Myasthenia gravis is due to a disorder of conduction at the myoneural junction which may be relieved by neostigmine or the closely related drug pyridostigmine.

Myopathy

The myopathies are a group of disorders of voluntary muscle which occur mainly in children and adolescents. A family history is often present. The affected muscles show progressive weakness and wasting. There are several different clinical varieties named according to the muscle groups involved. The facio-scapulo-humeral type is often recognizable by the fact that the zygomatic muscles are usually more markedly affected than the other facial muscles leading to weakness of retraction of the angles of the mouth and a characteristic 'transverse smile'.

HEAD INJURY AND CARE OF THE UNCONSCIOUS

Head injuries

Head injuries are either closed, in that the brain and its meningeal coverings are not penetrated, or are open, in that there is direct penetration and exposure of the cerebral tissues and their coverings. The major problem both in diagnosis and management is the recognition and assessment of the extent of intracranial damage.

Head injuries, although they may be caused by a high velocity missile as in war-time, are most frequently caused by blunt impact from solid objects and in civilian practice the large majority of these are related to car accidents. Indeed, over 60 per cent of all car accidents involve the head and in fatal accidents the percentage is over 70 per cent. Lastly, if a patient is admitted unconscious after an accident, there is a very high chance that he may be suffering from intracranial haemorrhage and brain damage.

Local injury to the skull and underlying brain may give rise to haemorrhage and subsequent infection, but the effects are generally less than those that follow the more generalised injuries associated with sudden acceleration or deceleration. Such injury may deform the brain within the skull and cause injury at a point opposite to that of the direct impact (contre-coup injury). In addition, the force may be transmitted to the vital central tissues and brain stem structures.

Injury to the head may be limited to the scalp, but may also involve the skull, the brain, or all three.

Injuries to the scalp

The scalp is a layered structure consisting of the hair and skin, the underlying fat, the aponeurotic layer and the sub-aponeurotic areolar tissue. Blunt injuries to the scalp thus tend to burst rather than crush the tissue and lacerations are very common. The coarse nature of the skin and the underlying aponeurosis is important in consideration of head injuries since they tend to hold open blood vessels in the fatty layer between them and haemorrhage is often profuse. Once haemorrhage is controlled and the tissues sutured, healing occurs very readily.

Skull fractures

Skull fractures are either linear, depressed, with some compression of underlying brain tissue, or compound with exposure of the bone. A skull fracture indicates that there has been a severe blow to the head, but is not necessarily an index to underlying brain damage which may be very severe even in the absence of fracture of the overlying bone.

A skull fracture which runs immediately across the middle meningeal artery or one of the venous sinuses may result in extradural or subdural haemorrhage and the patient must be particularly carefully observed for signs that may suggest the need for operation to relieve compression of the underlying brain.

Fractures of the base of the skull are not often seen on X-rays but depressed skull fractures are. It is important that the X-rays be carefully examined, since palpation is often misleading due to overlying haematoma. Fractures which extend into the nasal sinuses or mastoid air cells are really compound in nature, since they are in communication with the external surfaces of the body and infection is likely.

Injuries to the brain

Injuries to the brain may be classified as concussion, contusion or laceration. It is important to recognise that although they may occur on their own, they are frequently seen in combination.

Concussion

Concussion is a clinical syndrome which is recognised by immediate and transient loss of consciousness due to a blow to the head. It is usually accompanied by a period of amnesia (loss of memory) to events immediately preceding the injury and this is termed retrograde amnesia. In concussion there is usually no demonstrable permanent damage to the brain.

Contusion

This term implies a bruise within the brain. Contusions often occur along the base of the frontal lobes and posteriorly at the temporal lobe. There is underlying damage to the nerve tissues including the formation of local oedema and haematoma, and there may be ischaemia to brain tissue. If the injury is deep within the brain the results may involve a large mass of tissue.

Laceration

Severe injury to the head results in tearing of the brain tissue and this may occur at the point of application of a very considerable force to the head or at the directly opposite point (contre-coup).

Assessment and management

The assessment of a head injury is an emergency matter and early treatment important. Firstly, an adequate airway must be maintained and if necessary an endotracheal tube is passed. Secondly, it is important that there is a good blood supply to the brain. Although scalp lacerations may cause serious bleeding, shock is very rarely secondary to head injury alone and, if present, usually denotes haemorrhage within the thoracic cavity or the abdomen. Early control is essential.

Diagnosis

Having obtained the history of a blow to the head, the cause of unconsciousness is usually readily evident, but it must be remembered that other conditions may be associated with the patient's state. Thus, a diabetic in coma may present with head injury. Similarly, patients in hepatic coma or drug-induced coma may have initially fallen and struck the head. The most important condition requiring differential diagnosis is that of alcoholic coma. The examining clinician should be wary of not attributing coma to one of these associated causes, but should be absolutely certain to exclude severe head injury. Usually a clear history taken from the patient's relatives or the ambulance driver, assessment of the clinical status and appropriate special investigations will provide the necessary information. The patient is then assessed.

1. Symptoms and signs of head injury

A quick examination of the nervous system is important in order to establish a base line against which to measure subsequent events. The most important assessment is that of the level of consciousness.

a. Motor response. The patient's ability to move in response to command or stimulus is assessed and graded as to whether he responds to simple commands, shouted commands, localised painful stimulus or whether the response is abnormal. There may be no response at all.

b. Verbal response. The patient's ability to speak and his speech is assessed. Does the patient simple make odd noises or give confused answers, or are his answers completely intelligible and appropriate?

c. Level of consciousness. This is a difficult matter of judgement and especially if the patient is intoxicated or under the influence of drugs prior to injury. The ability to open the eyes is an important assessment in this regard. It should be noted whether the patient opens his eyes in response to commands or stimulus, or whether he is aware and opens the eyes spontaneously. In addition to this, there should be a careful note made of any complaint the patient may make of headache, of the period of retrograde memory loss (amnesia) and of course of any scalp lacerations or cranial deformity. Traditionally, it is important to assess the eyes of the patient especially if coma is evident. Pupillary size and their reaction to light is important and unequal size of the pupils, particularly unilateral dilatation of one pupil is a sign of raised intracranial pressure.

2. Investigations

In severe head injury and with a rapidly deteriorating level of consciousness, there may be no time for investigation. In such cases, the skull should be opened by means of surgical burr holes in order to allow rapid diagnosis of extracerebral haemorrhage, and it may be necessary to proceed to craniotomy (elevation of a segment of the skull) in order to alleviate pressure by evacuation of haematoma.

Skull X-rays

Skull X-rays should be obtained as soon as possible. The major information to be obtained relates to the presence or absence of a fracture and as to whether this crosses the line of one of the major vascular structures or breaches one of the paranasal air sinuses. The pineal gland which is calcified and radio-opaque in over 70 per cent of persons over the age of 20, may be detected and a shift of this gland to the right or the left on a good X-ray suggests an expanding intracranial haemorrhage.

Imaging of the brain. The brain may be imaged by means of:
1. A cerebral angiogram, the vessels of the brain being injected with contrast.
2. Radioactive isotopes may also be injected and the brain then imaged by means of a gamma camera.
3. An echo encephalogram may demonstrate midline shifts indicating the presence of an intracranial mass.
4. Air contrast studies allow the major ventricles of the brain filled with air to be visualised on a straight X-ray.
5. Finally, and most recently, computerised tomography allows very clear images of the skull and cranial contents and intracranial masses may be shown without hazard or discomfort to the patient.

Haemorrhage within the skull

The brain, like the pulp of the tooth, is enclosed within a rigid cavity and is thus incapable of expansion. For this reason, haemorrhage, particularly if progressive, is associated with severe effects, the major one being compression of the cerebral tissue. A rising intracranial pressure forces the brain down through the foramen magnum and produces pressure on the brain stem.

Intracranial haemorrhage may occur within the extradural space, the subdural or subarachnoid space, or within the cerebral tissue itself.

1. Subarachnoid haemorrhage

Blood in the spinal fluid is a common finding with head injuries. The bleeding arises often from superficial cortical vessels draining the cerebral cortex and quite large volumes of blood within the subarachnoid space may be relatively well tolerated. There may be headache, restlessness and signs of cerebral irritation, but this in itself is not a sign for surgical intervention.

2. Extradural haemorrhage

The most common cause of extradural haematoma is laceration of a branch of the middle meningeal artery and this is usually associated with skull fracture. The injury is common since the artery lies in a groove in the inner table of the temporal bone. Extradural bleeding may also occur as a result from laceration of dural sinuses.

It is important to recognise that extradural haemorrhage may be produced by a relatively minor blow to the head and there may have been no period of amnesia. Indeed, an initially unconscious patient may have a lucid interval. That is to say, he may become alert and then subsequently relapse into coma. The haematoma enlarges and compresses the brain, producing a contralateral hemiparesis or hemiplegia. If allowed to continue, compression of the brain results in compression of the brain stem, and in irreversible damage resulting in death. It is important to realise that every patient with a history of even a minor blow to the head and unconsciousness for even a brief interval must have a thorough neurological examination and a skull X-ray. If the X-ray shows a fracture, then careful monitoring of the level of consciousness (see above) and of vital signs is indicated. If the patient is admitted in coma with findings indicating unilateral cerebral compression (unilateral dilated pupils and hemiplegia), then immediate burr holes are necessary in order to relieve the pressure.

3. Subdural haematoma

Although extensive injury may result in an acute presentation within 24 hours, the symptoms of this condition usually develop more slowly than those associated with extradural haematoma. A gradually enlarging subdural haematoma may develop between one to three months after injury and an interval of up to six or seven weeks is quite common. The presentation is insidious and may develop after what has appeared to be a seemingly minor, perhaps forgotten accident. The leading physical sign is one of progressive mental or personality change and there may be associated cerebral signs and symptoms. This condition develops more frequently in infants and in the elderly. There should be a high index of suspicion in middle-aged persons with any history of head injury who have shown a progressive deterioration in mental acuity associated with headache.

4. Intracerebral haemorrhage
Intracerebral haemorrhage results from injury to a vessel within the brain tissue itself. Accumulation of haematoma produces no particularly classical clinical picture but may present as a space-occupying intracranial lesion. Such lesions are often associated with laceration and contusion of the brain and the patient's condition either becomes relatively stable or deteriorates progressively over days. A computerised tomographic scan is particularly valuable in diagnosis.

Cerebrospinal fluid leak
Leaks of cerebrospinal fluid through the nose (rhinorrhoea) or through the ear (otorrhoea) indicate a communication between the subarachnoid space or ventricular system (which contain the cerebrospinal fluid) and the nose and the ear. The particular hazard of such a fistulous opening is that it provides a pathway for the spread of infection leading to meningitis or brain abscess.

The leading clinical sign is a persistent clear, watery discharge from the ears or from the nose. Antibiotic prophylactic treatment is indicated and if the leak persists beyond 10 days to 2 weeks, then surgical repair of the torn dura is indicated.

Treatment of head injuries
1. Establish an adequate airway with tracheal intubation if necessary.
2. Provide respiratory assistance (by means of a respirator if necessary).
3. Control external haemorrhage and provide blood transfusion.
4. Assess the state of consciousness (see above).
5. If rapid deterioration is occurring, then carry out bilateral burr holes without further delay.

6. Counteract cerebral swelling by the administration of intravenous diuretic agents such as Mannitol and corticosteriod injections.
7. Provide antibiotic prophylactic treatment in the event of cerebrospinal fluid leaks.
8. If the patient's condition deteriorates, then this is an indication for specialised investigation such as angiography and CAT-scanning.
9. Compound fractures of the skull and penetrating wounds of the brain are clear indications for operation.

Prognosis
The prognosis and course of head injuries are related to the severity of intracerebral damage. The longer the period of unconsciousness and retrograde amnesia, the poorer the prognosis. Prognosis is very poor in an adult who presents with dilated fixed pupils and the signs of injury to the base of the brain.

The greatest improvement is likely to occur within the first 2 or 3 months but it should be noted that improvement following head injury can continue for 9 months or more.

Late disability is one of the most important aspects of head injury and includes physical handicaps as a result of weakness, dysphasia, blindness or paralysis or more mild forms of disability such as headache, difficulty in concentration, memory defect, dizziness and fatigue. Some patients develop epileptic fits during the posthead-injury period. Indeed, the physical and psycho-social results of head injury are a major health problem.

The unconscious patient
A depressed state of consciousness may be due to a large number of causes and may occur suddenly, for instance following concussion (see above) or more gradually as might occur with the gradual accumulation of an intracranial haematoma (see above) or, for instance, as a result of the overdose of a drug. Repeated neurological examination will establish not only the level of consciousness but its fluctuation. Depressed consciousness may be due to the following:
1. Trauma
2. Syncope as a result of transient cerebral ischaemia.
   Simple causes—vasovagal attack, postural hypotension.
   Serious causes—myocardial infarction, internal haemorrhage, Stokes-Adams seizure (p. 91).
3. A hypoglycaemic attack occurring in diabetes (p. 275).
   A non-convulsive epileptic seizure (p. 320).

A cerebrovascular catastrophe (p. 316).

In addition to these causes, there are many others, e.g. diabetic ketosis, uraemia, poisoning of various kinds and cerebral neoplasms.

The dentist will encounter but few of these in his practice, and for many of them complex investigations are necessary to establish a precise diagnosis. It is, however, important that the dental practitioner understands the care of the unconscious patient and also the action to be taken should a patient suddenly become unconscious while undergoing treatment.

Management of the comatose patient

The maintenance of an airway and control of coincident shock are the basic principles of the management of patients with a depressed level of consciousness.

Protection of the airway is perhaps the most fundamental procedure and attention to detail will avoid many complications. A patient without a good cough reflex is unable to protect his own airway. Furthermore, the tongue tends to fall back and obstruct the oropharynx. Aspiration of vomitus is a distinct risk.

The jaw should be pulled forward and the oropharynx cleared. An airway is maintained with an oropharyngeal tube, but it may be necessary to replace this with an endotracheal tube if there is no cough reflex. Tracheotomy may be necessary. Every effort must be made to reduce the likelihood of aspiration of gastric contents and to ensure unrestricted gas exchange at alveolar level.

A nasogastric tube should be passed in order to sample any ingested drugs and to remove gastric contents that might be aspirated into the lungs.

An intravenous line must be inserted in order to administer drugs and fluids to the patient. In prolonged unconscious states feeding may be carried out via a fine tube passed into the stomach. If gastric feeding is performed in this way, it should be always covered by an awareness on behalf of the staff of the dangers of aspiration.

An indwelling bladder catheter is used in order to assist with the assessment of fluid balance and the catheter must be carefully managed so as not to allow ascending infection.

The patient must be regularly turned and the skin cared for in order to prevent the development of pressure sores and passive movements must be performed by a physiotherapist. In addition, physiotherapeutic manoeuvres designed to keep the chest inflated and clear of secretions must be regularly carried out. The cause of coma must be diligently sought and treated.

Sudden loss of consciousness

If a dentist is faced with the problem of a patient who suddenly loses consciousness, the following are the most likely causes:

1. Syncope—usually as a result of a vasovagal attack, but sometimes due to a more severe cause.
2. A non-convulsive epileptic seizure.

In any event, the action to be taken is as follows:

1. The dental chair should be immediately lowered so as to allow the patient to lie flat and the patient should be rolled onto his side and, if possible, into a semi-prone position. Dentures and all foreign bodies, including dental instruments and cotton-wool rolls should be immediately removed from the mouth.
2. The mandible should be grasped and pulled forward so as to bring the tongue forward. The tongue is then grasped in a swab and also pulled forward so as to maintain the airway.
3. The dental suction apparatus should be used to clear any mucus or secretions from the patient's mouth.

At this point, any constricting clothing about the patient's neck is immediately loosened. An immediate assessment is then made as to whether the patient is recovering from a simple syncopal attack or whether it is necessary to summon the help of a qualified medical practitioner.

It is perhaps important to mention that general anaesthesia should not be administered in the sitting position in a dental chair. Syncopal attacks can occur while under the influence of anaesthesia and serious brain damage may result consequent on cerebral hypoxia.

18

Psychological disorders

Psychological disorders, not all of which are of serious import, are so common that it is inevitable that some dental patients will be suffering from them. The recent tendency to discharge many previously long-stay psychiatric patients to their homes has increased this likelihood. In this chapter a very brief account is given of the commoner psychiatric illnesses and also of some of the terms used when dealing with disordered function of the mind.

Disorders of the mind are traditionally classified into the psychoses, the neuroses and mental retardation but it should be appreciated that the boundaries between some psychotic states and some neurotic illnesses and indeed between neurotic traits and normality are sometimes difficult to define with certainty. Lack of precise understanding of the aetiology of many psychiatric illnesses is a distinct hindrance to precise classification and although some psychiatric illnesses have a recognisable cause such as organic brain damage or are related to some 'toxic' factor such as severe infection or drug abuse, in many instances of mental disorder there is, however, no discernible organic pathological change in the brain or recognisable causal factor.

With this background mental disorders will be considered under the following headings:-
1. Mental disorders associated with organic disease of the brain.
2. Mental disorders secondary to organic disease elsewhere or to metabolic, hormonal or deficiency states.
3. Alcoholism and drug abuse.
4. Functional psychoses.
5. Neurotic illnesses.
6. Personality disorders.
7. Mental subnormality.

MENTAL DISORDERS ASSOCIATED WITH ORGANIC BRAIN DISEASE

Obliterative disease of the cerebral vessels (cerebral arteriosclerosis) is the commonest organic brain disorder to result in mental abnormality. Other forms are cerebral tumours (primary or secondary), brain abscess, neurosyphilis (p. 26), encephalitis, and cerebral trauma. A special variety is the common but ill understood condition of senile dementia where there is a diffuse atrophy of brain with loss of nerve cells and fibres.

There are two principal clinical syndromes in this category of organic brain disorders, namely, delirium and dementia. Delirium is characterised by restlessness, irritability, marked anxiety, disturbed sleep or insomnia and auditory or visual hallucinations which may be terrifying to the patient. In dementia there is a progressive loss of the capacity of reasoning, inability to concentrate, inability to handle new information, loss of emotional control, narrowing of span of attention, a poor grasp of the abstract, and an inability to separate the important from the unimportant.

MENTAL DISORDERS SECONDARY TO ORGANIC DISEASE ELSEWHERE AND TO METABOLIC, HORMONAL AND DEFICIENCY STATES

The functioning of the mind may be markedly compromised by a variety of processes which have their origin in organs other than the brain. The mental derangement may be acute and potentially reversible (e.g., severe febrile illnesses) but if the cause is either not recognised or is untreatable then the damage to the mental processes may be permanent. Acute processes tend to produce confusion which may progress to delirium; chronic processes may produce mental retardation in the child and progressive dementia in the adult.

Acute confusional states and delirium may be produced by severe infection (e.g., pneumonia or typhoid), hypoxia (cardiac failure and respiratory disease), hypoglycaemia (e.g., due to inadvertent insulin overdosage), and other metabolic disorders such as hypocalcaemia, hepatic failure and uraemia. Important deficiency states include hypothyroidism and vitamin B deficiency.

ALCOHOLISM AND DRUG ABUSE

Alcoholism

The sense of relaxation and mild euphoria that follow consumption of a modest and socially acceptable amount of alcohol may not be unknown to the majority of students. Acute intake of larger amounts tends to lead to noisy and often aggressive behaviour and to a degree of disinhibition which is later regretted. Severe overdose can cause loss of consciousness during which serious complications such as pneumonia from inhalation of vomit or hypothermia may occur.

Chronic alcoholic dependence or addiction is a very common health problem. Perhaps as many as one million people in the United Kingdom have problems related to chronic excessive intake of alcohol and the number is probably increasing. A common pattern is drinking that commences in adolescence or early adult life and gradually escalates in an insidious manner without the individual being aware that he is becoming dependent on alcohol. It represents a form of psychological dependence usually with underlying emotional problems such as feelings of insecurity or inadequacy, lack of self-esteem, anxiety or depression. At particular risk are those concerned in the manufacture and sale of alcohol, commercial travellers and company directors, journalists, entertainers, those in the merchant navy and the armed forces, and doctors. Dependence on alcohol may produce social problems, psychological problems and physical problems. Detection in its early stages is obviously important, partly to prevent the development of complications and partly because at that stage management is rather more likely to be successful. The social problems may show as break-up of marriage after a period of time in which violence to the wife or children has occurred. The husband's sexual impotence (a complication of alcoholism) aggravates his feeling of inadequacy and contributes to marital unhappiness. The alcoholic is liable to be off work more frequently and absences on a Monday after weekend alcoholic bouts are particularly characteristic. He is more prone to be involved in road traffic accidents whether as a driver or a pedestrian. Psychological problems include depression, spells of amnesia during which he is unable to recollect recent events, delusions particularly of infidelity, and a gradual degeneration in moral standards with the result that many alcoholics become unreliable and untrustworthy. Acute alcoholic intoxication superimposed on chronic alcoholism can lead to delirium and in some cases a state of delirium, commonly termed delirium tremens, may develop following enforced abstinence from the usual daily intake of alcohol. The individual is extremely restless, commonly disorientated as to time and place, hallucinated often to a state of terror, and shows marked tremor, intense sweating and may experience severe muscle cramps and intense nausea and retching. Physical problems that may arise in the chronic alcoholic include peripheral neuropathy, gastritis and peptic ulcer, pancreatitis, cirrhosis of the liver, cardiomyopathy and macrocytic anaemia.

Early detection along with insight into the problem by the patient and a determination to do without alcohol in the future are essential for success. He may require hospitalisation in the initial stages and later may derive considerable support from membership of a body such as Alcoholics Anonymous or by firm adherence to a religious faith. Acute withdrawal symptoms such as delirium tremens require skilled hospital management involving adequate sedation with a drug such as promazine and correction of probable vitamin B deficiency.

Heroin and morphine addiction

Addiction to opiates, once uncommon in this country, is increasing. Even small doses of drugs can lead to dependence and the dependence is both physical and psychological. Tolerance is rapidly acquired and dependence increases as dosage increases. Most addicts tend to have been weak and rather inadequate and unhappy people before the addiction is acquired. Nevertheless it is a wise precaution to be extremely careful with administration of morphine in any individual who has a painful chronic disorder that is unlikely to progress to a fatal termination in a relatively short time.

Once addicted the addict will go to almost any lengths to acquire his necessary supply of drug. He becomes untrustworthy and may resort to crime. From the physical point of view he is prone to develop local infections due to lack of sterile precautions when injecting the drug, septicaemia and, of particular importance to the dentist, he is much more liable to acquire hepatitis virus B infection. Suspicion of addiction may be raised by tremors, restless movements, facial twitching, coryza, blood staining on the clothes from injections, injection marks particularly over veins, or multiple superficial venous thromboses.

Barbiturate addiction

Barbiturates are effective sedatives and used to be extremely widely prescribed for use during the day and as hypnotics at night. In recent years it has been realised that addiction is easily acquired and their chronic use can lead to confusion, defective judgment and loss of emotional control. Such patients can show dysarthria, tremor and be ataxic. The use of barbiturates is now frowned on in this country, their place being taken by preparations such as diazepam.

FUNCTIONAL PSYCHOSES

In contrast to the organic psychoses, the functional psychoses are characterised by a pathological state of mind producing gross distortion of reality without any discernible physical abnormality in the brain or underlying abnormality in other systems of the body. The two most important forms are the depressive, manic or manic depressive psychoses and the schizophrenic psychoses.

Depressive and manic psychoses

These are characterised by a profound and morbid disorder of mood without intellectual impairment. They are often referred to as the effective psychoses.

The depressive variety is characterised by loss of enjoyment of life, inability to concentrate, tearfulness, remorseless self critism, profound feelings of guilt and unworthiness and by suicidal ideas which are sometimes translated into action. Associated with these morbid thoughts are symptoms which may be mistakenly interpreted as indicative of a physical disorder; and indeed the patient not infrequently seeks medical advice for such symptoms rather than for the disorder of mood. The commonest symptoms are loss of appetite, loss of weight, disturbance of sleep (difficulty in getting off to sleep and early morning awakening), constipation, dryness of skin, diminution in sexual desire and amenorrhea.

The manic variety of the affective psychoses is characterized by a markedly abnormal elevation of mood which makes the individual very restless, agitated and over-active and leads him into a round of activities which he is unable to carry out efficiently and into which he has lack of insight. He may undertake financial or personal commitments he is later to regret or unable to meet and he is resentful of any advice that his actions are precipitate, ill judged and inappropriate.

Some patients, the manic depressives, may swing from one extreme of mood to the other or may display a mixed pattern of mood at the one time.

Management of the affective psychoses has been much improved by the availability of new psychotropic drugs which have powerful anti-depressant or tranquillising effects. The principal anti-depressant drugs are tricyclic preparations (e.g., imipramine and amitryptiline) which tend to be more effective and to have fewer side-effects than the monoamine oxidase inhibitors. Electroconvulsive therapy (ECT) is now much less widely used for the treatment of severe depression but it is still employed where there has been an inadequate response to anti-depressant drug therapy and particularly if there is a serious risk of suicide still present. The manic variety of the affective psychoses is often responsive to the tranquillizer drugs, particularly the phenothiazine group (e.g., chlorpromazine) and the diazepines (e.g., diazepam and meprobamate).

The schizophrenic psychoses

The term schizophrenia, which literally means split mind, is a common and very serious functional psychotic disorder which affects 0·8 per cent of the population. It usually commences between the ages of 15 and 25 years. Characteristic features include loss of initiative, withdrawal from social contacts, lack of emotional warmth, deterioration in intellectual capacity, and progressive disorder of thought processes. Hallucinations (especially threatening voices) are common, bizarre or paranoid delusions may be present, the individual may feel that he is under the control of external influences and that thoughts are being put into his mind. Phenothiazine drugs improve the symptomatology in many patients often quite dramatically and they may be able to return to the community, albeit to a sheltered pattern of life. Permanent and complete remission, however, probably does not occur in more than 25 per cent of patients. Relapses, often necessitating re-admission to hospital, and with an increasing deterioration in personality, are a common pattern and perhaps 25 per cent of patients will require long term care in psychiatric hospitals. The patient with schizophrenia is particularly at risk of suicide, especially in the early acute stages.

THE NEUROSES

The neurotic illnesses are much commoner than the psychoses and are less serious. Although the individual may develop quite disabling symptoms they tend to be an exaggerated form of many natural reactions (e.g., anxiety or fear of illness). Contact with the realities of every-day life is usually maintained and delusional ideas, hallucinations or profound disturbances of thought processes are absent.

Anxiety neurosis

The major feature in this disorder is excessive anxiety which may express itself in recurrent bouts of panic, in intense fear of illness (hypochondriasis), of choking (globus hystericus), of being in enclosed spaces (claustrophobia), of being in open spaces (agoraphobia), of mixing with people, or of animals. The patient is usually tense, sweats excessively, sleeps poorly, may have a tremor and commonly has tachycardia. In managing such patients it is obviously important to exclude organic disease, including thyrotoxicosis, and to provide re-assurance and support both medically and within the family. Sedation with a preparation such as diazepam is commonly employed.

Hysteria

The hysteric (from the Greek word for the womb, hystera, since this was considered the origin of the disorder) is usually an immature individual whose personality has not developed sufficiently to cope in a stable and constructive manner with the harsher realities, setbacks, and disappointments of life. When faced with problems hysterics tend to over-react, often in an extravagant and histrionic manner. They are often very suggestible and are easily hypnotized. Faced with difficulties they commonly indulge in childhood reactions such as denial or magical thinking and, like children, often look to others to solve their personal difficulties. At times of stress they may develop conversion symptoms (conversion hysteria) in which a physical illness is mimicked (e.g., paralysis of a limb, inability to speak, loss of sensation over part of the body, the apparent physical illness being quite unconsciously an honorable escape mechanism from an intolerable situation. Others may develop periods of amnesia as a reaction to unacceptable events (disassociation). As with anxiety states, it is important to demonstrate the absence of physical disease and to provide re-assurance and support.

Obsessional or compulsive neuroses

An obsession is a fixed idea or delusion that the individual cannot dispel from the mind even although it is recognised that it is irrational if not absurd. A compulsion is an irresistible urge to perform a particular act even although the individual knows that it is pointless if not harmful. Obsessions may take the form of ideas or images which haunt the mind, or phobias or of ruminations in which a problem or series of problems are turned over in the mind in an endless and senseless way. Compulsions can be very frightening and may involve acts of violence or may be harmless although bizarre. Many individuals with milder forms of obsessional/compulsive states are able to lead reasonably normal lives although they tend to be pre-occupied with detail, unimaginative, rigid in outlook and conscientious to a fault. If obsessional ideas are severe the patient may become very distressed and agitated or may become quite severely depressed and skilled psychiatric management will be essential.

PERSONALITY DISORDERS

The borderline between a normal personality and a personality disorder is almost always difficult to define and obviously may vary depending on the individual making the judgement. The adolescent punk rocker with strands of multi-coloured hair and safety pins in his nostrils considers himself one of his peer group, and therefore normal, whereas he is likely to be classified as distinctly odd by the conformist majority. It is wise to reserve the term 'personality disorder' for someone who over a period of years has a pattern of maladjustment to society which exceeds that of the social misfit or eccentric. It is also important not to make dismissive value judgments bearing in mind that many very gifted individuals who could be classified as having had a personality disorder have made enormous contributions to our cultural life.

Within the framework of personality disorders will be included many chronic alcoholics, sexual deviants, drug addicts and those with markedly anti-social traits who are considered to be psychopaths. A psychopath may conveniently be defined as someone who has a severe disorder of personality, emotional adjustment or maturation which leads him to behave in an extreme and often violent manner and which renders him unable to develop and sustain a non-destructive and productive social and emotional relationship. Aggressive behaviour, lack of feeling, lack of remorse, inability to learn from mistakes, and lack of trust are common features. The condition is more likely to be seen in individuals who have had periods of emotional and social deprivation in childhood.

MENTAL SUBNORMALITY

The commonest cause of mental retardation rendering the individual incapable of leading an independent existence is Down's syndrome or mongolism. This is due to trisomy of chromosome 21. Such children are mentally retarded and have stunted growth. The bridge of the nose is poorly developed, the eyes are slanting, the little finger is curved, the joints are hyper-extensible and the palms are broad. Mongol children are more likely to be born to older mothers (over 35 years) probably because of faulty chromosome production by the aging ovary.

Mongols, and other individuals who have severe mental retardation, frequently require to be cared for in institutions and the dentist should always remember that in such institutions the incidence of infection with hepatitis B virus is increased. Special precautions are, therefore, required when carrying out dental treatment in any such individuals.

Appendix

List of normal adult values in blood, serum or plasma of the more commonly measured substances

Where appropriate the values are given both in the International System of Units (S.I.) and in conventional units

	S.I. Units	Conventional Units
Bicarbonate	21–28 mmol/l	21–28 mEq/l
Bilirubin (total)	5–17 μmol/l	0·3–1 mg/100 ml
Calcium (total)	2·2–2·6 mmol/l	9–11 mg/100 ml
Chloride	95–105 mmol/l	95–105 mEq/l
Creatinine	35–115 μmol/l	0·5–1·4 mg/100 ml
Folate	3–20 μg/l	3–20 ng/ml
Glucose	4·0–5·5 mmol/l	80–120 mg/100 ml
Iron	10–34 μmol/l	55–190 μg/100 ml
Total iron binding capacity	45–72 μmol/l	250–400 μg/100 ml
Phosphorus (as inorganic phosphate)	0·8–1·4 mmol/l	3–4·5 mg/100 ml
Potassium	3·4–4·9 mmol/l	3·4–4·9 mEq/l
Sodium	136–144 mmol/l	136–144 mEq/l
Thyroxine (T$_4$)	55–144 nmol/l	5–11 μg/100 ml
Tri-iodothyronine (T$_3$)	0·9–2·8 nmol/l	65–175 ng/100 ml
Urate	0·1–0·4 mmol/l	2–7 mg/100 ml
Urea	2·5–7 mmol/l	15–40 mg/100 ml
LIPIDS		
Total Lipids	3·5–8·5 g/l	0·35–0·85 g/100 ml
Total Fatty Acids	3·6–18 mmol/l	100–500 mg/100 ml
Cholesterol (total)	3·6–7·8 mmol/l	100–300 mg/100 ml
Triglycerides	0·3–1·7 mmol/l	25–150 mg/100 ml

	S.I. Units	Conventional Units
PROTEINS		
Total Serum Protein	—	65–85 g/l
Albumin	—	35–55 g/l
Globulins	—	22–33 g/l
Fibrinogen	—	1·5–4·0 g/l

Index

DATE DUE

Demco. Inc. 38-293